# Health Norms and the Governance of Global Development

This book maps the emergence of health in global development discourse and governance since 1990. It argues that health norms have emerged, diffused, and subsequently become internalised through the various direct and indirect negotiation processes that created the global development goals.

Covid-19, Ebola, and HIV/AIDS are prime illustrations of the fact that health is supremely political. Governments – whether they are local, national, international, or multilateral – make decisions about their policy responses, coordinate their response, and channel the necessary resources. Such decisions are informed by local and global conditions as well as sets of values, norms, and standards that determine policy and interventions. As states and regions become more interconnected, the politics of health are increasingly relevant to the sustainable future envisioned by global governance. This book explains how considerations of global health have come to inform and infuse the United Nations development agenda. It identifies processes, actors, institutions, and interactions in global health by analysing two related case studies: the Millennium Development Goals and the Sustainable Development Goals.

Providing an overview of, and insights about, the context of global development thinking and practice, the subtleties of global health, and global health governance, this book is an innovative contribution to the literature. It is suitable for students and scholars of global health, development studies, and international relations.

**Anders Granmo** was educated at universities in Norway and South Africa. He is a lecturer and researcher, focusing on issues related to global health governance.

**Pieter Fourie** teaches political science at Stellenbosch University, South Africa. He has worked in the field of global health since the late 1990s, including at UNAIDS, the AIDS Foundation of South Africa, and he has taught at universities in South Africa and Australia.

# Routledge Studies in Public Health

www.routledge.com/Routledge-Studies-in-Public-Health/book-series/RSPH

# Health Norms and the Governance of Global Development

## Development

The Invention of Global Health

Anders Granmo and Pieter Fourie

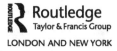
Routledge
Taylor & Francis Group

LONDON AND NEW YORK

First published 2021
by Routledge
2 Park Square, Milton Park, Abingdon, Oxon OX14 4RN

and by Routledge
52 Vanderbilt Avenue, New York, NY 10017

*Routledge is an imprint of the Taylor & Francis Group, an informa business*

*British Library Cataloguing-in-Publication Data*
A catalogue record for this book is available from the British Library

*Library of Congress Cataloging-in-Publication Data*
Names: Granmo, Anders, author. | Fourie, Pieter, 1972– author.
Title: Health norms and the governance of global development : the
    invention of global health / Anders Granmo and Pieter Fourie.
Description: Abingdon, Oxon ; New York, NY : Routledge, 2021. |
    Series: Routledge studies in public health | Includes bibliographical
    references and index.
Identifiers: LCCN 2020041217 (print) | LCCN 2020041218 (ebook) |
    ISBN 9780367625658 (hardback) | ISBN 9781003109716 (ebook)
Subjects: LCSH: World health—Economic aspects. | World
    health—Political aspects. | Public health—International cooperation. |
    Sustainable development—International cooperation.
Classification: LCC RA441 .G74 2021 (print) | LCC RA441 (ebook) |
    DDC 362.1—dc23
LC record available at https://lccn.loc.gov/2020041217
LC ebook record available at https://lccn.loc.gov/2020041218

ISBN: 978-0-367-62565-8 (hbk)
ISBN: 978-1-003-10971-6 (ebk)

Typeset in Goudy
by Apex CoVantage, LLC

We dedicate this book to the work and legacy
of Mahbub ul Haq.

# Contents

# Figures

# Tables

# Boxes

# Abbreviations

| | |
|---|---|
| AIDS | acquired immunodeficiency syndrome |
| ARV | antiretroviral |
| AU | African Union |
| CARICOM | Caribbean Community |
| CHAIR | Centre for Health and International Relations |
| CHGA | Commission on HIV/AIDS and Governance in Africa |
| CIA | Central Intelligence Agency |
| CSD | Commission on Sustainable Development |
| CSDH | Commission on Social Determinants of Health |
| DAC | Development Assistance Committee |
| ECOSOC | United Nations Economic and Social Council |
| EID | emerging infectious disease |
| EU | European Union |
| FAO | Food and Agriculture Organization |
| FCTC | Framework Convention for Tobacco Control |
| GDI | gender development index |
| GDP | gross domestic product |
| GFC | global financial crisis |
| GHG | global health governance |
| GPA | Global Programme on AIDS |
| HDI | human development index |
| HDR | human development report |
| HIV | human immunodeficiency virus |
| HLP | high-level panel of eminent persons |
| HLPF | high-level political forum on sustainable development |
| HRP | Special Programme of Research, Development and Research Training in Human Reproduction |
| IBRD | International Bank for Reconstruction and Development |
| ICPD | International Conference on Population and Development |
| IDGs | International Development Goals |
| IFI | international financial institution |
| IHRs | International Health Regulations |
| IMF | International Monetary Fund |

| | |
|---|---|
| IO | international organisation |
| IOM | Institute of Medicine |
| IPCC | Intergovernmental Panel on Climate Change |
| IR | international relations |
| IWHC | International Women's Health Coalition |
| LDC | least developed country |
| LMIC | low- and middle-income country |
| MDG | Millennium Development Goal |
| MSF | Médecins Sans Frontières |
| NGO | non-governmental organisation |
| NSRT | North-South Roundtable |
| OAU | Organisation of African Unity |
| ODA | official development assistance |
| OECD | Organisation for Economic Co-operation and Development |
| OWG | Open Working Group |
| PEPFAR | President's Emergency Plan for AIDS Relief |
| PRSP | poverty reduction strategy paper |
| R2P | responsibility to protect |
| SAP | Structural Adjustment Programme |
| SARS | Severe Acute Respiratory Syndrome |
| SDG | Sustainable Development Goal |
| SPA | Special Programme on AIDS |
| SPC | Secretariat of the Pacific Community |
| THS | Transforming Health Systems |
| TRIPS | Trade-Related Aspects of Intellectual Property Rights |
| UDHR | Universal Declaration of Human Rights |
| UHC | universal health coverage |
| UN | United Nations |
| UNAIDS | Joint United Nations Programme on HIV/AIDS |
| UNCED | United Nations Conference on Environment and Development |
| UNDA | United Nations development agenda |
| UN-DESA | United Nations Department of Economic and Social Affairs |
| UNDP | United Nations Development Programme |
| UNDRIP | United Nations Declaration of the Rights of Indigenous Peoples |
| UNESCO | United Nations Educational, Scientific and Cultural Organisation |
| UNFCCC | United Nations Framework Convention on Climate Change |
| UNFPA | United Nations Population Fund |
| UNGA | United Nations General Assembly |
| UNIATF | United Nations Interagency Task Force on the Prevention and Control |
| UNICEF | United Nations Children's Fund |
| UNSC | United Nations Security Council |
| UNSTT | United Nations System Task Team on the Post-2015 Agenda |
| U.K. | United Kingdom |

| | |
|---|---|
| U.S. | United States |
| WHA | World Health Assembly |
| WHO | World Health Organization |
| WSSD | World Summit on Sustainable Development |
| WTO | World Trade Organization |

# 1 Why we wrote this book, and how to read it

## Introduction

Covid-19, Ebola, and HIV/AIDS have all recently illustrated that health is supremely political. Few other issues in international relations or in global development so dramatically and directly determine who dies, who lives, who benefits, who pays, and who governs global affairs. Governments – whether they are local, national, international, or multilateral – need to make decisions about their policy responses, coordinate such responses, and then channel the necessary resources. Such governance decisions are informed by local and global conditions as well as sets of values, norms, and standards that determine policy thinking and programmatic interventions. As states and regions become more interconnected, the politics of health are increasingly relevant to the sustainable future envisioned by global governance.

Given the immediacy of global health concerns, how and why has health emerged in global development and policy thinking since the end of the Cold War? Who are its main champions, and which values determine the contemporary global health agenda? How can governments (rich and poor) and multilateral institutions use the new global health development agenda to enhance their own agency?

This book traces and explains the emergence of health in global development discourse and governance since 1990. The book explains how considerations of global health have come to inform and infuse the United Nations development agenda. We identify processes, actors, institutions, and interactions between the spheres of development thinking and international relations. We do this by analysing two discrete but closely related and historically sequential case studies: the Millennium Development Goals and the Sustainable Development Goals. We provide an overview of and insights about the context of global development thinking and practice, the subtleties of global health, and global health governance.

The book includes a short history of development practice and discourse, an introduction to the complex field of global health, and the relationship between them. We find that health norms have emerged, diffused, and subsequently become internalised through the various direct and indirect negotiation processes that created the policies formalised as global development goals. The book underscores the topicality and increasing traction of global health within international relations and, conversely, the utility of international relations for understanding contemporary global health and development challenges.

## A brief history of modern inequality

In December 2014, the United Nations (UN) published its *Synthesis Report of the Secretary-General on the Post-2015 Agenda* (UNGA, 2014a). In it, the trajectory of globally coordinated development efforts for the following 15 years was outlined. The new paradigm includes a fresh set of goals, titled the 'Sustainable Development Goals' (SDGs). These goals are envisioned to make up the framework that now carry forward the torch passed by the underachieving preceding framework, the Millennium Development Goals (MDGs). The multifaceted story of the evolution of these development frameworks is one of triumphs and defeats, of steps taken forwards and then backwards over the past several decades. However, the conversation concerning the impetus for, as well as the proper conduct of, what is now known as *global development* is not new. Older still is a narrative inextricably connected to it – namely, one concerning the *unequal* reality of human existence.

In 1887 the author Edward Bellamy published *Looking Backward: 2000–1887*, a piece of social commentary in the guise of speculative fiction, in which the protagonist wakes up in the distant future, year 2000. Rather than being described as rife with futuristic technology, the defining quality of the new millennium for Bellamy was a socialist utopia:

> The fear of want and the lust of gain became extinct motives when abundance was assured to all and immoderate possessions made impossible of attainment. There were no more beggars nor almoners. Equity left charity without an occupation. . . . Humanity's ancient dream of liberty, equality, fraternity, mocked by so many ages, at last was realised.
>
> (Bellamy, 1951, pp. 233–234)

Bellamy died in 1898, in blissful ignorance of the actual future. Indeed, French economist Thomas Piketty's hard-hitting *Capital in the 21st Century* (2014) recently reminded us that the world remains an unmistakably unequal place. The fact that the world is made up of a few *haves* and many *have-nots* has long been known.

While this reality has been acknowledged for centuries, the perceived reasons for inequality have undergone a number of paradigmatic shifts. From initially being viewed as natural and expected, ideas about the origins of – and *panacea* for – inequality have evolved dramatically. Today, an effort to mitigate this global situation is one of the largest-scale international initiatives in history, reaching its zenith with the SDGs. This project is commonly known as *development*, an infamously ambiguous concept that has different meanings and policy implications for the different people, organisations, and entities that constitute this multifaceted industry. However, in the minds of most people today, *development* approximates the following broad definition:

> Development means making a better life for everyone. In the present context of a highly uneven world, a better life for most people means, essentially, meeting basic needs: sufficient food to maintain good health; a safe, healthy place in which to live; affordable services available to everyone; and being treated with dignity and respect.
>
> (Peet & Hartwick, 2009, p. 1)

As suggested, these aspirations, values, and norms have been established over time. Development theorist Gilbert Rist's *The History of Development: From Western Origins to Global Faith* (2008) traces the seeds of present development thought at least as far back as Aristotle. However, it was only by the early 20th century that several factors converged to set the scene for what was to become the massive undertaking by the international community that continues to grow in scope and ambition. By the end of the 19th century, the great nations of Europe were enjoying the pinnacle of their power, laying claim to about 85% of the world (Greig, Hulme, & Turner, 2007). However, the perpetuation of this situation was already in doubt. It became untenable when these various colonial empires destroyed each other's capabilities in World War I, which coincided with a wave of rebellion in the colonies as well as the growth of liberal (and sometimes more humanitarian) sentiments domestically. By the end of World War II, all these material and ideational factors had grown in scope and significance. Additionally, the Western world's new hegemon, the United States (U.S.), lacking significant colonies, explicitly buttressed the process of decolonisation; the final years of World War II and the period immediately following it would lay the most significant groundwork for the way development was to be pursued in the decades to follow.

In 1944 a meeting was held in the New Hampshire town of Bretton Woods that was to have great implications for the future of the global economy. Its attendees included 44 of the richest nations of the world, convening to address their common financial challenges in an increasingly economically interdependent world. The meeting led, among other things, to the creation of the International Monetary Fund (IMF) and the International Bank for Reconstruction and Development (IBRD), which came to be known as the World Bank. The institutionalisation of the Bretton Woods system coincided with ideational realities such as an increased emphasis on the importance of universal human rights in what was becoming a truly global community. As Greig et al. (2007, p. 66) suggest,

> A constellation of forces came into alignment to create 'development' as an intellectual and practical project. These included Western responses to the experiences of economic depression and global conflict, the emergence of postcolonial independent states, the onset of the Cold War and the structure of the postwar global economy.

These factors culminated in a specific moment viewed by some (Escobar, 1995; Rist, 2008) as the one that sparked the development project. In January 1949 newly re-elected U.S. President Harry S. Truman, in his inaugural address, somewhat surprisingly spoke about the need for prosperous states to help those who are worse off and that those who are able *should* be willing. With a few choice words, Truman had proposed a norm that suggested an obligation for all affluent states; in the same moment, Truman created a binary describing the developed and the underdeveloped world. Escobar (1995, p. 4) comments:

> The Truman doctrine initiated a new era in the understanding and manage-ment of world affairs, particularly those concerning the less economically accomplished countries of the world. The intent was quite ambitious: to bring about the conditions necessary to replicating the world over the features that characterised the 'advanced' societies of the time – high levels of industriali-sation and urbanisation, technicalisation of agriculture, rapid growth of mate-rial production and living standards, and the widespread adoption of modern education and cultural values.

Almost immediately, economists became influential in planning the development project. Many of these were inspired by important economic events in recent his-tory, including the American rehabilitation from the throes of the Great Depres-sion a decade before and, more recently, the rebuilding of Europe after the war with the help of the Marshall Plan. They believed that similar steps could be taken to help the large portion of the world now labelled 'underdeveloped'. They were further convinced that laissez-faire economic approaches perpetuated inequality and instability in the economy, and there was an overarching sense that state-regulated, planned management of economics would be the appropriate method to facilitate the development of the rest of the world – a strategy championed by economist John Maynard Keynes.

In the 1950s, these economists, along with other social scientists, designed a development discourse that would later be known as *modernisation theory*. The assumption was that by "playing catch-up" (Greig et al., 2007, p. 73), underde-veloped countries could gain equality with the developed world and work towards the goal of, ideally, emulating the Western model of modernity and progress. Pro-ponents of modernisation theory imagined an evolutionary line of society that stretched from traditional to modern, consisting of different stages of economic growth (Rostow, 1956). Strikingly, Rostow's stages of modernity are reminiscent of Karl Marx's own emphasis on material dialectics, the decisive difference being that while Marx envisioned conflict and eventual downfall of societies after pass-ing through technological stages, liberal modernisation proponents, such as Ros-tow, saw these stages as a sequence of new horizons, each leading naturally and painlessly closer to idyllic modernity.

For adherents of modernisation theory, the rationale behind development was to enable traditional societies to start their trajectory towards modernity. Not only was this intellectually satisfying for Western leaders and technical experts, but it also provided an ideational and policy template in which to work:

> The practical advantage of this model was that by comparing poorer countries with the Western model, the attributes that a society 'lacked' could be determined. Policies could then be derived that removed 'obstacles' that lay in the path of historical development. . . . Modernisation theorists used historical comparison to discover the *missing* ingredients that were necessary for all countries to achieve future modernity.
>
> (Greig et al., 2007, p. 74, original emphasis)

In short, the perceived reason for the existence of inequality in the paradigm of modernisation was simply the backwardness of the underdeveloped countries, not only in terms of industrialisation and technology, but also in culture – all of which needed to be modernised.

In 1961 the UN realised that in spite of their efforts since the end of World War II, global inequality was actually on the rise. The organisation decided to name the 1960s the *Decade of Development*, in which its member states were urged to intensify their efforts to ensure economic growth. The idea of planned growth still held 'an exalted position' (Arndt, 1978, p. 55) in development policy, which is reflected in the rhetoric of the development decade resolution document (UNGA, 1961). By the late 1960s, however, not much had changed in terms of global inequality. This led to the development of counter-theories, particularly evident in the form of the neo-Marxist *Dependency Theory*, most notably espoused by its leading theorist, André Gunder Frank (Frank, 1966, 1967). This view proposed that the underdeveloped world in a capitalist system would necessarily stay undeveloped, because "European and US development was predicated on the active *under*development of the non-European world, that is, making it less developed than it had been" (Peet & Hartwick, 2009, p. 166, original emphasis). Indeed, the countries in the global periphery had actually experienced a decline regarding their positions in terms of trade. Essentially, they were exporting primary goods at a low price to the core while importing manufactured goods back at a high price. The reality was that the periphery was not at all catching up to the core; the inequality gap was widening.

Still optimistic, the UN named the 1970s the *Second Decade of Development*, lamenting and admitting the failure to reach the goals set in the preceding 10 years. While some of the ideational concerns associated with the dependency school were recognised in the UN resolution document this time around, not many changes were made in terms of policy. Again, the objectives of the decade were ambitious, albeit somewhat naive in its reliance on the generosity of its more affluent member states. Regardless, the efforts of the 1970s were thwarted by a series of interconnected events that led to the decade's two 'oil shocks', which were to have significant repercussions for the global economy in the 1980s, and which heralded a new era for international development. Indeed, crushing debt was the reality for many Third World countries at the beginning of the 1980s. Debts totalled approximately $600 billion in 1982, having increased almost 10-fold since 1970 (Greig et al., 2007). Meanwhile, the UN launched its *Third Decade of Development*, which again bemoaned the lack of progress during the previous decade, and noted the difficult economic climate characterising the international economy as being "in a state of structural disequilibrium" (UNGA, 1981, p. 107).

Enter the international financial institutions (IFIs). The stifling debt of the non-oil-producing developing countries led most of them to apply for loans from the World Bank and the IMF – loans that came with conditionalities, later termed the Washington Consensus–inspired Structural Adjustment Programmes (SAPs). Essentially, these conditions compelled recipient states to change their national economic policies towards neoliberalism. The directives entailed trade liberalisation, privatisation, and enhanced rights for foreign investors. These reforms, which Escobar (1995, p. 57) characterised as "draconian", meant that state-led development, protectionism, and alternatives to untrammelled capitalism were now effectively extinct; the neoliberal norms prescribed by the IFIs also achieved the acquiescence of the UN, apparent in the organisation's objectives and policy measures for the *Third Decade of Development*. This led many (see Escobar, 1995; Easterly, 2001) to characterise the 1980s as a 'lost decade' for development. It "was one of falling growth rates, declining living standards and deepening poverty" (UNGA, 1990, p. 125). The number of countries placed in the UN's category of 'least developed' increased from 24 in 1972 to 47 in 1991. In fact, the 1980s were so dire that it led many development experts to consider the development project to be over: "[t]he last 40 years can be called the age of development. This epoch is coming to an end. Time is ripe to write its obituary" (Sachs, 1992, p. 1). Indeed, the 1990s was an uncertain decade for the future of development, and scholars were already planning for a post-development world (see, for example, Escobar, 1995; Esteva & Prakash, 1998; Rist, 2008).

The UN, however, had no intention of accepting this. Introducing its *Fourth Decade of Development*, the end of the Cold War led to much optimism in the international development community. As the bipolar ideological tension was one of the factors which had motivated states to engage in the disastrous development project in the first place, this might seem counter-intuitive, but the idea was that funds that had thus far been spent on military resources could now be reallocated, and the Global South might "be able to cash in on the 'peace dividend'" (Rist, 2008, p. 197). The strategies of the *Fourth Decade of Development* were once again unsuccessful. Among other indicators, this was illustrated by the fact that official development assistance (ODA) fell to an all-time low in the 1990s. To most, the *Decade of Development* resolutions had lost all credibility by this time (Greig et al., 2007).

However, the 1990s were significant in development discourse for two reasons. First, the decade saw the introduction of the human development paradigm and the related publication of the first *Human Development Report* (HDR), which shifted development focus from economic outcomes to a more nuanced picture – a fresh mainstream view articulated with phrases like "the link between economic growth and human progress is not automatic" (UNDP, 1990). Second, several momentous conferences and summits took place, the combined effects of which the UN itself claims "generated an unprecedented global consensus on a shared vision of development" (UN, 2007, p. iii). Something significant had changed: by the 1990s norms and institutions based on the *human development paradigm* were emerging, presaging an initiative to meaningfully address global poverty and inequality.

## The Millennium Development Goals and the Sustainable Development Goals

The eventual products of these conferences and summits were the *Millennium Development Declaration* and with it, the MDGs (Table 1.1), which were adopted by all 189 UN member states after the Millennium Summit in September 2000. Often called a 'roadmap for global development', these eight goals targeted diverse areas across the sphere of development, such as poverty, equality, health, and education. Each of the goals had specific sub-goals that were to be measurable by a total of 48 indicators, with the stated ambition that all of them be fulfilled by the end of the year 2015.

The validity and utility of the MDGs as an agenda-setting ideational framework for international development were contested from the get-go. Gilbert Rist, for example, criticised the division of the development agenda into separate goals, arguing that they were in fact mutually exclusive and contradictory, making the full framework all but impossible to achieve (Rist, 2008). Vandemoortele summarises the criticisms directed towards the MDGs:

> They are too limited in scope; their definition is too narrowly focused on the social sectors; their sectoral fragmentation leads to vertical silos; their emphasis on quantification is excessive; and they omit fundamental objectives contained in the Millennium Declaration, such as peace and security, human rights, democracy and good governance.
>
> (Vandemoortele, 2011, p. 9)

Regardless, the status of the MDGs as the guiding light towards which all development projects should strive quickly became a reality. As a World Health

*Table 1.1* The MDGs

| | |
|---|---|
| **Goal 1** | Eradicate extreme hunger and poverty |
| **Goal 2** | Achieve universal primary education |
| **Goal 3** | Promote gender equality and empower women |
| **Goal 4** | Reduce child mortality |
| **Goal 5** | Improve maternal health |
| **Goal 6** | Combat HIV/AIDS, malaria, and other diseases |
| **Goal 7** | Ensure environmental sustainability |
| **Goal 8** | Develop a global partnership for development |

Organization (WHO) report suggested, "[t]he MDGs have gained widespread acceptance in rich and poor countries alike. They are seen to provide an overarching framework for development efforts, and benchmarks against which to judge success" (WHO, 2005a, p. 7).

In hindsight, the stated targets were overly ambitious, and the results by the UN itself characterised as "insufficient and uneven" (UNGA, 2014a, p. 7). Though neither futile nor totally ineffective, the MDGs were largely unsuccessful in attaining their original objectives in spite of this broad-based support. By the end of the first decade after the Millennium Summit, it had become clear that in spite of significant progress in certain areas, the goals that had been set at the inception were not likely to be met. Indeed, the UN (now grown to 193 members) was preparing for the next step by at least as early as 2011, made explicit by the establishment by Secretary-General Ban Ki-moon of the *UN System Task Team on the Post-2015 UN Development Agenda* (UNSTT).

The year after saw the hosting of a large-scale conference held in Rio de Janeiro, called the *UN Conference on Sustainable Development*, designed to develop and set up future International Development Goals. In the wake of this, an outcome document titled *The Future We Want*, along with the reports submitted, *inter alia*, by the task team, laid the basis for an Open Working Group (OWG), which in July 2014 proposed a total of 17 new goals with 169 associated targets: the SDGs, which were formally adopted in 2015. The SDGs inherited and expanded on the role of the MDGs as the road map for global development from 2016 through 2030, all with newfound ambition:

> In addition to reinforcing the commitment to the unfinished MDGs, the SDGs break new ground with goals on inequalities, economic growth, decent jobs, cities and human settlements, industrialisation, energy, climate change, sustainable consumption and production, peace, justice and institutions.
>
> (UNGA, 2014a, p. 10)

The period between the inception of the MDGs and the creation and adoption of the SDGs was highly eventful in terms of international dynamics in general and within development in particular. The conception of the MDGs and indeed the UN itself was a result of norms associated with liberal cosmopolitanism, and the magnitude of the effects of globalisation has grown exponentially. Since 2000 these effects have included the further heterogenisation of the global governance discourse and political economy, including increased power of new actors, ranging from emerging state powers to the rise of nongovernmental juggernauts. Adding to this flux is an ever-increasing interdependence resulting from growing border-crossing issues such as health and climate, major advances in science and technology in all fields, and an increasingly fragile and interconnected global economy, as illustrated by the global financial crisis (GFC) of 2008.

## Global health, sustainable development, and international relations

Health is a principal theme in the discourse surrounding development and inequality. In fact, ways to measure health are among the more quantifiably assessable indicators by which development progress can be judged (Murray, 2007). Additionally, the aggregated improvement of health status is considered essential because health is not only the result of developmental progress, it is also an essential ingredient and determinant of further development (see Strauss & Thomas, 1998). Aside from the often-mentioned battles against poverty and hunger, the most salient theme in the MDG framework was the ubiquitous importance of issues related to health. Indeed, three of the eight goals explicitly referred to specific health concerns, while the remaining five could be, to varying extents, placed within the category of *social determinants of health* (Marmot & Wilkinson, 2005).

International cooperation on health issues has existed since the early 19th century, initially in efforts to quarantine diseases, based on national self-interest by the states involved. The formation of the WHO in 1948 placed the norm of '*health for all*' on the UN's agenda, sowing the seeds for what would later be known as *global health*. Nevertheless, health was typically not a specific focal point in early development discourse. While there was an awareness of the poor health conditions in the underdeveloped world, the focus on modernisation expected that the improvement of health, along with everything else, would automatically follow once the financial and technical means for progress were in place – few or no targets were set for health as an objective in and of itself.

The late 1960s and the 1970s saw health positioned in the global development limelight for the first time (Hall & Taylor, 2003). There was great optimism and even a sense of triumph over nature when smallpox was eradicated after global vaccination efforts in 1977. The year after, the *Declaration of Alma-Ata* (WHO, 1978) was adopted after a conference held in today's Kazakhstan. In short, the *Declaration* established that inequality existed not only broadly in terms of modernity, but more tangibly in terms of health – a fact that was described in the resulting publication as "politically, socially and economically unacceptable and . . . therefore, of common concern to all countries" (WHO, 1978, p. 1). Furthermore, the *Declaration* stipulated that all should have the health levels required to 'lead a socially and economically productive life' by the year 2000 and thus urged efforts directed towards the establishment of primary health care throughout the world. The *Declaration of Alma-Ata* was a milestone for health, for development, and for health *in* development for a number of reasons:

> Although billed as a primary health-care revolution, the content was much wider – a comprehensive philosophy for development. It presented a shift in thinking that saw health not merely as a result of biomedical interventions but also an outcome of social determinants. Motivated by the call for social justice, Alma-Ata identified the key principles of equity and community

participation supported by health promotion, intersectorial collaboration and appropriate use of resources. According to Halfdan Mahler, WHO's Director at the time, Alma-Ata was 'one of those rare occasions where a sublime consensus between the haves and the have-nots in local and global health emerged'.

(Lawn et al., 2008, p. 919)

However, the prescriptions of the *Declaration of Alma-Ata* were not heeded for long (Hall & Taylor, 2003). As mentioned, the 1980s are known by many as development's 'lost decade', and the normative admonishments of the *Declaration of Alma-Ata* were not spared the consequences of the global recession; the *Declaration's* initial momentum was quickly abandoned. The SAPs of the 1980s effectively closed down such initiatives by proscribing state involvement in the name of neoliberal norms and forcing states to cut social spending across the board, health being no exception. Under the IFIs' supervision, an explicit institutionalised link between health and development was again undermined. In large part, as a consequence of this, the WHO's credibility and influence suffered over the course of the last two decades of the 20th century, only to regain a certain measure after the turn of the millennium. This still has significant consequences. As Jeremy Youde suggests, "[I]ts previous position as the unquestioned leader of international health efforts is no longer tenable. Thanks to the organisation's weakening during the 1970s and 1980s and the emergence of a host of new organisations, the architecture of global health governance is significantly more crowded" (Youde, 2012, p. 45).

In health (perhaps more than in any other aspect of development) the playing field has changed significantly since 2000. Certain international non-governmental organisations (NGOs) now share the upper echelons of global health governance with major international organisations (IOs), illustrated by the creation of the so-called Health-8.[1] Other pertinent factors influencing this change include the controversial power of pharmaceutical companies, the rise of emerging powers that compete for increased influence in the global governance sphere, and the ever-increasing mobility of disease.

Furthermore, global health is political, a fact that has increased with the momentum of globalisation: infectious disease travels with people and animals, and unless states elect to close their borders entirely, they can no longer be concerned only with the health status of their own citizens living within their own borders. Davies, Elbe, Howell, and McInnes (2014) have suggested that the increasing intersection between global health and global politics has the potential to be mutually beneficial and enlightening. First, the insights of IR can help to illuminate the significant political dimension of global health and its governance, as it has become clear "that global health is anything but simply a technical pursuit: health policies, practices and outcome occupy politically contested spaces" (Davies et al., 2014, p. 829).

Conversely, investigating the myriad aspects of global health can contribute new perspectives to the topics and methodologies of IR, rooted in the combination of novelty and significance for the actors and issues traditionally studied – namely, states. For example, there is increasing contestation whether health is – or should be – more aptly placed within the sphere of *high politics* (security) or *low politics* (justice). Further areas of interest include the related significance of novel foreign policy tools such as health diplomacy or the tension between humans and states as the focal point of global security concerns. All these themes are central to an analysis regarding two of the most momentous undertakings in the history of global health governance – the MDGs and the SDGs – and the evolution of these agendas.

## How do we make sense of this?

In this book we apply insights from the *constructivist tradition* of IR theory to identify, define, and explain the complexity set out earlier. The core rationale behind this choice is that the constructivist approach focuses explicitly on *processes* and how these are shaped and carried out by complex social interactions. In particular, constructivism is helpful in investigating how identities and interests can be modified over time as responses to social processes interact with material developments. Furthermore, the perspective is unique in its focus on how changes in meanings and values translate to changes in behaviour.

Constructivist IR theory emerged in the late 1980s as a serious alternative to mainstream and traditional 'rational' thinking within the field (Wendt, 1992). Positivism – that is, the belief that human interaction (in which international politics is included) is subject to a set of objective laws, of which its actors are mere products and over which they exercise no control – is represented in IR theory by the classic theoretical views of Realism and Liberalism. Along with their contemporary neo/structural varieties, these views assert that the intractable overarching reality of international politics is anarchic (meaning that there is no single global government), and that this reality necessarily and utterly dictates actors' behaviours.

Adopting insights from a diversity of disciplines in the social sciences (Adler, 2002; Guzzini, 2000; Katzenstein, Keohane, & Krasner, 1998), constructivists emphasise the way in which actors continuously construct reality rather than how actors are affected by an objective reality that exists outside of them. The core argument is that because international politics happens within the inherently social world of human relations, its constructs cannot be observed and measured as if they were neutral material objects with universally acceptable answers. Constructivism views reality along the lines of anthropologist Clifford Geertz's articulation: "man is an animal suspended in webs of significance he himself has spun" (Geertz, 1973, p. 5). This view holds that actors and their peers are, wittingly or not, the perpetual architects of a structure that is constantly being redrawn. In IR, constructivists are interested in unravelling these webs of significance by identifying the ideas, values, norms, knowledge, and practices that underpin them and that ultimately dictate the realities of global relations. In essence, constructivists are interested in human *ideas* rather than in the so-called immutable inevitability of human nature or other supposedly innate characteristics of world politics (Wendt, 1999). They focus on ideational rather than on only material causality; rejecting the dogmas of objectivity, universal truths, and innateness, constructivism emphasises instead the importance of inter-subjectivity (i.e. shared beliefs) – malleable and continuously renegotiated – governing the way in which its adherents behave (Ruggie, 1998).

Several subtypes of IR constructivist thought exist (see overviews provided in, for example, Jackson & Sørensen, 2013; Wendt, 1999). For the purposes of our analysis, select contributions comprise the theoretical foundation: from James March, Johan Olsen, and particularly, from Martha Finnemore and Kathryn Sikkink, all influenced by institutionalist sociology (for overviews, see DiMaggio & Powell, 1991; Finnemore, 1996). The institutionalist perspective describes the mechanisms behind – and emphasises the importance of – inter-subjective social constructs termed *institutions*. An institution is defined "as a relatively stable collection of practices and rules defining appropriate behaviour for a specific group of actors in a specific situation" (March & Olsen, 1998, p. 948). It further focuses on *institutionalisation* – that is, the process by which these institutions are constructed, diffused, and integrated. With regard to organisations, Finnemore (1996, p. 329) explains that institutionalism emphasises cultural aspects, rejecting the Weberian notion that organisations are "rationalised bureaucratic structures . . . the most efficient and effective way to coordinate the complex relations involved in modern technical work". In terms of this view, organisations of all sizes are also inherently social actors and are therefore informed by a set of cultural values that legitimises some behaviours and rejects others.

That is not to say that organisations such as the UN cannot act with some autonomy and be entrepreneurs and propagators of norms themselves: they certainly can, and do. Finnemore, along with colleague Michael Barnett, has characterised international organisations (IOs) – a category in which the UN is perhaps the most commonly known representative – as "the 'missionaries' of our time" (Barnett & Finnemore, 1999, p. 713). Indeed, they suggest, IOs are imbued with a powerful legitimacy that enables them to shape behaviour on a global scale both directly and indirectly, often through processes of the concentric spheres of *conference diplomacy* (Groom, 2013), *commission diplomacy* (Evans, 2013), and *summit diplomacy* (Dunn, 1996; Melissen, 2003). However, the idea is not to suggest that organisations, like all actors, make decisions and changes in a vacuum of pure rationality, but rather in relation to a plethora of social variables and influences:

> History is created by a complicated ecology of local events and locally adaptive actions. As individuals, groups, organisations, and institutions seek to act intelligently and learn in a changing world involving others similarly trying to adapt, they create connections that subordinate individual intentions to their interactions. The locally adaptive actions that constitute that ecology are themselves based on subtle intertwinings of rational actions based on expectations of consequences and rule-based action seeking to fulfil identities within environments that influence but do not uniquely require actions.

Expectations, preferences, identities, and meanings are affected by human interaction and experience. They coevolve with the actions they produce.

(March & Olsen, 1998, p. 969)

For March and Olsen, the behaviour of any actor is always rule based, since appropriate behaviour is conducted in ways prescribed by the relevant institutions, lest the actors risk losing their legitimacy: "[a]ction involves evoking an identity or role matching the obligations of that identity or role to a specific situation" (March & Olsen, 1998, p. 951). Indeed, actors behave "in accordance with rules and practices that are socially constructed, publicly known, anticipated, and accepted" (1998, p. 952).

Integral to Finnemore's work is a theme that permeates all the aforementioned aspects of global transformation characterising the subject matter at hand – namely, the notion of *norms* and their role in informing and constituting institutions. Finnemore and Sikkink, in their influential article 'Norm Dynamics and Political Change' (1998), argue for the significance of norms and morality in the world of international politics. The authors define a norm as "a standard of appropriate behaviour for actors with a given identity" (1998, p. 891), suggesting that norms act as significant determinants in limiting the actions taken by the actors of the international arena in any given context. Following this, it is argued that an understanding of the social institution of norms – and how these are constantly and continually renegotiated – can give great insight into the processes that determine behaviour and decision-making. The authors further lament the (at the time) complete lack of norm-based research and suggest the open possibility of doing so: "because norms by definition embody a quality of 'oughtness' and shared moral assessment, norms prompt justifications for action and leave an *extensive trail of communication* among actors that we can study" (1998, p. 892, our emphasis). Indeed, it is in the study of the dynamics and evolution of these shared moral assessments in which the value of this view is found for the subject matter of this book.[2]

The most celebrated aspect of the contribution of the aforementioned article lies in its description of the institutionalisation process of norms, termed the *norm life cycle*. The life cycle is divided into three stages: (1) *norm emergence*, (2) *norm cascade*, and (3) *norm internalisation*.

In short, it aims to follow the evolution of a norm from its inception, through its diffusion and finally to its full-fledged adoption. Following its evolution since 1989, this frame is useful for reviewing the life cycles of norms of various origins, sizes, and significances pertaining to global health in development. The value of

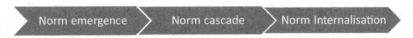

Norm emergence  ›  Norm cascade  ›  Norm Internalisation

*Figure 1.1* Summary of the norm life cycle

(Source: Finnemore & Sikkink, 1998, p. 896).

this framework is that it provides a way to trace elements of meaning as they evolve from idea to practice. Focusing on norms thus offers a lens through which the effects of a changing world to a global agenda-setting organisation can be traced: "norm language can help to steer scholars toward looking inside social institutions and considering the components of social institutions as well as the way these elements are renegotiated into new arrangements over time to create new patterns of politics" (Finnemore & Sikkink, 1998, p. 891).

In sum, this book utilises these constructivist perspectives in combination. We do this to trace how norms emerged, cascaded, and have become internalised to subsequently influence and make up the institutions that informed the decision- and policy-making of the health-related targets of the MDGs and the SDGs, respectively.

## The structure of the book

The present chapter provides a brief account of the book's broader context. It prefaces several aspects and concepts that will be more thoroughly explored in subsequent chapters. Most notably, these include the context that has precipitated today's development agenda, the basics of global health and its relation to IR, and a brief overview of the analytical framework that guides our analysis.

Chapter 2 provides context for the current UN development agenda by offering one version of its 'ideational genealogy'. With 1989 as its starting point, the chapter explores various normative developments relevant to the evolution of the MDGs and the SDGs. For the former framework, these anchor points refer mostly to the contents of a range of conferences and summits and their respective outcome documents as well as to the publication of the annual human development reports (HDRs), which began in 1990. The lead-up to the post-2015 agenda is treated in a slightly different manner and focuses more on the performance of the MDGs, as well as other global events and developments considered pertinent, before providing an account of the far more structured process that eventually produced the SDGs. The chapter's main purpose is to set the ideational stage for the book as a whole, perhaps most significantly by presenting an account of the normative axioms that guide the UN development agenda and explaining the processes through which these were introduced and cemented. The chapter provides the wider context of the development agendas that comprise the case studies; as part of this process, it introduces several central concepts and ideas, such as the human development paradigm.

Contextualising is also the purpose of Chapter 3, which explores the nexus of health and IR. More specifically, it introduces the basic concepts associated with global health and global health governance, setting the stage for subsequent chapters. Most pertinent is the introduction of the various actors involved in global health, and the categorisation of norms related to the respective rationales of state security and human security. The main aim of the chapter is to present the political dimensions of health governance, including health development efforts, and to identify the actors and variables relevant to the norm analyses that feature in Chapters 5 and 6. The chapter also situates this study within an expanding sub-field that connects health and IR.

Chapter 4 provides an account of the normative mechanics that precipitated the institutionalisation of the human development paradigm. The chapter also introduces the concept of the *meta-norm* and places the human development paradigm within the concept's description and definition. The chapter has two main objectives. First, it provides supplementary context to the intrinsic characteristics of the two development agenda case studies; it postulates that the human development paradigm constitutes the normative backbone of both the MDGs and the SDGs and thus establishes the foundation for the two framework and health norm-specific chapters that follow. The second objective of the chapter is a normative exploration that sets the stage for the more specific norm life cycles of the health norms that feature in Chapters 5 and 6. It identifies and explores the overarching normative institution that sets the standards of appropriateness for the MDGs and the SDGs while also establishing the prerequisite conditions for the evolution of the specific norms and institutions more directly related to the health development goals of the two frameworks.

The first health norm life cycle examinations appear in Chapter 5, in which the health goals of the MDGs are scrutinised. Building on the technical, theoretical, and contextual content of the preceding chapters, the three health-specific MDGs are viewed through the lens of the norm life cycle and its three stages, particularly emphasising the first stage of norm entrepreneurship and framing. The three MDGs in question contain norms related to children's mortality, maternal mortality, and communicable diseases, respectively. The purpose of the chapter is to identify the leading health norms of the framework and to determine the rationale and basic motivations behind their institutionalisation. The chapter positions these rationales within the interest-categories of human security and state security. Furthermore, the chapter identifies norm entrepreneurs and picks up the thread from the previous chapter regarding the trajectories of health norms in global development policy.

Chapter 6 has a similar function to the preceding chapter, focusing on the post-2015 development agenda, as signified by the SDGs. The first half of the chapter is dedicated to further normative contextualisation, with a particular focus on the meanings associated with the concept of sustainable development and its relationships with health. One particularly important aspect of sustainable development – that of inclusivity – is given special treatment in the chapter, due to the heavily publicised and clear normative implications it has for the development agenda at large and for health development more specifically. In the second half of the chapter, the two health-normative novelties of the SDGs, identified as (1) the prevention and treatment of non-communicable diseases and (2) the pursuit of universal health coverage, are discussed. Again, there is a greater focus on the first stage of the norm life cycle, as the meanings and framings of health norms are considered most pertinent to our research questions. The purposes of the chapter are similar to those of Chapter 5 – namely, to identify norm entrepreneurs and to further understand health-normative trajectories as they relate and interconnect with the development agenda on the one hand and global health politics on the other.

## Notes

1 The Health 8 (H-8) is an informal group of eight health-related organisations comprising WHO, UNICEF, UNFPA, UNAIDS, GFATM, GAVI, the Bill & Melinda Gates Foundation, and the World Bank.
2 There are, of course, always competing epistemologies and conceptual frameworks available – particularly, in the broad church that is Constructivism. In particular, see critical realist approaches (the work on norm circles in particular) (Archer & Elder-Vass, 2012; Elder-Vass, 2015).

# 2 How ideas have evolved in the United Nations development agenda

The purpose of this chapter is to contextualise the setting within which health norms in the UN development agenda have evolved since 1989. Health-focused development efforts, though significant, are part of this much larger system. The UN development agenda, as a whole, is a system of thought and a system of practice, permeated with ideas and norms that have been woven together, pulled apart, and rewoven since the inception of the organisation itself and, in particular, since the beginning of the 1990s. To explain how health has come to achieve such prominence within the contemporary global development project, one needs to understand how the UN development agenda itself emerged. This chapter provides such an understanding through presenting a history of the ideational and practical underpinnings of this environment and, in the process, creates a road map of some of the social and political influences that steered its evolution.

The chapter is divided into three separate sections, each focusing on and describing a chronological period. The first section focuses on the 1990s, generally viewed as the most explicitly formative years of the current development agenda. The second component of the chapter investigates more closely the lifespan of the MDGs from 2000 to 2015, covering their conception, implementation, performance, and conclusion. The third and final section describes the process of the construction of the post-2015 development agenda and the goals associated with it, the SDGs. The period stretches from 2010 to 2016, thus partially overlapping with the timeline of the previous section.

## The seminal 1990s

The focus of this book is the period between 1989 and 2015–2016. This does not mean, however, that the 44 years between the establishment of the UN and the beginning of our timeframe are irrelevant. They are, in fact, absolutely essential for understanding the world today. However, a more detailed view of the period 1945–1989 is omitted because we lack the space to do it justice, and the 1990s, the 2000s, and the 2010s have greater immediacy.

This section presents the continued evolution of the UN development agenda, focusing on a significant period of that process – namely, the 1990s. It focuses on the major ideas and norms that informed and spurred major international meetings and summits, which, in turn, further solidified these ideas and translated them into policy. We aim to give an account of how these norms culminated in the 2000 Millennium Summit and the subsequent creation of the MDGs.

### 1990–1991: initial origins

The publication in 1990 of the first *Human Development Report* (HDR) by the United Nations Development Programme (UNDP) is often considered a pivotal moment in global development. This 200-page publication explicitly aimed to shift the UN development agenda's paradigm from an economic focus that largely emphasised growth to what was referred to as a *human* focus:

> People are the real wealth of a nation. The basic objective of development is to create an enabling environment for people to enjoy long, healthy and creative lives. This may appear to be a simple truth. But it is often forgotten in the immediate concern with the accumulation of commodities and financial wealth.
>
> (UNDP, 1990, p. 9)

This report effectively heralded a new approach for global development: its goals were to be centred around *human development indicators*, of which financial goals were to be considered as contributing factors to the whole rather than being primary ends of development. Instead, there was to be an emphasis on people's *freedom of choice* – an idea most prominently championed by two of the report's most influential co-authors, Amartya Sen and Mahbub ul Haq, both of whom worked as advisors to the UNDP at the time. Haq, in particular, was to become the main norm entrepreneur for the coming development era – though other individuals were also highly influential and integral to this process. This process is covered in greater detail in Chapter 4. The new paradigm included further non-economic factors such as health, knowledge, and freedom from violence. Furthermore, variable social- and contextual-specific factors were also to be integrated as well as a range of other new indicators. Already in its opening paragraphs, the report is remarkably ambitious with regard to its own future significance:

> The Report is of a seminal nature. It makes a contribution to the definition, measurement and policy analysis of human development. It is the first in a series of annual reports. It opens the debate. Subsequent reports will go into further detail regarding the planning, management and financing of human development.
>
> (UNDP, 1990, p. iii)

In hindsight, the first HDR was indeed influential. While the initial academic responses to it were rather lukewarm, characterised by a blend of scepticism and hopefulness (see, for example, Hopkins, 1991; McGillivray, 1991), it was, along with its new human-centred development paradigm, quickly adopted by UN member states – developed and developing alike. The annual HDRs would have a powerful voice within the discourse of global development thinking in the next decade. In 2004, the UNDP proudly published *Ideas, Innovation, Impact: How Human Development Reports Influence Change*, in which they emphasised the popularity and significance of the endeavour: "since 1992, more than 500 national and sub-national HDRs have been produced by 143 countries, in addition to 28 regional reports. The launch of a report is frequently a high-profile regional or even international event" (UNDP, 2004, p. 1).

This rapid adoption of the ideas that the HDR(s) suggested did not occur in isolation; the timing and impact of the first HDR took place in a very specific global context. The previous decade had been disastrous in terms of developmental progress, and the SAPs had not been successful (in hindsight, perhaps rather detrimental), and the venture of development as a whole was in desperate need of revision. One observer goes as far as suggesting that the human development paradigm was more of an ignoble attempt to save the dwindling reputation of global development writ large than a revolution in thought:

> What use was 'development' unless it was 'human-centred'? Why had it taken so long to make this obvious point? Had development previously been 'inhuman'? But the point, of course, was to rehabilitate a largely discredited concept by giving it a spiritual boost that it would be in bad taste to refuse.
>
> (Rist, 2008, p. 205)

Regardless of the extent of the accuracy of such claims, the previous decade had also provided a significant change in all global relations, as the end of the Cold War had brought a number of changes to global dynamics in general (see Fukuyama, 1989). One significant change was the new perspectives and realities surrounding the theme of security. As the Cold War came to an end, the notion of *security* began to dilute, from focusing mainly on military threats (particularly, weapons of mass destruction) to encompassing several alternative variables (Buzan, 1997). As one contemporary scholar noted at the time, "[t]he security structures of the old bipolar, Cold War Europe are increasingly anachronistic in an era of deepening interdependencies and East-West cooperation" (Hyde-Price, 1991, p. 189). In the study of international relations, this 'widening' (Buzan, 1997) of the concept of security had slowly gained traction over the course of the 1980s, as critical and constructivist alternatives questioned the fundamental assumptions of the traditional *rationalist* paradigms (Wendt, 1992). As the unpredicted end of the Cold War became a reality, this more nuanced view of security increasingly solidified. A new and more pluralistic concept of security became a reality for policymakers and scholars alike, as the threat of military destruction was at least partially replaced by other less obvious threats. These non-military sources of threat include "domestic poverty, educational crises, industrial competitiveness, drug trafficking, crime, international migration, environmental hazards, resource shortages, global poverty, and so on" (Baldwin, 1995, p. 126). As one observer suggests:

> Alongside this expansion of the security agenda has developed a feeling that 'security' can no longer be conceived of simply as the 'absence of insecurity', any more than 'peace' can be regarded as 'the absence of war'. 'Security' should be considered more positively, as requiring the building of a more just and humane world in which human beings are better able to realize their aspirations and potential.
>
> (Garnett, 1996, p. 14)

Embedded in these circumstances, notions of interdependence and the recognition of the existence of common interests that defy national borders also made their impression on the UN's development agenda towards the end of the 1980s. Traditional perspectives of several disciplines were increasingly inconsistent with – and apparently unable to explain and predict – empirical reality. For those in charge of global development planning, signs that the primacy of purely economically focused programmes was undergoing a fundamental shift were starting to show. Economic growth, however achieved, was no longer considered the panacea to fuel and optimise global development. A widening of the scope of what constitutes *development*, and indeed a reimagining of the very goal of development, was underway.

The most significant action of the 1980s in the spirit of this newfound perspective came in the form of the *General Assembly's Resolution 44/228* (UNGA, 1989). Echoing ideational roots dating back to the UN Conference on Human Environment in Stockholm held in 1972, and inspired by the *Report of the World Commission on Environment and Development: Our Common Future* (Brundtland, 1987), the resolution "[d]ecides to convene the United Nations Conference on Environment and Development, which shall be of two weeks' duration and shall have the highest possible level of participation, to coincide with World Environment Day, on 5 June 1992" (UNGA, 1989, p. 152).

While this conference was in its early stages of planning, 1990 was already well underway. This specific year has been characterised as a "year [that] marked a watershed in the evolution of ideas about international development and poverty reduction" (Hulme, 2010b, p. 16). One of the major anchor points in the new development paradigm was a renewed perspective on poverty and poverty reduction that came about partly as a result of the disappointing results of the SAPs. In June, the World Bank released its annual *World Development Report* (World Bank, 1990). This report is considered particularly significant, as it provided a framework for measuring poverty, including the definition of characterising those living on less than $1 per day to be in extreme poverty, an amount that was applicable to about 1.1 billion people at the time.

In March of the same year, a smaller-scale conference was held in Jomtien, Thailand, named the World Conference for Education for All. Written in the spirit of the new human development paradigm, the background paper to the

---

**Box 2.1  Terminology**

**Summits and conferences:** Summits are extraordinarily large-scale meetings that are mainly attended by heads of states or governments. They differ slightly from conferences, which are often attended by *representatives* of governments, such as relevant ministers. Summits also differ from conferences in that they are more heavily publicised in the media and have more gravity of significance about them.

**Declarations:** Have the purpose of outlining the intentions and aspirations of the parties involved. Typically, a declaration is *not* legally binding – although there are some significant exceptions to this: for example, the 1948 *Declaration of Universal Human Rights*.

**Programmes/plans of action:** Often accompanying *Declarations*, these documents typically provide specific means of implementation, policy implications, and recommendations pertinent to the sentiments agreed upon at the relevant conference.

**Conventions:** Agreed upon by parties, usually after multilateral negotiations, conventions are considered to be a source of international law. Conventions typically cover specific matters – for example, the UN Convention on the Law of the Sea of 1982.

(Source: The authors).

---

conference reaffirms the integral importance of education as a contributing factor to development. The main fruits of this conference were its adoption of the *World Declaration on Education for All* and, in particular, its practical *Framework for Action to Meet Basic Learning Needs*. The *Declaration* reaffirmed the status of education as a human right as well as its integral part in personal and social lives and in creating a safer, more prosperous, and peaceful world and thus in optimising development efforts. The *Framework* describes the practical implementation of the ideas set out in the *Declaration* and is one of the pioneering documents in terms of setting time-bound intermediary and long-term goals. A decade later, these goals would inspire much of the language for MDGs 2 and 3.

Similarly, the second conference on the least developed countries (LDCs), held in September 1990 in Paris, produced a *Programme of Action* that would prove a precursor to how the MDGs would finally be formulated more than a decade later. The conference, with 150 governments represented among its attendees, had the main object of reviewing the progress of the LDCs in the preceding decade and, in particular, the effect of the economic policies that were so widespread in the 1980s: the SAPs. Subsequently, the purpose was to agree upon concrete goals and strategies that were meant to ensure a greater sense of progress in the 1990s.

Again, there is optimism and ambition tinged with the sentiments of the emerging human development paradigm in the UN's official statement post-conference:

> The various elements of the Programme should be viewed as essential components of the overall strategy for economic and social progress for the developing world. The Programme represents a qualitative step forward which goes beyond the Substantial New Programme of Action for the 1980s for the Least Developed Countries, adopted in 1981, and contains many novel features. One notable aspect concerning actions at the national level relates to the emphasis placed on the need for development to be human-centred and broadly based.
>
> ("Outcome on Least Developed Countries", n.d., para. 2)

Along with the *Programme for Action*, the conference also resulted in the *Paris Declaration* (not to be confused with the *2005 Paris Declaration* on aid effectiveness), which acts as a pledge of commitments from the attending member states to contribute as much as possible in achieving the goals set out in the *Programme for Action*.

That health was another significant component in the new development paradigm became clear at another important event in 1990, an event that would prove to be another ideational antecedent to the MDGs. The World Summit for Children held in New York was, in several ways, responsible for setting the tone for the range of other issue-specific summits that would be held throughout the decade. At the time, it was considered to be the largest convocation of world leaders so far in history: 159 governments were represented as well as 45 non-governmental organisations (NGOs). Its focus was ambitiously manifold, with goals in health (generally for children and mothers), education, nutrition, and human rights all on the agenda. Again, a *Declaration* and a *Plan for Action* followed in the wake of the conference, also the largest in sheer scale of its kind up until that point in history. The conference is still remembered fondly by the UN's development history database:

> The goals established at the 1990 World Summit for Children have had an extraordinary mobilizing power, generating a high level of commitment on behalf of children around the world, and creating new partnerships between Governments, NGOs, donors, the media, civil society and international organizations in pursuit of a common purpose.
>
> (UN, 1997, para. 2)

The Children's Summit came to be very significant because it pioneered many 'firsts' in the context of global development coordination. It was the first meeting of this scale that intended and managed to identify specific goals across a broad spectrum of issues with quantifiable targets, while also taking care to ensure the necessary political commitment of the attending states. As Hulme observes, it also "established the notion that 'global summits,' that is large meetings of national leaders, could motivate processes leading to real improvements in human welfare" (Hulme, 2010a, p. 35). In the UN's own words, the Children's Summit

> served as an important organizational model for global mobilization. Its involvement of world leaders and its establishment of time-bound, measurable goals were pioneering endeavours, helping to mobilize resources and commitment and shape new initiatives with clear aims and directions.
>
> (UN, 1997, para. 3)

1991 was a far quieter year in terms of development-focused UN conferences. Indeed, no large-scale meetings were held that year, directed by, or in any way under the auspices of, the UN. The most significant events were (1) the second annual HDR (UNDP, 1991) and (2) the announcement of the 1990s as the Fourth Decade of Development (UNGA, 1990). The HDR was centred on firming the position and legitimacy of the human development paradigm (including the HDI measurements) in global governance. The main conclusion of this edition was that the main culprit for what it classifies as 'human neglect' is not the lack of financial resources, but of political commitment. That is to say that while there are sufficient funds to ensure a steady path to fulfilling human development, the funds are not being put to their full potential: "much current spending is misdirected and inefficiently used. If the priorities are set right, more money will be available for accelerated human progress" (UNDP, 1991, p. 1). In addition, the report emphasises that economic growth be viewed not as meaningless to development, but rather as a significantly integral part of the holistic human development project.

The resolution that proclaims the beginning of the UN's Fourth Decade of Development is full of lamentations in its introduction. The lament is directed towards the woefully unsuccessful previous decade and effectively reads as a litany of all that had gone wrong. In its section on priorities for the 1990s, it echoes the trending sentiments of the day: a continued focus on economic growth is still emphasised, but poverty alleviation, environmental issues, and human rights and resources are also underlined. Generally, the human development paradigm's sentiments, particularly those discussed in the 1991 HDR, influence the resolution:

> The decade of the 1990s must witness a significant improvement in the human condition everywhere and establish a mutually reinforcing relationship between economic growth and human welfare. The need to strengthen this relationship is, in fact, a principal theme for the current Strategy. It has not only to be reflected in the national efforts but must also be promoted by the international community through financial and technical support.
>
> (UNGA, 1990, p. 131)

By the conclusion of the decade's first two years, the tone had already been set for the 1990s in terms of the global development endeavour. Ideas that had been evolving towards the later years of the 1980s were now being adopted and becoming evident in policies and statements. Summits and conferences as forums in

which specific facets of development could be discussed in-depth with the participation of all member states and which produced specific plans of implementation
that had concrete and time-bound goals were becoming the *modi operandi* for performing and evolving the normative, theoretical, and practical aspects of the project. This trend had become especially clear after the Children's Summit. These
two years had also seen the explicit adoption and solidification of the human
development paradigm. The language of the outcome documents of the various
summits and that of the announcement resolution of the Fourth Decade of Development reflect this clearly. Additionally, the ideas set out in the annual HDRs supplemented this process by innovating new approaches and ideas for development
and refining and expanding on the ideas of the human development paradigm.

### 1992–1995: consolidation

1992 was another significant year for the further evolution of the ideas in development that would eventually lead up to the creation of the MDGs. Of particular
significance was the United Nations Conference on Environment and Development (UNCED), also known as the Earth Summit, held in Rio de Janeiro.
The preparations for the conference had already started a few years before, and
the original impetus had existed for 20 years. The preparatory period preceding the
Earth Summit was the most extensive yet, "unique in its size, scope, level of
participation, and process" (Grubb, 1993, p. xiii). This included substantial contributions from, above all, the 172 attendees representing governments, which took
the form of reports outlining the present and future of their specific environmental
concerns. Additionally, the preparatory period saw unprecedented significant contributions from NGOs.

In practice, the emphasis of the conference was more on environment than
on development. However, it held major significance for both these interconnected spheres of global governance. UNCED yielded five agreements signed
by all attending governments: the *Rio Declaration on Environment and Development*, *Agenda 21*, *the Framework Convention on Climate Change* (UNFCCC), *The
Convention on Biological Diversity*, and the *Forest Principles*. The two conventions
were considered successes by reason of sheer magnitude and then particularly the
UNFCCC, which would prove to be an antecedent to the Kyoto agreements five
years later. Additionally, a number of new international institutions were created
resulting from these agreements:

> The conventions on climate change and biodiversity created new bodies for
> scientific and technical advice relating to the treaties and their implementa-
> tion. Other new organizations whose creation was motivated by the UNCED
> process, though not created formally by governments at UNCED, include
> the Planet Earth Council and the Business Council for Sustainable Develop-
> ment. Worldwide, a number of national NGOs and umbrella NGOs also were
> formed as citizens organized to participate in UNCED.
>
> (Haas, Levy, & Parson, 1992, p. 7)

The most significant institution created was the Commission on Sustainable Development (CSD), mandated by *Agenda 21*. Its responsibilities included reviewing and monitoring progress in the implementation of *Agenda 21*,

> and activities related to the integration of environmental and developmental goals throughout the United Nations system through analysis and evaluation of reports from all relevant organs, organizations, programmes and institutions of the United Nations system dealing with various issues of environment and development, including those related to finance.
>
> (UN, 1992, Institutional Structure section, para. 38.13)

Against this background, the CSD was to communicate its findings and subsequent recommendations to the General Assembly through the UN Economic and Social Council (ECOSOC). In addition, the CSD was to collect input from NGOs and also act as a facilitator in the conversation between the UN system and various non-governmental actors. The CSD convened annually until its disbandment in 2012.

The norms and ideas set out in the *Rio Declaration* and *Agenda 21* duo had a significant bearing on the future of development thinking. The *Declaration*, though not immune to criticism – and perhaps not living up to what was envisioned prior to the summit – was nonetheless received with a great deal of optimism. In short, the *Declaration* comprises 27 principles outlining the views of the 'international community' with regard to future environmental and developmental issues. *Agenda 21* is a much more detailed, 350-page 'action' plan designed for helping IOs, NGOs, and states practically fulfil their part of the principles outlined in, above all, the declaration but also in the aforementioned conventions. However, the implementation of the various policies of the action plan remains voluntary and therefore was not as widely adopted as had been the stated ambition prior to the summit. From a larger perspective, the UNCED agreements, particularly the *Declaration* and *Agenda 21*, added significant volume and momentum to the snowball of summitry that was beginning to characterise the decade. With regard to mass coordination of both normative principles and of practical quantifiable goals and methods for achieving the ideals set out in the principles, UNCED was doubtlessly the most significant event to date. In the words of one observer writing the year after, the preparatory process, execution, and products of UNCED, and specifically the *Rio Declaration*, would serve as "a new basis for international cooperation" (Porras, 1992, p. 245).

1992 also produced another *Declaration*, a product of the International Conference on Nutrition, directed by the World Health Organization (WHO). Signed by the 159 government representatives present at the conference, the *World Declaration on Nutrition* is one that announces an intention "to eliminate hunger and all forms of malnutrition" (WHO, 1992, p. 9). Emphasising that access to proper food is a human right, the *Declaration* further proposes that the problem lies not with the amount of food in the world, but in its inequitable distribution. The appended *Plan of Action* provides guidelines for a number of actors, including governments both affected and non-affected by hunger issues, the private sector and local communities, and multilateral institutions and NGOs.

The 1992 HDR focuses on optimising global markets for the purpose of maximising human development and particularly for reducing poverty. It suggests that developing countries should invest in their capacity to compete in the global market place. In this respect, the 'Asian tigers' are referred to as examples of developing countries that have been able to create a competitive edge for themselves in the global market. The report also suggests changes in the foundation of the global markets, including a restructuring of the IFIs and suggesting that a Summit on Social Development be held under the auspices of the UN. This summit became a reality in Copenhagen in 1995 and is discussed in more detail later.

The year 1993 was a relatively quiet year in terms of conferences and summits, with one significant exception. In June, the World Conference on Human Rights was held in Vienna. Attended by representatives from 171 governments, the purpose of the conference was to take stock of the global human rights situation since the adoption of the *Universal Declaration of Human Rights* 45 years earlier. The conference was somewhat marred by a degree of controversy in its preparation and execution. The original impetus for the conference had come in the spirit of the aforementioned enthusiasm that swept the globe around the end of the Cold War. By 1993, however, much of this optimism had waned (see Boyle, 1995). In the period before the conference, the preparatory committees struggled to find common ground on which all member states could agree. Indeed, attendees were politely forbidden to speak to specific human rights violations of which some of the attending states were guilty at the time, including China, Liberia, and those involved in the conflict in the Balkans. Nevertheless, the conference did achieve a degree of success in terms of adding to the mentioned snowball of global development coordination through summitry and conferences. It had an impressive array of participants from diverse spheres of the global communities, including 800 NGOs. A large number of academics and national institutions were represented – totalling 7,000 participants for the conference. The *Vienna Declaration* (UN, 1993) was released as the product of the conference, along with a *Programme of Action*, signed by all participating governments. These agreements were intended to strengthen and enhance international cooperation in order to secure human rights for all. Not only development but also certain contemporary global issues such as terrorism are considered to fall within the scope of human rights. Development is viewed in the *Vienna Declaration* as a human right, reaffirming the *right to development*, as was originally recognised and outlined by the Organisation of African Unity (OAU)[1] in 1981 and subsequently adopted by the UN five years later in the *Declaration on the Right to Development* (UNGA, 1986) – now reiterated with a stronger tinge of the human development paradigm:

> The World Conference on Human Rights reaffirms the right to development, as established in the Declaration on the Right to Development, as a universal and inalienable right and an integral part of fundamental human rights. As stated in the Declaration on the Right to Development,

the human person is the central subject of development. While development facilitates the enjoyment of all human rights, the lack of development may not be invoked to justify the abridgement of internationally recognized human rights. States should cooperate with each other in ensuring development and eliminating obstacles to development. The international community should promote an effective international cooperation for the realization of the right to development and the elimination of obstacles to development. Lasting progress towards the implementation of the right to development requires effective development policies at the national level, as well as equitable economic relations and a favourable economic environment at the international level.

(UN, 1993, pp. 3–4)

These and similar sentiments in the *Vienna Declaration* attempt to solidify the interdependent connection between human rights and development, further amplifying the individual and communal responsibility of signatory governments to contribute in a coordinated development agenda.

The theme of the 1993 HDR (UNDP, 1993) is people's participation in development. In short, it insists that policy measures should actively aim to include the beneficiaries of development, identified as people, into employment and entrepreneurship. This was meant to reinforce the view of people as essential resources rather than as passive recipients of development or victims of underdevelopment. Among the general suggestions of the report are the development of new partnerships between state and market, emphasising that a balanced symbiosis between the two rather than a separation is the ideal. It also speaks to the growth and spread of democracy as integral to a real sense of participation, as well as the importance of enabling international cooperation in order to optimise people-centred development (Haq, 1995).

The same year, the World Bank added extra weight to the position of health in development with economically focused arguments that generally framed health as an investment that would result in economic productivity and accelerate development. The contents of the *World Development Report 1993: Investing in Health* (World Bank, 1993) largely revolves around identifying the respective roles of governments and the market with regard to this investment endeavour. It concludes with a suggestion of a three-pronged approach:

First, governments need to foster an economic environment that enables households to improve their own health. . . . Second, government spending on health should be redirected to more cost-effective programmes that do more to help the poor. Government spending accounts for half of the $168 billion annual expenditure on health in developing countries. Too much of this sum goes to specialized care in tertiary facilities that provides little gain for the money spent. . . . Third, governments need to promote greater diversity and competition in the financing and delivery of health services.

(World Bank, 1993, p. iii)

Yet to fully embrace the essential assumptions of the burgeoning human development paradigm, the World Bank's emphasis still lay more with the economic implications of health improvement; its inherent merit is also mentioned, but the report is void of explicit reference to capabilities and human development.

Like the year preceding it, 1994 was a calm year in terms of large-scale UN events on development. The only notable high-level meeting was the International Conference on Population and Development (ICPD) held in Cairo in September. Although the attendees at the ICPD discussed a broad spectrum of themes, it gained most of its significant media attention because of its controversial subject matter of maternal health and, specifically, family planning.[2] Despite the fact that the Holy See and certain Islamic states very publicly challenged any agreements on that particular topic, the conference ended in agreements that included these themes. Universal education; reduction of infant, child and maternal mortality; and access to sexual health services were central themes in which specific goals were agreed upon by the 179 governments attending – including the active discouragement of female genital mutilation. These goals are specified in ICPD's subsequent *Programme for Action*, which suggests policy implications and a plan for implementation.

The 1994 HDR is one of the more distinguished and discussed of the series. This is owing to its emphasis on and definition of *human security*. Offering an alternative paradigm that challenged the traditional notions of the state as the referent object for security, human security had become increasingly popular – particularly since the end of the Cold War. The 1994 HDR is largely credited for formulating the concept and ideas behind it and its links with development (MacLean, Black, & Shaw, 2006). As initially outlined in the report, human security entails the concepts of *freedom from want* and *freedom from fear*. It is defined in these terms:

> Human security can be said to have two main aspects. It means, first, safety from such chronic threats as hunger, disease and repression. And second, it means protection from sudden and hurtful disruptions in the patterns of daily life – whether in homes, in jobs or in communities. Such threats can exist at all levels of national income and development.
>
> (UNDP, 1994, p. 23)

The 1994 report is confident about the success of this new concept of security: "The idea of human security, though simple, is likely to revolutionize society in the 21st century" (UNDP, 1994, p. 22). Similarly, Haq confidently commented a year after the report's publication that "the emerging concept of human security will lead to many fundamental changes in thinking" (Haq, 1995, p. 40). The concept sparked a number of theoretical debates within development as well as within IR and in areas where these overlap – this is discussed in further detail in Chapter 3. In terms of its effect on the UN development agenda, the human security perspective acted as yet another building block on which the foundation of the human development paradigm was strengthened. However, as the report stresses, human security and human development are interlinked, but not strictly the same thing. Human development is a broader concept of which human security is only one integral aspect. However, without human security, human development is in serious jeopardy.

The years from 1992 to 1994 were highly consequential in both shaping and illustrating the direction in which the UN development agenda was moving. The 1992 Earth Summit solidified the role of the summit and that of the significance of their products, with its range of ideas manifested in documents that are still influential to this day. This is particularly true of its *Declaration* and, to an even larger extent, *Agenda 21* – a document that would later explicitly be a source of inspiration in the process of creating a post-2015 agenda 20 years later. While the Earth Summit integrated and developed ideas that had been opened up in Stockholm in 1972 prior to present challenges, the 1993 World Conference on Human Rights did the same, reaffirming the right to development and merging these older sentiments with the ever-growing human development paradigm. Furthermore, the 1994 HDR was the most significant instalment since the first edition of the series, and it presented scholars, politicians, and policymakers with a new view on security that would be compatible with the human development paradigm. Although the lasting impact of this idea is debatable (Paris, 2001), it challenged norms that were once thought undisputable and contributed significantly to the discourse of security.

## 1995–1999: the millennium approaches

The year 1995 is commonly remembered as one of the most noteworthy years in the context of the evolution of the UN development agenda. Most significant was the World Summit for Social Development held in Copenhagen in March: a summit requested in the 1992 HDR. Setting new records in terms of attendance of world leaders in history, the summit had a broad focus on various development themes, particularly poverty, employment, and social integration. The summit's products, the *Copenhagen Declaration* and the *Programme of Action*, are saturated with ideas of the human development paradigm. The *Declaration* opens its section on 'Principles and Goals' in this manner:

> We heads of State and Government are committed to a political, economic, ethical and spiritual vision for social development that is based on human dignity, human rights, equality, respect, peace, democracy, mutual responsibility and cooperation, and full respect for the various religious and ethical values and cultural backgrounds of people.
>
> (UN, 1995a, p. 6)

The conference covered a broad array of themes. Among the issues discussed that subsequently led to goals agreed upon were the eradication of poverty, the achievement of full employment, gender equality and equity, the attainment of universal and equitable health care and the strengthening of international development cooperation. Another consequence of the conference was a new role for the UN Commission for Social Development, originally established in 1946. The commission was meant to act as a follow-up to the conference and still convenes annually to discuss issues and themes in the sphere of social development. Essentially, the purpose of the commission, 46 members strong, is to ensure the implementation of the principles and goals agreed upon at the conference, in a way similar to that in which the aforementioned CSD monitors progress of the implementation of *Agenda 21* and the *Rio Declaration* of 1992. In essence, the *Copenhagen Declaration* further solidified the ideas of the human development paradigm in all strands of the development endeavour in a very explicit way, while firmly placing the eradication of poverty as the most essential goal of development.

The other major conference of 1995 was September's Fourth World Conference on Women held in Beijing. As had been the case with the previous women's conferences, its purpose was to achieve a greater sense of equality for women globally. Leading up to the conference, the issue of sexual and reproductive health was once again publicly criticised by the Holy See. Regardless, the conference went ahead without major complications and produced the *Beijing Declaration* and a *Platform for Action*. The *Declaration* reaffirms the principles that guide the agenda of the conference – namely, the empowerment of women in terms of equal rights and opportunity. The language of these agreements is heavily centred on a discourse of inherent human rights and of the integral importance of women in the global development project as well as in contributing to the attainment of global peace. The *Platform for Action* is a detailed account of the situation for women and 'the girl child' in the world at the time; of areas of concern; and finally, of suggested policy measures.

The 1995 HDR (UNDP, 1995) also focused on mitigating gender disparities and ensuring women's rights, which it views as integral to the realisation of human development. With the slogan "human development, if not engendered, is endangered" (UNDP, 1995, p. 1), this report carries with it much of the same phraseology as the products of the Beijing Women's Conference. It emphasises the many areas globally where women are underappreciated, abused, generally mistreated, and underestimated as a consequence of their gender, all the while showing how this is detrimental to the human development project. The report also introduces the *Gender Development Index (GDI)* as a basis for measuring gender (in)equality.

One significant 'external' publication appeared in late 1995. Haq's *Reflections on Human Development* explores the author's "intellectual journey – and the world's – through a profound transition in development thinking in recent decades" (Haq, 1995, p. xvii). The Pakistani economist, the main intellectual and practical architect behind the human development paradigm and the founder of the HDRs, writes about the philosophical and technical underpinnings of the paradigm, its current success, and its future utility. Haq reiterates and expands on the ideas presented in the HDRs that had been published up to that point, succinctly contextualising their sentiments into realistic policies that would replace existing ones – arguing in some detail for the reasons why this would make sense, from both a financial and developmental perspective. The book also includes a sub-stantial argument for the legitimacy of the HDI as a global monitoring tool. These ideas are expanded upon in greater detail in Chapter 4.

The most significant event for global development discourse in 1996 was the World Food Summit held in November in Rome, with 10,000 participants and representatives from 185 countries attending the event. The agenda was to discuss the response to one of the most challenging and salient global problems: world hunger and malnutrition. The Food Summit created a platform for the interna-tional community to debate the ways in which to best go about this endeavour and to renew commitments from the attending states. The *Rome Declaration on World Food Security* reaffirms the universal human right of access to safe food and defines the concept of *food security*.[3] It also lists all the negative physical and social consequences of hunger and reiterates food security's integral importance to the human development paradigm. The declaration's *Plan of Action* subsequently out-lines the practical implications of the results of the summit. The *Plan of Action* provided the UN's Food and Agriculture Organization's (FAO) Committee on World Food Security with a new mandate to monitor the progress of the goals set out in the *plan*.

In June, a smaller event took place in Istanbul. The UN Conference on Human Settlements (nicknamed Habitat II) was focused on the issue of adequate and safe shelter for all. Habitat II, planned during the Earth Summit four years earlier, explicitly recognised the connection between adequate housing and development. The outcomes of the conference can be found in its agreements, which comprise the *Istanbul Declaration* and the *Habitat Agenda*. These documents are framed within the human development paradigm and recognise the connection among various global challenges. In certain passages, nearly all aspects of the develop-ment project are summed up:

> As human beings are at the centre of our concern for sustainable devel-opment, they are the basis for our actions as in implementing the Habitat Agenda. We recognize the particular needs of women, children and youth for safe, healthy and secure living conditions. We shall intensify our efforts to eradicate poverty and discrimination, to promote and protect all human rights and fundamental freedoms for all, and to provide for basic needs, such as education, nutrition and life-span health care services, and, especially, ade-quate shelter for all. To this end, we commit ourselves to improving the living conditions in human settlements in ways that are consonant with local needs and realities, and we acknowledge the need to address the global, economic, social and environmental trends to ensure the creation of better living envi-ronments for all people. We shall also ensure the full and equal participation of all women and men, and the effective participation of youth, in political, economic and social life. We shall promote full accessibility for people with disabilities, as well as gender equality in policies, programmes and projects for shelter and sustainable human settlements development.
>
> (UN, 1996, para. 7)

Indeed, the *Declaration* and *Agenda* explicitly refer to the outcome documents of previous summits, taking inspiration from them and forming a holistic view of the settlement problem that includes concerns about health, nutrition, human rights, and more. Habitat II produced a new mandate for the United Nations Centre for Human Settlements (UNCHS), originally created after Habitat I in 1978. Its new responsibility was to act as a supporting and monitoring body for the implementation of the Habitat Agenda.

The same year saw a contribution to the global development discourse from a thus far unmentioned source: namely, the Organisation for Economic Co-operation and Development (OECD). The OECD's Development Assistance Committee (DAC) is a forum for discussing themes that relate to aid and development for the OECD members: a membership that includes the majority of the world's largest donor states. As Hulme (2009) suggests, aid agencies were struggling in the mid-1990s because fund allocation from national budgets towards ODA was decreasing:

> Ministers of International Development or Development Cooperation found themselves increasingly marginalised and the bureaucrats heading aid agencies found themselves engaged in the thankless tasks of defending their organisations and downsizing. The environment for aid was not propitious.
>
> (Hulme, 2009, p. 13)

In 1995 the DAC held a high-level meeting in Paris with the intent of reviewing the state of aid, assessing its utility, and making plans for the future. The eventual result was a 1996 DAC report titled *Shaping the 21st Century: The Contribution of Development Co-operation*. This 20-odd-page document was significant not only because it expressed the sentiments of the world's largest donors but also because it pioneered a realistic and rational framework of specific goals and deadlines for reaching these goals. It covered most, if not all, the themes of development challenges – but lacked a proper plan of action. These goals became known as the *International Development Goals* (IDGs). Although they did not receive much public attention, they were significant in an immediate sense in setting the agenda for certain OECD countries' strategies for ODA in the coming years. However, aside from specialised agencies, the IDGs were generally not particularly well followed up on or acted upon by their creator states. On the other hand, "drawing up the IDGs had unleashed a genie – the idea that an authoritative list of concrete development goals could be drawn up and used as a mechanism to rapidly reduce global poverty" (Hulme, 2009, p. 21). Fukuda-Parr and Hulme (2009) credit the IDGs with contributing to the emergence of what they call the *super-norm*[4] of poverty eradication. Interestingly, the IDGs were heavily inspired by goals originally formulated in the various UN conferences that had taken place earlier in the 1990s. This interchange of ideas would continue in the future, as a series of circumstances over the next years led to the IDGs greatly influencing how the MDGs would eventually come into being.

The 1996 edition of the HDR "explores in detail the complex relationship between economic growth and human development" (UNDP, 1996, p. iii). It concludes that there is no automatic link between the two, as many countries that have experienced economic growth have simultaneously experienced deterioration in terms of their HDI score. However, there is a potential symbiosis of economic growth and human development that needs to be realised in order to truly optimise the effort within the paradigm. The report is principally directed towards countries, recommending and outlining policy implications that, in theory, would allow economic growth to act as a contributor to human development.

Finally, 1996 saw the commencement of operations for the Joint United Nations Programme on HIV/AIDS (UNAIDS). HIV/AIDS had, by this time, largely become recognised as the most severe epidemic facing the developing world; its role in negatively affecting global health outcomes, and development progress in general, was to be a central topic in health development from this point. The trajectory of the disease's normative and practical position within the UN development is mapped in more detail in Chapters 3 and 5.

The years 1997 and 1998 were relatively quiet in terms of conferences and large-scale events, as the UN was slowly beginning to plan and build its forthcoming plans for the new millennium. The UNDP's HDR of 1997 was focused on poverty eradication. As the report alludes to in its introduction, the problem of poverty was perhaps the most discussed topic over the course of the 1990s, highlighted by the aforementioned 1995 Copenhagen Summit on Social Development. Now, this goal had also become the focal point of human development:

> [The] UNDP has made the eradication of poverty its overriding priority. As the principal antipoverty arm of the United Nations, it is well placed to work with other parts of the UN system, especially its sister organizations and agencies at the country level, to assist states in their programmes to eradicate poverty. Already, UNDP is working with more than 70 countries to follow up on the commitment made at Copenhagen.
>
> (UNDP, 1997, p. iii)

The report insists that the eradication of poverty is not a figment of utopian imagination. With the right policies implemented in the right ways (i.e. within the frames of the human development paradigm), it is a tangible and realistic goal. Subsequently, it spends most of its more than 120 pages convincing the reader of this point. For the UNDP, poverty is by now defined in terms of the human development paradigm and is meant to refer to "the denial of choices and opportunities for a tolerable life" (UNDP, 1997, p. 5). Subsequently, the policy recommendations are approached holistically and include several other major themes in development such as gender equality, general education, and health for all.

In 1998, the HDR keyword of the year was *consumption*. The report (UNDP, 1998) investigates the various forms and consequences of the massive rise in consumption seen in the 20th century. In the report and, by extension, the human development paradigm, consumption is viewed as a double-edged sword. On the one hand, increased consumption has benefitted the livelihoods of hundreds of millions of people: they are better fed, they are better sheltered from hot and cold weather, and they enjoy the manifold benefits of a stable supply of electricity. However, the distribution of consumption on a global scale is hopelessly unequal. Indeed, the report concludes, while one part of the world is over-consuming well beyond their needs and to the point of depleting global resources, another part is at the opposite end of the spectrum. Additionally, the inconvenient side effects of the dominant minority's excessive consumption often fall directly on those in poverty. Among these side effects, the report mentions pollution and the general degradation of the environment. In short, the UNDP is urging an increased sense of austerity in an increasingly interdependent world for the sake of sustainability. Additionally and relatedly, this report includes a meditation on the positive and negative effects of globalisation. The idea of the need to think globally and act locally is central in this report, as it tries to balance the responsibility of the international community with that of individual states, regions, and civil societies.

In 1999, the renowned economist Amartya Sen published his hugely influential book *Development as Freedom*. From the first sentences, one is immediately reminded of the theme of the 1998 HDR: "We live in a world of unprecedented opulence, of a kind that would have been hard even to imagine a century or two ago. . . . Yet we also live in a world with remarkable deprivation, destitution and oppression" (Sen, 1999a, p. 15). Sen, awarded the Nobel Prize in Economic Sciences the year before, uses the book to propose the expansion of freedom as both the ends and the means of development, giving freedom a dual role as both *constitutive* and *instrumental* in the development process. As expected from his background as a central figure in the evolution of the human development paradigm, Sen explicitly distances himself from 'narrower views of development' that focus primarily on economic growth, modernization, and technological advances. What is meant by 'freedom' in this framework is a multifaceted concept that involves a range of social, economic, and political factors that, in aggregate, constitute greater or lesser degrees of total "'capabilities' of persons to lead the kind of lives they value – and have reasons to value" (Sen, 1999a, p. 50). Furthermore, he argues that these different freedoms reinforce each other and are thus highly interdependent, which argues for the need of a holistic approach. As for the instrumental aspect of freedom in development, Sen suggests that:

> The second reason for taking substantive freedom to be so crucial is that freedom is not only the basis of the evaluation of success and failure, but it is also a principal determinant of individual initiative and social effectiveness. Greater freedom enhances the ability of people to help themselves and also to influence the world, and these matters are central to the process of development.
>
> (Sen, 1999a, p. 51)

The ideas outlined in this work had already been influential for some time, owing to Sen's prestigious position in the UNDP but were now truly well known by nearly all those connected with the global development project. They were received with general acclaim and propelled Sen's status further as one of the leading minds in global development thinking (see Pressman & Summerfield, 2000; Streeten, 2000).

Finally, 1999 saw the release of the 10th instalment of the HDR. This edition, dedicated to the memory of the recently deceased Mahbub ul Haq, is a further exploration of the various consequences of globalisation. Specifically, it focuses on

> those marginalized by globalization, and calls for a much bolder agenda of global and national reforms to achieve globalization with a human face. It cautions that globalization is too important to be left as unmanaged as it is at present, because it has the capacity to do extraordinary harm as well as good.
> (UNDP, 1999, p. v)

The report attempts to set an agenda for the future of global governance and particularly its necessary role for the future in reducing inequality. In terms of globalisation, this entails making sure that the benefits of the phenomenon are distributed more equitably while at the same time taking steps to minimise the negative side effects associated with the process.

The five years preceding the turn of the millennium were a testament to the power of the ideas that had been consolidated in the first half of the decade. The World Summit for Social Development in 1995 is perhaps the best example, as the norms of the human development paradigm informed its broad focus. Encompassing nearly all aspects of development, the outcome documents from this summit formalised a human-centred agenda across the board. The women's conference in the same year ensured that a gendered perspective was also integrated into the development agenda – a process that was further cemented with the publication of the 1995 HDR. The two major conferences of 1996 (the World Food Summit and Habitat II) developed important new idealistic anchor points and practical goals pertaining to their areas of concern, all framed within the now near-omnipresent and all-permeating human development paradigm. Additionally, the paradigm was further explored and legitimised with the publications of its two greatest minds, as Haq's (1995) and Sen's (1999a) books both were well received and highly influential, leading to further adoption of human development norms and sentiments (see, for example, Gasper, 2000; Gore, 2000).

Further, the latter half of the 1990s saw the crystallisation and internalisation of the super-norm of poverty eradication as the unequivocal main focus of the global development effort, as evidenced by the UN's conference outcome documents and by the DAC's IDGs. These goals were to become an example of how to formulate global development goals on the scale that the MDGs would later aim for. The HDRs of the final years before the millennium were topical for the present and the future, including poverty eradication, sustainable consumption, and the effort to steer globalisation into a force for good. These processes, along with those described earlier, combined to reach a critical mass as the millennium drew nearer.

## The creation, implementation, and efforts to salvage the MDGs

This section gives an account of the 15 years of the lifespan of the MDGs, from their inception and initial implementation through various tweaking processes that tried to secure their completion.

### 2000–2001: setting the stage

The planning for the relevant events that were to take place in the year 2000 had started at least as early as in 1998. In *Resolution 53/202* (UNGA, 1998), adopted in December 1998, intentions were made clear to begin a process of renewing the UN for the new millennium: the 55th session of the UN General Assembly (UNGA) was designated for mapping out this purpose. The same *resolution* had also announced the Millennium Summit, which was to be held in September 2000. Subsequent resolutions outlined the organisation and rough schedule of the summit and, most significantly, produced a draft of the seminal *Millennium Declaration*. The draft included discussions about foundational principles and values that were to inform a renewed UN. The organisation's future role in global peace and security is outlined, and the future of efforts in development is discussed. In the latter section, a wide array of the themes that concern development are covered, as it reiterates the UN's intention of continued and intensified work on alleviating poverty in particular, as well as addressing inequality, gender inequities, malnutrition, health problems, and many other areas.

As part of the UN renewal process and as preparation leading up to the summit, the organisation published an 80-page document titled *We the Peoples: the Role of the United Nations in the 21st Century*, authored by the then Secretary-General Kofi Annan. Its opening few sentences begin, as the HDRs also tend to do, on a positive note. People, Annan states, generally live longer and healthier lives and are better educated than in the past; they have access to better nutrition and information. However, as the HDRs also invariably do, Annan shifts his focus to the less fortunate:

> There are also many things to deplore, and to correct. The century just ended was disfigured, time and again, by ruthless conflict. Grinding poverty and striking inequality persist within and among countries even amidst unprecedented wealth. Diseases, old and new, threaten to undo painstaking progress. Nature's life-sustaining services, on which our species depends for its survival, are being seriously disrupted and degraded by our own everyday activities. The world's people look to their leaders, when they gather at the Millennium Summit, to identify and act on the major challenges ahead. The United Nations can succeed in helping to meet those challenges only if all of us feel a renewed sense of mission about our common endeavour. We need to remind ourselves why the United Nations exists – for what, and for whom. We also need to ask ourselves what kind of United Nations the world's leaders are

prepared to support, in deeds as well as words. Clear answers are necessary to energize and focus the Organization's work in the decades ahead. It is those answers that the Millennium Summit must provide.

(Annan, 2000, p. 5)

*Globalisation* is central theme in this publication. Much in the spirit of the most recent HDRs, the idea furthered by Annan is that the UN should work to ensure that the effects of globalisation are directed towards being beneficial for all of the world's population rather than "leaving billions of them in squalor" (Annan, 2000, p. 6). *We the Peoples* was intended as preparatory reading for the attendees of the Millennium Summit, as it outlines and identifies the most salient issues that were to be discussed. It is divided into chapters that cover the gamut of contemporary global challenges: 'governance and globalization', 'freedom from want', 'freedom for fear', 'sustaining our future', and finally 'renewing the United Nations'.

The 'freedom from want' chapter is directly devoted to how Annan and the UN envision the future of development in the 21st century. Poverty, education, employment, health (particularly, HIV/AIDS), settlements, trade, ODA, and other themes are all covered at some length, and the chapter gives an indication of areas upon which the renewed UN will focus, as well as how it will approach these issues, in the immediate future. The final pages of *We the Peoples*, titled 'For consideration by the summit', include three lists of targets, covering the areas of development, war, peace and security, and the renovation of the UN envisioned for the 21st century. The development section comprises 19 goals that cover all the areas of the 'freedom from want' chapter. Significantly, many of these goals are quantifiable and were set to be fulfilled within a proposed period of time. These most envisaged their end point in 2015, a year that would symbolise both hope and subsequent lack of progress and – finally – renewal for the UN's development agenda.

*The millennium summit and drawing up the MDGs*

The scope of the Millennium Summit was enormous, covering the plethoric range of themes mentioned in *We the Peoples*. Despite the fact that the reputation of the UN as the undisputed leader of global governance had declined over the last decade or so,[5] there was massive anticipation before the event. The months preceding it, however, were slightly chaotic – perhaps because of the sheer scale of its focus as well as its large number of stakeholders. The summer of 2000 was characterised by "frantic negotiations about what should finally go in to the *Millennium Declaration*" (Hulme, 2009, p. 33). The OECD countries had hopes that the wording of the *Declaration* would approximate their own IDGs. Other stakeholders and interest groups, such as the remaining members of the UN; countless NGOs; business corporations; and other social interest groups were all vying for influence. As Hulme suggests, the disparities between *We the Peoples* and the *Declaration* can to an extent reflect how the UN was influenced by various groups to modify or reprioritise certain points. For example, direct references pertaining to infant, child and maternal mortality, absent from Annan's preparatory document, were included in the *Declaration* after a lobbying competition between women's health organisations and the Vatican, a point of normative contention returned to in Chapter 5.

In the end, on 8 September 2000, the *Millennium Declaration* was unanimously approved by all the attending states (of which a record 149 were represented by their heads of state, making the Millennium Summit the hitherto largest gathering of state leaders in world history). In terms of its section on development, where poverty reduction stands as the undisputed *leitmotif*, the *Declaration* essentially worked as a prototype for the MDGs. As was the case in *We the Peoples*, 2015 is given as a deadline year for the goals that are mentioned (with the exception of 2020 for improvement of the lives of 100 million slum dwellers). After the Millennium Summit had been convened and deemed successful, the challenge of implementing the sentiments agreed upon in the *Declaration* followed. In UNGA *Resolution 55/162: Follow-up to the Outcome of the Millennium Summit*, it is stated that the body "[recognises] the necessity for creating a framework of implementation of the Millennium Declaration" (UNGA, 2000a, p. 1). It was extremely important for Annan and the UN that this be done quickly, while the momentum of the Millennium Summit was still alive. As Vandemoortele writes:

> Each global conference or world summit produces a declaration which captures the public's attention for a while but quickly recedes into oblivion. This occurred again in September 2000 when the Millennium Summit issued the Millennium Declaration. For several months, the document was quoted in countless speeches, reports and articles. But after a while the attention started to fade. It was then that the idea arose to place selected targets contained in the Millennium Declaration into a free-standing category in order to rescue them from oblivion. They came to be known as the Millennium Development Goals.
>
> (Vandemoortele, 2011, p. 4)

In practice, this process turned out to be slightly untidy and far from straightforward, as the UN and its agencies found itself in negotiations with the IFIs, various NGOs, and particularly, with the DAC. The latter, integral to the realisation of the world envisioned by the *Millennium Declaration* (UNGA, 2000b), proved to be a thorn in the side for Annan and the UN during the making of this implementation plan. As Hulme (2009) indicates, the OECD countries, in spite of signing the *Declaration*, wanted the wording of the goals to be all but identical to those of the IDGs originated by the DAC in 1995 – with support from the IFIs. They did not see a reason to develop new indicators for new goals when the ones that they had perfected for five or six years were already there. Meanwhile, the UN was in a pickle: Annan desperately wanted to have one set of coordinating goals for global governance led by the UN and did not want to compete with the DAC's IDGs. At the same time, he had to follow through on his promise from the Millennium

Summit, and simply adopting the IDGs as its framework would have been less than satisfactory.

After some reportedly resentful meetings, most of which were held in private, the two parties seemed to have come to agreement by the middle of 2001. In *Road Map towards the Implementation of the United Nations Millennium Declaration*, published in early September, Annan makes reference to consulting with the Bretton Woods institutions as well as with the OECD in the final process of designing and defining the MDGs. Finally, after being laid out in detail in a section of this report, the MDGs were published in their entirety in the last pages of the document: 8 goals, 18 targets, and 48 indicators (see Table 1.1). The list of MDGs as a product of the Millennium Summit and *Declaration* were actually products of a much longer conversation and, particularly, one carried through the conferences and HDRs of the decade preceding it. The human development paradigm–saturated norms and values that had cascaded throughout these summits, along with their implementation plans, combined with the experienced and hands-on mind-sets of the IFIs and the DAC to realise the final version of the MDGs (see Figure 2.1).

### 2002–2004: progress, results, and signs of trouble

Now was the time to monitor progress and see whether or not the goals would be reached by the 2015 deadline. Several steps had been taken over the years to ensure that this would become a reality. As early as 2002, the *Millennium Campaign* was launched, designed to encourage and facilitate citizen participation in the endeavour to reach the goals. This initiative seemed to be the result of cracks already starting to show in the implementation processes of the MDGs. Indeed, Kofi Annan and UNDP administrator Mark Malloch Brown, who had been a central figure in the MDG negotiations, along with the organisation at large, came to realise that member states were not contributing nearly enough resources to the cause they had committed to a mere two years earlier. An example is that of the U.S., who was overtly opposed to some of the MDG requirements. The Goal 8 clause that 0.7 per cent of gross national income should go to

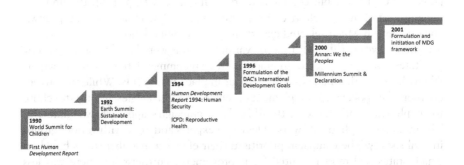

*Figure 2.1* Key moments and publications, 1990–2001

ODA was not, Washington argued, part of the original *Millennium Declaration*. In their view, they had signed the *Declaration*, not the MDGs. In practice, the Millennium Campaign was tasked with the purpose of mobilising 'partners for action'. In various ways, the idea was to encourage member states to give more to the cause. These included activities in negotiations and lobbying, engaging with intergovernmental and governmental agencies, NGOs, and mobilising the media to gain extra support.

Also in 2002, the *Millennium Project* was created. This initiative, likewise commissioned by Annan and Malloch Brown, was created to bring together specialists from an array of fields in order to develop the best strategies in the quest for achieving the MDGs. The Millennium Project acted as an independent advisory body to the UN and was headed by the famous economist Jeffrey Sachs. After nearly three years of research, the Millennium Project presented its findings in the publication *Investing in Development: A Practical Plan to Achieve the Millennium Development Goals*. In its introduction, the process of the project is outlined:

> The UN Millennium Project has been a unique undertaking. Its 10 task forces, Secretariat, and broad array of participants from academia, government, UN agencies, international financial institutions, nongovernmental organizations, donor agencies, and the private sector created a worldwide network of development practitioners and experts across an enormous range of countries, disciplines, and organizations.
>
> (Sachs, 2005, p. x)

The 10 task forces mentioned were each in charge of a theme about which they produced specific reports and recommendations. In essence, the report provided an overview of what *was* and what *was not* working on the road towards the MDGs and subsequently also provided a framework of recommendations for how to alter the trend and thus ultimately succeed in reaching the goals within the timeframe. In the author's own words, "it outlines ways to put the Goals on the fast-track they require and deserve" (Sachs, 2005, p. 11).

Though they shared common ancestry, the Campaign and the Project were very different endeavours in terms of approach and method. While the two were supposed to be "discrete but complementary" (Hulme, 2010a, p. 156), the underlying mind-set of the two clashed almost immediately. The project was a top-down engagement, in which selected experts made recommendations on *poverty reduction strategy papers* (PRSPs)[6] that for various reasons were largely not adopted by the states that were targeted. In practice, these recommendations were incompatible with PRSPs that had already been put in place by the IFIs. While the project envisioned its policies to complement or replace these strategies, most states chose to simply stick with those of the IFIs. The campaign's approach was different. The initiative emphatically worked less with experts and more with various groups in civil society. The campaign prioritised their efforts in member states based on which states had most potential for improvement. Furthermore, there was less concern with global policy strategies than with country-specific initiatives – and the campaign seldom sought credit for achievements, in stark contrast to the bravado associated with the publication of the project's report.

Renewing commitment and refining the implementation structure of the MDGs did not stop there. While alternative multilateral *fora* also convened to help the process,[7] 2005 saw the first major MDG-focused event since the Millennium Summit in the form of the World Summit, again held in New York. Six months before the meeting, Annan published *In Larger Freedom*, which hinted towards the substance that was to be discussed. As was the case in *We the Peoples*, the section on development was titled 'Freedom from Want'. The publication urges member states to pick up the pace: "[t]he MDGs can be met by 2015 – but only if all involved break with business as usual and dramatically accelerate and scale up action now" (Annan, 2005, p. 1). This was an appeal for improvement directed towards developing and the developed countries alike, and admonished all states to 'accelerate' their efforts. Additionally, there were hints of growing concerns about environmental sustainability in the development section and an explicit prescription to mobilise research in order to combat climate change.

Of the 191 concurrent member states that attended the World Summit, 170 were represented by their heads of state, making it the largest gathering of world leaders to date. In short, this summit was a follow-up to the Millennium Summit and had a similarly broad array of themes on its agenda. The conclusions of the summit were unanimously agreed upon and published in its outcome document. The document came to draw most of its subsequent fame and discussion for its adoption from the controversial norm concerning the responsibility to protect (R2P). In terms of development, the document reiterates member states' motivation for fulfilling the MDGs. However, it is also full of amendments and recommendations due to the lack of progress towards the goals of the MDG framework in its first 'trimester'. In this vein, two main overarching and interlinked sentiments were emphasised, both of which had already been alluded to in Annan's *In Larger Freedom* (2005). First, developing country governments needed to show a greater sense of responsibility for the development of their countries. Second, developed countries needed to contribute substantially more ODA.

Many of the perspectives and policy recommendations of the World Summit's outcome document are derived from two seminal 2002 conferences: the International Conference on Financing for Development held in Monterrey, Mexico, and the World Summit on Sustainable Development (WSSD) held in Johannesburg, South Africa. The former, sponsored by the UN and attended by a large number of heads and ministers of governments, along with the respective heads of the UN, the IMF, the World Bank, and the World Trade Organization (WTO), produced the *Monterrey Consensus*. This outcome was later called a "landmark global agreement" (UN, n.d.[b], para. 2), particularly because of the unprecedented level of direct, overt, and concrete cooperation between the biggest actors in global governance. In a similar vein to *In Larger Freedom* and the sentiments expressed at the World Summit, the *Monterrey Consensus* concluded that the progress towards 2015 had been too slow and particularly emphasised the mutual responsibilities of developing and developed countries. Again, the developing countries were asked to improve and intensify their policies and to show greater initiative in terms of governance, while the developed countries were implored to improve and intensify their support, "especially by opening their markets and providing more and better aid" (Qureshi, 2005, p. 224). The *Monterrey Consensus* draws up strategies for how developed as well as developing countries can address specific challenges and make improvements in the various areas of concern within development.

The WSSD, which gained some notoriety due to the non-attendance of US President George W. Bush, was convened to discuss matters pertaining to the future of sustainable development. Its primary themes were the eradication of poverty, the protection of natural resources, and changing unsustainable patterns of consumption. For example, agreements included restoring the world's depleted fish stocks as well as greatly reducing the rate at which biological diversity was being lost. Health was also a major feature in the WSSD's products: the *Johannesburg Declaration* and the *Johannesburg Plan of Implementation*. While the WSSD received mixed reviews and was not generally perceived to have been successful (Seyfang, 2003), the policy recommendations outlined in these products did affect subsequent agendas, such as the one produced by the 2005 World Summit.

### 2006–2010: *pessimism and crises*

By 2008 it was increasingly clear that reaching the targets of the MDGs within the next seven years was unrealistic. In September, the UN hosted a high-level meeting in New York. The intention of the meeting was to 'rally' member states for the purpose of strengthening their commitment to the fulfilment of the MDGs. The situation was, in fact, rather dire. As UN Secretary-General Ban Ki-moon writes in a background note to the meeting,

> At midpoint towards 2015, the achievement of the Millennium Development Goals has been uneven, and we face nothing less than a development emergency. While many developing countries are on track to achieving a few of the Goals, large disparities persist across and within countries. On current trends, no African country is likely to achieve all of the Goals.
>
> (Ban, 2008, p. 2)

Many academic observers had also been casting doubt on the feasibility of reaching the goals by 2015 (see, for example, Berg & Qureshi, 2005; Clemens, Kenny, & Moss, 2007). The outcome of the high-level meeting indeed included new commitments from several member states, mostly in terms of increasing both the quantity and quality of their aid contribution. Another document, titled *MDG Action Points* (UN, 2008), was published as an addendum to the aforementioned background note. This document points to specific policy measures that need to be taken in order to speed up the processes that may lead to the success of the MDG deadlines.

September 2008 in New York also happened to be *ground zero* of the global financial crisis (GFC), which had devastating ripple effects across the globe. Following this, it was initially widely believed that contributions towards development in the form of ODA would decrease (see Griffith-Jones & Ocampo, 2009). While the short- and medium-term decreases were less severe than had been feared, the growth in ODA since the turn of the century slowed down significantly (Johri, Chung, Dawson, & Schrecker, 2012). This was the opposite of what had been envisioned for the last half of the MDG's target period, and there was a real fear that the crisis would have a dire effect on global development efforts. Indeed, the UN convened the *Conference on the World Financial and Economic Crisis and Its Impact on Development* in June 2009, at which discussions centred around the present – and potential future – adverse impacts the crisis could have. Aside from the question of decreasing ODA, other factors potentially detrimental to the development of LDCs in particular, included deceleration of growth and trade, stark decrease in revenue from tourism, the contraction of world trade, and a reduction in private capital inflows, among many others. In the immediate aftermath of the 2008 GFC, millions of individuals lost their livelihoods and, by extension, millions of families lost their homes. Unemployment rates rose globally as businesses were bankrupted. One study suggests that the crisis significantly increased suicide rates across Europe and the Americas (Chang, Stuckler, Yip, & Gunnell, 2013). However, the massive negative effect the GFC was expected to have on ODA output was never realised. In fact, 2013 marked a new all-time high in ODA from OECD countries. Several studies have been done on the relationship between foreign aid commitment and large economic shocks, and results remain inconclusive – owing, for example, to the heterogeneity of donor states (see Dabla-Norris, Minoiu, & Zanna, 2015; Jones, 2015). For Dodds, Laguna-Celis, and Thompson (2014), the GFC acted as a catalyst that ultimately allowed for the comeback of sustainable development in the lead-up to the construction of the post-2015 development agenda, a point which is further discussed in Chapter 6. The HDRs also started to increasingly feature climate and sustainability as subjects of primary concern (see Table 2.1).

Whether or not the feared impact of the GFC was a deciding factor in the increasingly clear and impending failure of reaching the goals, a new meeting was convened in 2010 to address how to speed up the effort. Leading up to the meeting, the UN in June published *The Millennium Development Goals Report 2010*. The report did little to hide the fact that the MDG effort was struggling:

> Though progress has been made, it is uneven. And without a major push forward, many of the MDG targets are likely to be missed in most regions. Old and new challenges threaten to further slow progress in some areas or even undo successes achieved so far.
>
> (UN, 2010, p. 4)

However, the report does suggest that the goals were still attainable through coordinated effort. It subsequently explores each of the goals in detail, addressing the progresses and shortcomings in the road towards achieving them. A few months earlier, Secretary-General Ban Ki-moon had published a report similarly outlining

*Table 2.1* List of human development reports published after 2000

| Year | Title |
| --- | --- |
| 2000 | Human rights and human development |
| 2001 | Making new technologies work for human development |
| 2002 | Deepening democracy in a fragmented world |
| 2003 | MDGs: A compact among nations to end human poverty |
| 2004 | Cultural liberty in today's diverse world |
| 2005 | International cooperation at a crossroads: Aid, trade and security in an unequal world |
| 2006 | Beyond scarcity: Power, poverty and the global water crisis |
| 2007/8 | Fighting climate change: Human solidarity in a divided world |
| 2009 | Overcoming barriers: Human mobility and development |
| 2010 | The real wealth of nations: pathways to human development |
| 2011 | Sustainability and equity: A better future for all |
| 2012 | (No publication) |
| 2013 | The rise of the South: Human progress in a diverse world |
| 2014 | Sustaining human progress: Reducing vulnerabilities and building resilience |
| 2015 | Work for human development |
| 2016 | Human development for everyone |

successes and shortfalls, which also included a substantial section containing "specific recommendations for action" (Ban, 2010, p. 1). These two publications would set the agenda for the September 2010 UN Summit on the MDGs. The summit (alternatively referred to as a high-level plenary meeting), held at the UN headquarters in New York, was largely a review of MDG progress meant to create new commitments to a plan of accelerated effort/action. Its outcome document, *Keeping the Promise: United to Achieve the Millennium Development Goals*, reaffirms the member states' commitment to the achievements of MDGs and the principles underpinning them, before subsequently outlining a detailed 'action agenda' for each of the goals.

However, 2010 was the beginning of the end of the belief of actually achieving the MDGs from the perspective of the UN. Ten years into the project, grand ambition was slowly changing into a looming sense of pessimism. The overarching narrative of the MDG effort was now mixed; it had become slightly less about predicting grandiose global improvements and more about limiting the extent of a now seemingly inevitable non-fulfilment. The language in the reports and outcome documents of 2010 still included phrases like 'inspiring examples of progress from every region' and allusions to a hope of achieving the goals through concerted efforts. But while negative trends and pessimistic sentiments are downplayed, paragraphs are also spent lamenting the challenges that have hindered *sufficient* progress – reminiscent of the lamentations seen in the Decade of Development resolution documents of the 1970s, 1980s, and 1990s. Arguably, the very need to organise summits for mobilisation due to underwhelming results both in 2008 and 2010 could be seen as tell-tale signs that there was an increasing sense of pessimism and concern permeating the upper echelons of the UN development system. Indeed, they were already beginning to look towards the future and to start the process of shaping the agenda for a post-MDG era of international development coordination.

In 2015, the UN published its final *Millennium Development Goals Report*, in which the relative failure of the endeavour was at least partially admitted:

> Although significant achievements have been made on many of the MDG targets worldwide, progress has been uneven across regions and countries, leaving significant gaps. Millions of people are being left behind, especially the poorest and those disadvantaged because of their sex, age, disability, ethnicity or geographic location. Targeted efforts will be needed to reach the most vulnerable people.
>
> (UN, 2015, p. 8)

The document concludes, however, that concerted global action for development *works*. Further, it looks towards the future with a newfound optimism and is full of praise for the new agenda that will fill the role of the MDGs from 2016 onwards.

## The construction project of the post-2015 development agenda

In September 2015 the UN held a summit for the adoption of the post-2015 development agenda. In a draft resolution submitted by the president of the UNGA the month before, it is proudly stated that:

> This is an Agenda of unprecedented scope and significance. It is accepted by all countries and is applicable to all, taking into account different national realities, capacities and levels of development and respecting national policies and priorities. These are universal goals and targets which involve the entire world, developed and developing countries alike. They are integrated and indivisible and balance the three dimensions of sustainable development.
>
> (UNGA, 2015, p. 3)

This assertive statement was the result of an ambitious and complex process. Unlike the process of creating the MDGs, which involved "a group of mostly UN experts" (Vandemoortele, 2012, p. 5), the process to construct the post-2015 UN development agenda explicitly involved a myriad of actors and various interest groups, governments and civil societies, experts and laymen:

> The Goals and targets are the result of over two years of intensive public consultation and engagement with civil society and other stakeholders around the world, which paid particular attention to the voices of the poorest and most vulnerable. This consultation included valuable work done by the Open Working Group of the General Assembly on Sustainable Development Goals

and by the United Nations, whose Secretary-General provided a synthesis report in December 2014.

(UNGA, 2015, p. 3)

In this section we provide an abridged account of this process. It had been clear for some time that 2015 was not meant to be the end point of the UN's development efforts – a sentiment that had grown in significance upon the relative failure of the MDGs. The 81st and very last paragraph of the *2010 MDG Summit Outcome Document* requests that the secretary-general "report annually on progress in the implementation of the Millennium Development Goals until 2015 and to make recommendations in his annual reports, as appropriate, for further steps to advance the United Nations development agenda beyond 2015" (UNGA, 2010, p. 29). Ban Ki-moon's establishment of the *UN System Task Team on the Post-2015 UN Development Agenda* (UNSTT) in September 2011 was the first response to this request.

The request was the impetus for several unfolding processes. While the secretary-general was assembling the team, other non-governmental entities were also beginning the process of looking towards the future in the hopes of influencing the outcome of the post-2015 agenda. One example is *Beyond 2015*, an association of more than 1,300 NGOs that started cooperating towards common interest shortly after the 2010 summit. In February 2011-Beyond 2015 had already developed strong ideas as to what the process of creating this new agenda should be:

> Given the recognition of how much potential influence a post-2015 framework could have, the process of agreeing a successor to the MDGs will take place in the full glare of public scrutiny. The UN should harness this energy to develop a successor framework in a participative way, through extensive consultation and deliberative engagement.
>
> (Beyond 2015, 2011, p. i)

Beyond 2015 and initiatives like it started spawning in the attempt to influence the process. Beyond 2015 initially comprised five NGOs in three countries – a number that had grown to 262 NGOs in 65 countries in little over a year. This type of NGO 'coalition' was symptomatic of how smaller non-state actors pooled their resources to increase their influence over the course of the consultation process. These were influential also with regard to health, as are discussed in greater detail in Chapter 6.

## The post-2015 preparatory process – the arduous path to the SDGs, 2011–2016

The following section features a timeline of the contribution of several entities mandated by the UN system in order to form the post-2015 development agenda. While some of the initiatives started earlier than others, much of their work was done contemporaneously and often in direct or indirect contact with each other.

For the sake of structural practicality, we present these parallel processes consecutively rather than in an overlapping fashion. The events and meetings described in the section are integral results or impetuses – consequential for, or informed by, the work of the various groups. Though not an exhaustive list, the most relevant groups for the purpose of this study are the already mentioned UNSTT, the high-level panel of eminent persons (HLP), and the Open Working Group (OWG).

## The UN system task team

The mandated task team was soon up and running. In short, it was led by the UN Department of Economic and Social Affairs (UN-DESA) and the UNDP and was intended to provide preparations for the new agenda by initiating multi-stakeholder consultations. The UNSTT consisted of representatives from UN entities as well as from international organisations, totalling a number of more than 50 experts. Its role was to provide official consultation in the process of creating a post-2015 UN development agenda.

The task team's first output was the June 2012 publication *Realizing the Future We Want for All: Report to the Secretary-General* (UNSTT, 2012), just in time for the UN Conference on Sustainable Development (also referred to as Rio+20) in Rio de Janeiro. The report is tentative in nature and makes few, if any, concrete recommendations as to the nature of a post-2015 agenda in terms of goals or indicators. Rather, it keeps a bigger perspective, providing the context within which such recommendations will eventually be constructed. In this process, the report picks up a theme reminiscent of HDRs of the late 1990s and of Kofi Annan's *We the Peoples* (2000), making sure that globalisation will ultimately be a force for good for all. An additional main theme is the unsustainable and uneven patterns of consumption and resource use characterising present human existence on the Earth: "[b]usiness as usual thus cannot be an option and transformative change is needed. As the challenges are highly interdependent, a new, more holistic approach is needed to address them" (UNSTT, 2012, p. i). It states that this holistic approach will be underpinned by the three core values of *human rights*, *equality*, and *sustainability*. These core values would heavily influence the more specific approach to health development adopted by the SDGs, as is explored in Chapter 6.

In its first chapter, the report explores the successes and shortcomings of the MDGs at some length – in a sense describing what they would suggest keeping or discarding (see Table 2.2). In terms of the strong points of the MDG framework, emphasis is put on the strength of concrete, specific, and time-bound goals. The report further commends other characteristics of the original framework:

> Its simplicity, transparency and multi-dimensionality helped rally broad support for the goals and their achievement, and the emphasis on human development shifted policy attention well beyond the economic growth objectives that dominated previous agendas. The Rio+20 Outcome also recognizes these as features to be retained in a future development agenda.
>
> (UNSTT, 2012, p. 6)

*Table 2.2* Suggestions of the first UNSTT report

| Stated as keeping | Improvement suggestions |
|---|---|
| The intention of unifying a pursuance of various **developmental objectives, within the principles of peace, security, and human rights. Priority lies with protecting the poor, the destitute, and the vulnerable.** | Should keep its focus on 'ends' (i.e. the goals), but should also be more explicit about providing guidelines to the 'means' dimension without being overly prescriptive. |
| The concrete form of goals, targets, **and indicators should be realistic and credible, but also ambitious.** | Collective goals are beneficial, but one-size-fits-all approaches should be avoided. Flexibility is needed so that approaches can be customised according to context. |
| Main approach should keep its focus on human **development and poverty eradication, but also on new challenges such as combating climate change and rectifying inequality within countries.** | Focus should be broadened significantly, as some issues were not covered adequately in the MDGs or, in some instances, at all. |
| The effort to create a truly global partnership for **development (MDG 8) must be intensified, and goals towards the effort should be more precisely defined.** | A more inclusive consultation process should be facilitated in the development of the agenda. |

Conversely, there were also characteristics of the MDGs that the task team did not want repeated in the post-2015 agenda, both in terms of the design of the goals themselves and in terms of implementation. In the first sense, the goals may have been too limited and limiting, which caused aspects of development not included in the framework to be neglected. Furthermore, the global focus of the goals sometimes negatively affected the ability of the implementers to sufficiently consider local contexts. There had also been a general lack of commitment and action from the international community, making it difficult for developing countries to take sufficient strides towards achieving the goals – although the local governments of many developing countries also were to be blamed. This alludes in particular to the shortcomings in the attempt to achieve a true global partnership for development, as envisioned in MDG 8.[8]

Several obstacles are identified as impeding 'the future we want for all'. Globalisation, the report notes, has sped up since the turn of the millennium. As a consequence, the world has become more interdependent than before, a process that is both exponentially growing in scope and in seemingly perpetual acceleration. The pitfalls of such a high degree of interdependence became all too evident during the 2008 GFC, the 2007 world food price crisis, the more recent Euro crisis, and controversial refugee influxes into Europe. While millions have been 'lifted out of poverty' since 2000, global and local inequality gaps have actually widened. Demographics are also changing. The developed world is aging, and the demographic proportion of the elderly population of its countries is generally growing while there is a current surplus of young people in developing countries – all factors that contribute to various new challenges pertaining to economies, job markets, and health care systems globally (Magnus, 2012).

One major theme is the currently unsustainable consumption patterns and their consequences, particularly the concerns related to certain dwindling resources and the many challenges associated with global warming:

> Growth of population, income, energy and resource use, waste and pollution have come at the cost of unprecedented use of natural resources and environmental degradation. Almost half of the Earth's forests are gone, groundwater sources and fish stocks are being rapidly depleted, and land degradation and ocean acidification are worsening. Biodiversity has been enormously reduced, and carbon dioxide emissions increased by 40 per cent between 1990 and 2008, to reach dangerous climate destabilizing concentrations of close to 30 billion tonnes a year.
>
> (UNSTT, 2012, p. 16)

Finally, there is the subject of conflict. Although the world is generally less violent than ever before (Gleditsch, Pinker, Thayer, Levy, & Thompson, 2013), violence and insecurity still affect the daily lives of many of the world's population. This has significant consequences that impede any development process, including unemployment, undernourishment, child mortality, bad mental health, lack of clean drinking water, and more.

In this context, the task team wanted a post-2015 UN development agenda "that seeks to achieve inclusive, people-centred, sustainable global development" (UNSTT, 2012, p. 21). The pillars of such an agenda are summed up as follows:

> The values and principles affirmed in the Millennium Declaration and its seven key objectives remain a solid foundation for addressing today's and tomorrow's global development challenges and should therefore be used to help shape the post-2015 UN development agenda. This can be done in a focused manner by building a framework that: (i) is based on the three fundamental principles of human rights, equality and sustainability; and (ii) orients key goals along the four, highly interdependent dimensions of inclusive social development, environmental sustainability, inclusive economic development, and peace and security. These core dimensions are consistent with the notion of 'freedom from want' for present and future generations, building on the three pillars of the sustainable development concept (economic, social, environmental), and that of 'freedom of fear'.
>
> (UNSTT, 2012, p. 22)

The remainder of the report details what these three fundamental principles and the subsequent four dimensions mean and, against this background, offers some 'key considerations'. They suggest that the agenda should beware of three pitfalls. The first of these is *overloading*, meaning that the agenda should be concrete, clear, and measurable – which is argued to have been one of the major strengths of the MDG framework. Second, the agenda should *neither be too prescriptive nor too vague*, as a balance of external (global) governance and local (national) initiative and responsibility is considered to be essential. Third, the agenda should *not be donor-centric*. This means that there needs to be an inclusion of all countries in the design of the agenda, in an attempt to create a truly global partnership for development.

Over the course of its report, the task team seems determined to ensure a process that is open to and inclusive of all stakeholders. This is further emphasised in one of the closing sections of the task team's report, titled 'proposed road map'. It is introduced as follows:

> The proposed road map is based on a two-step approach for supporting Member States to develop the post-2015 UN development agenda. The first step, from now through the special event, is to promote an open, inclusive and transparent consultation process, to take stock and encourage contributions from a wide range of stakeholders. The second step, from the special events through 2015, is to intensify efforts to achieve intergovernmental consensus, while sustaining an open and inclusive process.
>
> (UNSTT, 2012, p. 48)

The task team's second report, titled *A renewed global partnership for development* was submitted in March 2013. It reviews the state of the current global partnerships for development (as elaborated upon in MDG 8) in order to provide recommendations for improvements with regard to these partnerships in the post-2015 development agenda. In the report, it is made clear that the post-2015 development agenda faces new challenges:

> The world has changed fundamentally since the adoption of the Millennium Declaration. It is faced with new challenges and opportunities, many of which require collective action. The renewed global partnership for development underpinning the post-2015 development agenda will need to evolve with the changing development landscape to enable transformative changes. To do so effectively, it should build on the strengths of the current global partnership for development while going beyond its present framework. Most importantly, it will have to be based on a strong commitment to engage in collective actions with a clear distribution of tasks between developed and developing countries.
>
> (UNSTT, 2013, p. v)

In short, the recommendations toward this endeavour in the new agenda point out that all countries realise and accept that they have a common but diverse set of responsibilities. This necessarily entails the inclusion of developing countries into multilateral institutions that administer important areas such as global trade agreements. Indeed, the task team suggests, developing countries as well as non-governmental agents should be included to a much greater degree in all processes with regard to the governance of development. Resulting from this is the further necessity of strengthened accountability mechanisms, keeping close track of progress to ensure that all parties are fulfilling their commitments.

The conclusions of the task team's reports were indicative of the underlying and overarching sentiments that would make up the complexion of the final post-2015 agenda. It laid out definitions of cornerstones of the new framework, particularly its focus on inclusiveness. While praising its trailblazing achievements, the reports also made explicit the shortcomings of the MDG agenda and subsequently attempted to outline how the new agenda must learn from both these aspects of the past. It further solidified a new emphasis on sustainability as central to the new agenda as well as the need to include all stakeholders in the process of constructing the new agenda.

### The high-level panel of eminent persons

The HLP was another group assembled by the secretary-general requested in the outcome document of the 2010 MDG Summit. The panel's members – a versatile blend of leaders from governments, civil society, and the private sector – were selected in July 2012. It comprised 27 members and was co-chaired by President Yudhoyono of Indonesia, President Johnson-Sirleaf of Liberia, and UK Prime Minister Cameron. The panel had, by the end of November 2012, agreed to 24 'framing questions' that would guide their work. The sub-themes for these questions were (1) lessons learned and context (from the MDG processes and implementation), (2) the shape of a post-2015 development framework, (3) themes and content of a new framework, (4) partnership and accountability for development, and (5) shaping global consensus for the goals.

After holding meetings in New York, London, Monrovia, and Bali, the panel submitted its final report to the secretary-general in late May 2013, titled *A New Global Partnership: Eradicate Poverty and Transform Economies through Sustainable Development* (HLP, 2013). Their approach is made clear early on, explicitly intending to draw on the best from the *Millennium Declaration* and the MDGs while being mindful of the essential need to consider present challenges and of looking towards the future, particularly increasing the environmental emphasis. In the process, the panel engaged with a broad spectrum of actors in their work:

> So the Panel asked some simple questions: starting with the current MDGs, what to keep, what to amend, and what to add. In trying to answer these questions, we listened to the views of women and men, young people, parliamentarians, civil society organisations, indigenous people and local communities, migrants, experts, business, trade unions and governments. Most important, we listened directly to the voices of hundreds of thousands of people from all over the world, in face-to-face meetings as well as through surveys, community interviews, and polling over mobile phones and the internet.
>
> (HLP, 2013, p. vi)

*Table 2.3* The main recommendations of the HLP

|   | Title | Description/summary |
|---|-------|---------------------|
| 1 | 'Leave no one behind' | Literally no one in the world should be denied universal human rights and basic economic opportunities. Goals should focus on reaching excluded groups in particular, in order to completely eradicate world poverty and hunger. |
| 2 | 'Put sustainable development at the core' | Unsustainable consumption patterns must be stopped as soon as possible. The developed countries are implored to lead the charge in this matter. |
| 3 | 'Transform economies for jobs and inclusive growth' | The panel calls for a 'quantum leap' in economic opportunities, meaning that everyone should have an equal chance of being an entrepreneur, of investing and trading. |
| 4 | 'Build peace and effective, open, and accountable institutions for all' | Peace and good governance should be recognised as essential for well-being. There should also be a universally increased transparency, while values such as freedom of speech and the media and rule of law are seen as ends as well as means. |
| 5 | 'Forge a new global partnership' | Suggests the need for a truly global circle of empathy, where common interests are recognised and strived for in solidarity. All goals should be pursued by means of a united engagement of all relevant actors, including, but not limited to, governments. |

The report's main conclusion is that the post-2015 development agenda is universal in nature, and that it should be driven by five significant, highly interdependent shifts, summarised in Table 2.3:

The report concludes by providing a set of 12 targets, titled *Universal Goals, National Targets*, reflecting the oft-mentioned central dynamic between global concerns and local contexts. In general, the goals reflect the sentiments expressed earlier in the sense that some of the proposed goals are very similar to those of the MDGs, while others are new or at least more contemporary, presenting new goals and solutions for issues in sustainability and governance in particular.

The aforementioned five points are repeated nearly verbatim in the 2013 MDG Review Summit outcome document; they are characterised as "key elements for the emerging vision for the development agenda beyond 2015" (UNGA, 2013b, p. 13). Further, as the outcome documents proceed to a list of "transformative and mutually reinforcing actions" (UNGA, 2013b, p. 13), these correspond largely to the HLP's list of *Universal Goals, National Targets* – the contours of the SDGs were already beginning to take form a full year before the OWG's deadline.

### Rio + 20 and the open working group

These sentiments were also central at the 2012 United Nations Conference on Sustainable Development in Rio de Janeiro, also known as Earth Summit 2012 or simply 'Rio + 20'. The summit was the third UN conference focusing on sustainable development – succeeding UNCED in 1992, and WSSD in 2002 – and was argu-ably the most important milestone for the post-2015 process (Dodds et al., 2014). Rio+20 was a massive 10-day affair that included participation from 192 UN member states, representatives from the private sector, NGOs, civil society groups, and others. The conference gained much of its attention in the media for the large demonstrations surrounding it in the city and its consequently massive security precautions involving around 15,000 military and police officers. Its significance in setting the scene for the development of the post-2015 agenda is considerable. *Agenda 21*, the aforementioned outcome document from the first Rio Earth Sum-mit of 1992, was, to a large extent, the foundation for discussion as the summit assessed progress towards the goals and principles of *Agenda 21* and discussed the framework's place in the future of international development.

The outcome document of Rio+20 was titled *The Future We Want* and was adopted as Resolution 66/228 (UNGA, 2012a). It is a 50-odd-page document com-prising 283 points that prescribe guidelines to the process of developing an agenda for sustainable development in the post-2015 era. The document emphasises the importance of keeping in mind and balancing the three dimensions of sustainable development[9] – namely, economic, social, and environmental considerations:

> The institutional framework for sustainable development should integrate the three dimensions of sustainable development in a balanced manner and enhance implementation by, inter alia, strengthening coherence and coordi-nation, avoiding duplication of efforts and reviewing progress in implement-ing sustainable development. We also reaffirm that the framework should be inclusive, transparent and effective and that it should find common solutions related to global challenges to sustainable development
>
> (UNGA, 2012a, p. 14).

Speaking more directly to the practical implementation of realising and improve-ment in these dimensions, prescriptions for the principles on which the SDGs should rest are also outlined:

> Sustainable development goals should be action-oriented, concise and easy to communicate, limited in number, aspirational, global in nature and univer-sally applicable to all countries, while taking into account different national realities, capacities and levels of development and respecting national poli-cies and priorities. We also recognize that the goals should address and be focused on priority areas for the achievement of sustainable development, being guided by the present outcome document. Governments should drive implementation with the active involvement of all relevant stakeholders, as appropriate.
>
> (UNGA, 2012a, p. 47)

*Inter alia*, the document mandates the creation – and prescribes the tasks and form – of the OWG. It provides a date and time for its constitution, which is 'no later' than the opening of the 67th session of the UNGA (September 2012). It stipulates that the OWG should be made up of "thirty representatives, nominated by Member States from the five United Nations regional groups, with the aim of achieving fair, equitable and balanced geographical representation" (UNGA, 2012a, p. 47). After they have decided their methods for working and found ways to involve input from all various stakeholders as well as from relevant experts from the scientific community, civil society, and the various UN agencies, "it will submit a report, to the Assembly at its sixty-eighth session, containing a proposal for sustainable development goals for consideration and appropriate action" (UNGA, 2012a, p. 47). Furthermore, the next paragraph asks the secretary-general to spark the discussion by providing the OWG with an *initial input* document. He is also requested to "ensure all necessary input and support to this work from the United Nations system, including by establishment of an inter-agency technical support team and expert panels, as needed, drawing on all relevant expert advice" (UNGA, 2012a, p. 47).

Shortly after Rio+20, an important meeting for the construction of the OWG took place in October 2012, at what was characterised as a 'special event of General Assembly's Second Committee'.[10] The event acted as a precursor for the OWG thematic sessions that were to follow. There were presentations by scholars, practitioners, and policymakers, followed by an ensuing discussion. Among the topics of discussion was the possibility of two or more sets of goals to be used in different contexts where applicable: poverty eradication as the main focus of the agenda, the need for global collective action in surmounting the looming environmental challenges, the importance of processes ensuring greater gender equality, and other areas of concern. Another major point discussed was the importance of including perspectives from the poor in the conversation, thus supporting the now increasingly integral sentiment of having an open and inclusive post-2015 agenda-setting process. The same sentiment was expressed for including input from civil society and the private sector – without going as far as providing answers as to how this could be best accomplished.

In mid-December 2012, the secretary-general submitted an 'initial input document'. "It offers a synthesis of the input received to a questionnaire sent to Member States and is presented as an input to the work of the Open Working Group on Sustainable Development Goals" (UNGA, 2012b, p. 1). The main message of this input document is the result of this questionnaire, responded to by 63 member states, the answers of which were intended to lay the basis for the forthcoming OWG agenda discussions. The results as presented in Ban's report gave a good indication of how the member states viewed the upcoming agenda-setting process at the time and to which key areas the majority of them attributed top priority for the post-2015 agenda. These key areas include the retention of the eradication of poverty as the highest priority for the agenda, while priority areas associated with the human development paradigm are also seen as integral. Added to this is a concern for negative environmental conditions and the potential consequences of these for human well-being: The suggestion is that the agenda should constitute, "in short, a shared vision . . . of achieving universal and equitable human development while respecting the Earth's ecological limits" (UNGA, 2012b, p. 19).

Further, some member states had suggested clustering related themes with the purpose of creating crosscutting and holistic goals, such as, for example, gender equality and equity. Each goal should also, according to the answers, balance the three aforementioned dimensions of sustainable development. Sentiments concerning the balance between the global nature of the goals and flexibility that would be able to lend itself to context-specific local tailoring when and where necessary, were also discussed. The outcome documents of the two previous Earth Summits (*Agenda 21*, the *Rio Principles*, and the *Johannesburg Plan of Implementation*) are stated as ideal for providing guidelines for the process, coupled with innovative new solutions to problems that had been inadequately covered in these documents and others. Significantly, there was a general consensus that there should be a single development agenda with a single set of goals: namely, the SDGs.

The *Special Event towards Achieving the Millennium Development Goals* was scheduled for September 2013, at the opening of the UNGA's 68th session. In March, the OWG had its first session (a total of 14 sessions were held); the last one of which was concluded in July 2014. A progress report produced about a year into the process describes in broad terms what the OWG was concerned with during these sessions:

> The Group's work has been organized into two main phases. The first phase focused on stock-taking, collecting views of experts, Member States and other stakeholders, from its first meeting in March 2013 through its eighth meeting in February 2014, when members of the Group deliberated on the main themes, including those identified in the Rio+20 outcome document's Framework for Action, and how they might be reflected in a set of sustainable development goals (SDGs). In the second phase, from February through September 2014, the Group will prepare a report to the 68th session of the [UNGA] mandated by the United Nations Conference on Sustainable Development containing a proposal for SDGs.
>
> (OWG, 2014, p. 5)

The Special Event, held in September 2013, fell between the 4th and 5th sessions of the OWG. In its short outcome document, the OWG is only mentioned explicitly in one paragraph, acknowledging the group 'with appreciation' of its work towards formulating the SDGs – before encouraging and urging that these processes be completed by September 2014. The OWG was well within this deadline and submitted its final report in July 2014, including the proposed list of 17 SDGs (UN, 2014).

The first three pages of the OWG's report is made up of 18 introductory paragraphs with the aim of explaining the ideational rationale behind the list of SDGs. These paragraphs are recognisable in that they are, in large part, a reiteration of many of the main points of the outcome document that mandated the creation of the OWG in the first place: the Rio+20 summit. As with the MDGs, the primacy of striding towards poverty eradication is introduced immediately. Next, the endeavour of the OWG and the post-2015 agenda in general is framed within a cosmopolitan human development paradigm, reminding one of the new framework's early 1990s origins:

> People are at the centre of sustainable development and, in this regard, in the outcome document, the promise was made to strive for a world that is just, equitable and inclusive and the commitment was made to work together to promote sustained and inclusive economic growth, social development and environmental protection and thereby to benefit all, in particular the children of the world, youth and future generations of the world, without distinction of any kind such as age, sex, disability, culture, race, ethnicity, origin, migratory status, religion, economic or other status.
>
> (UN, 2014, para. 4)

Many of the conventions, declarations, and programmes of action discussed earlier are given explicit credit as antecedents to the SDGs. Indeed, the Rio+20 outcome document affirms that the aim is full implementation of all these mentioned. The *Charter of the UN*, International Law, and the *Universal Declaration of Human Rights* are also mentioned as additional and foundational guidelines for the agenda. It also repeats the sentiment that developing countries are responsible for their own progress, while developed countries must commit to assist as much as possible. Similarly, it reiterates that while the goals are global targets, each individual country will have to set its own national targets within the framework, in order to accommodate local contexts.

In October of that year, the UNGA published an addendum to the OWG's report, including both praise and slight reservations. The latter were primarily raised by the Holy See and most predominantly Catholic countries towards anything pertaining to family planning. Other countries and groups also had relatively minor reservations about the suggested SDGs, but the feedback was generally positive. Some of the feedback specifically focuses on the benefits of the process, an example being praise from the representatives of Guatemala:

> It should be highlighted that the outcome of the Open Working Group was developed under a process that was open, transparent and somewhat different from the traditional format of negotiations that we know so well in the United Nations. At the beginning, we all expected that negotiations would be carried out behind closed doors, only with the designated members; however, this process included every delegation of the United Nations and it also received contributions from civil society. Now, we have a proposal that emerged from a universal process and the goals are also universally applicable.
>
> (UNGA, 2014b, p. 12)

In *Resolution 68/309*, the UNGA marks the conclusion of the efforts of the OWG, and "decides that the proposal . . . shall be the main basis for integrating sustainable development goals into the post-2015 development agenda, while recognizing that other inputs will also be considered, in the intergovernmental negotiation process at the sixty-ninth session of the General Assembly" (UNGA, 2014c, p. 1).

### The 68th session of the general assembly – 'setting the stage!'

The MDG review event marked the start of the 68th session of the UNGA and was to be the first of several events related to the post-2015 agenda organised by the UNGA during this session; the entire year-long session was given the theme 'The post-2015 development agenda: Setting the stage!':

> The central objective of each event and/or debate is to enable Member States to begin the elaboration of the priority areas for the post-2015 Development Agenda through in-depth deliberations on the chosen topics, in a participative and interactive manner, and to make concrete contributions to the ongoing process of developing sustainable development goals in these areas within the overall context of the post-2015 development agenda.
>
> (Ashe, 2013, p. 1, para. 7)

These meetings covered a versatile array of themes, all focused on how these respective specific themes would fit into the post-2015 agenda. Water, sanitation, and sustainable energy; the role of women and youth; the role of new partnerships, of South-South Cooperation, of Human Rights and the Rule of Law; the role of information and communications technologies for developing countries – all were discussed in the various meetings. The final session took place in September and was labelled a 'high-level stock-taking event'. The event was meant to provide "an opportunity to identify possible inputs to the synthesis report of the Secretary-General, to the work of the 69th session of the General Assembly, and to the elaboration of the post-2015 development agenda itself" (UNGA, 2014d, p. 2). The products of the events would later be incorporated into the secretary-general's synthesis report.

In the summary document published in the wake of the 'stock-taking' session, several 'key messages' were identified and summarised. Most of the themes that arose during discussion at the final event reflected the work and results of the OWG, that is to say the SDGs. The attitudes of most of those attending the stock-tacking event had emphasised sentiments that were now essentially part and parcel of the post-2015 agenda. Adjectives such as *visionary, transformative, inclusive, ambitious, transparent, monitorable*, and *accountable* were used to describe the ideal post-2015 development agenda. Implementation and financing were also discussed at some length, but the ideational foundation had found stability. So had the key areas of concern – namely, those of poverty, inequality, gender equality, health, and sustainability.

---

### Box 2.2    The Sustainable Development Goals

1  End poverty in all its forms everywhere
2  End hunger, achieve food security and improved nutrition, and promote sustainable agriculture
3  Ensure healthy lives and promote well-being for all at all ages
4  Ensure inclusive and equitable quality education and promote lifelong
   learning opportunities for all
5  Achieve gender equality and empower all women and girls
6  Ensure availability and sustainable management of water and sanitation for all
7  Ensure access to affordable, reliable, sustainable, and clean energy
   for all
8  Promote sustained, inclusive, and sustainable economic growth; full
   and productive employment; and decent work for all
9  Build resilient infrastructure, promote inclusive and sustainable industrialisation, and foster innovation
10 Reduce inequality within and among countries
11 Make cities and human settlements inclusive, safe, resilient, and
   sustainable
12 Ensure sustainable consumption and production patterns
13 Take urgent action to combat climate change and its impacts
14 Conserve and sustainably use the oceans, seas, and marine resources for
   sustainable development
15 Protect, restore, and promote sustainable use of terrestrial ecosystems,
   sustainably manage forests, combat desertification, and halt and reverse
   land degradation and halt biodiversity loss
16 Promote peaceful and inclusive societies for sustainable development;
   provide access to all; and build effective, accountable, and inclusive
   institutions at all levels
17 Strengthen the means of implementation, and revitalise the global
   partnership for sustainable development

---

### The high-level political forum on sustainable development

In addition to the OWG, the Rio+20 outcome document also mandated the creation of another group:

> We decide to establish a universal, intergovernmental, high-level political
> forum, building on the strengths, experiences, resources and inclusive par-
> ticipation modalities of the Commission on Sustainable Development, which

would subsequently replace the Commission, as well as the decision that the high-level political forum should follow on the implementation of sustainable development and should avoid overlap with existing structures, bodies and entities in a cost-effective manner.

(UNGA, 2012a, p. 16)

The CSD, as described earlier, was originally created after the'92 Earth Summit, as a means to follow up on the implementation of that conference, and particularly that of *Agenda 21*. The High-Level Political Forum on Sustainable Development (HLPF) was now created to carry the same responsibility with regard to the Rio+20 *Outcome* Document, replacing the previous commission. As the CSD had done for 20 years, the HLPF was scheduled to meet annually at a ministerial level to discuss the state of the implementation of the agenda. Furthermore, the HLPF would also meet every four years at the UNGA with the purpose of promoting the implementation of sustainable development and address challenges that arose; the meetings would produce a declaration meant to aid and amplify policies. For these purposes, HLPF is explicitly open to suggestions by all member states as well as from NGOs. Essentially, the idea behind the creation of the forum is to make sure that the issue of approaching the implementation of sustainable development measures throughout the post-2015 agenda is constantly being refined and deliberated upon by all stakeholders as well as of reviewing the progress of the mentioned implementation efforts. This is not limited to the Rio+20 Outcome Document, but for "all the outcomes of the major United Nations conferences and summits in the economic, social and environmental fields, as well as their respective means of implementation" (UNGA, 2013a, p. 4). The forum should also facilitate the sharing of experiences and best practices concerning sustainable development, with the goal of creating "system-wide coherence and coordination" (UNGA, 2013a, p. 4).

In summary, the role of the forum is to ensure that the three dimensions of sustainable development are integrated in a balanced way, both throughout the process of creating the new agenda and in implementing it after its realisation. With regard to the former of these, the forum "has an important role to play in providing the political leadership needed to reach agreement on a post-2015 agenda that will advance sustainable development in an integrated and universal manner, as well as in guiding and reviewing implementation" (UNGA, 2013c, p. 4).

Before the aforementioned September 2015 summit, the HLPF met twice more under the auspices of ECOSOC. One meeting was held in late June and early July 2014 and was centred around optimising the final year of the MDG efforts as well as helping to 'chart the way' towards the impending start of the new agenda. With regard to the latter, the meeting's product (the *Ministerial Declaration* of the HLPF), the language of the OWG, and the HLP reports of the special 68th session of the UNGA and of the general human development paradigm are restated. The importance of people, men, women, and children alike being at the centre of development, as well as central themes such as sustainability and prioritisation of technological innovations, is particularly reiterated, as is the importance of an open and transparent process and that the central theme of poverty eradication will retain its role of primacy. Also restated is the HLPFs role in the coming agenda: the forum

> shall conduct regular reviews, starting in 2016, on the follow-up to and implementation of sustainable development commitments and objectives, including those related to the means of implementation, within the context of the post-2015 development agenda, and further reiterate that these reviews shall: be voluntary, while encouraging reporting, and shall include developed and developing countries, as well as relevant United Nations entities; be State-led, involving ministerial and other relevant high level participants; provide a platform for partnerships, including through the participation of major groups and other relevant stakeholders; and replace the national voluntary presentations held in the context of the annual ministerial-level substantive reviews of the Council.
>
> (United Nations Economic and Social Council, 2014b, pp. 4–5)

By now it had become clear that the role of the HLPF is to spearhead the implementation and review of the SDGs. At its next and third meeting in June–July 2015, the discussion was wholly dedicated to how the forum would organise its work once the implementation of the post-2015 development agenda got underway. Once again, the prioritisation of the eradication of poverty coupled with sustainability was given strong emphasis. Essentially, the HLPF's future role was to be the platform that looks at the 'big picture'; it will continuously review the progress of the SDGs and will be working on recommendations for optimising implementation – all the while attempting to balance a sense of predictability to the agreed framework with a flexibility for the various challenges that might arise over time.

A number of common threads can be found in the complex composition of input groups and events as described earlier, coming together to form a consensus of what eventually formed the post-2015 development agenda process. As a whole, the process was in large part a process (1) of balancing the good parts of the MDG framework in terms of both ideas and implementation and (2) of updating the ideas and action areas for present and future challenges and optimising and improving on implementation measures. One significant shift was on a process level. This was the explicitly inclusive approach for the construction of the new agenda, which stood in stark contrast to the rather top-down approach seen in the creation of the MDGs – an approach that had faced significant criticism by development experts, member states, NGOs, and others. On a different level was the ever-present challenge concerning the dynamic between addressing local needs while still maintaining a global view – a challenge solved by making the global goals malleable to local contexts to a larger extent than had previously been the case. In this vein, the responsibilities of local govern-ments have grown.

In terms of prioritisation, the global super-norm of poverty eradication contin-ues to be the centre of gravity around which the other development focus areas revolve. However, the heavily increased emphasis on themes pertaining to the *leitmotif* of sustainability marks the greatest shift in focus. This does not mean that the areas prioritised by the MDGs would now be neglected, but that the project has grown in scope and complexity, and is indeed more challenging. The impact of the new principal norm of sustainability is illustrated by the aforementioned attempt of the *mainstreaming* of the three dimensions of sustainable development on the entire organisation of the UN.

## The synthesis report, the 2015 summit, and final touches

In December 2014, Secretary-General Ban Ki-moon, via the UNGA, published his *Synthesis Report: The Road to Dignity by 2030: Ending Poverty, Transforming All Lives and Protecting the Planet*, a report that was presented for consideration to member states and that had the purpose of outlining the post-2015 vision that would be negotiated and adopted at the special summit planned for September 2015. The UN also opened up online mechanisms for civil society groups and NGOs to send in responses to the report that would subsequently be taken into consideration in the final negotiations.

Generally, the ideational agenda had been more or less completed by the turn of 2015, and it was "agreed that the agenda laid out by the OWG is the main basis for the post-2015 intergovernmental process" (UNGA, 2014b, p. 15). The fol-lowing months featured negotiations to finalise all the parameters of the agenda, culminating in the September 2015 UN *Summit for the Adoption of the Post-2015 Development Agenda*, which, aside from minor discussions, was more of a formal-ity in terms of actual content, the details of which had been developed over the course of the processes described earlier (see Figure 2.2).

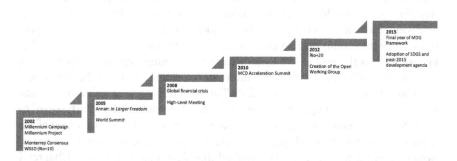

*Figure 2.2* Key moments and publications, 2002–2015

In these goals and targets, we are setting out a supremely ambitious and transformational vision. We envisage a world free of poverty, hunger, disease and
want, where all life can thrive. We envisage a world free of fear and violence.
A world with universal literacy. A world with equitable and universal access
to quality education at all levels, to health care and social protection, where
physical, mental and social well-being are assured.

(UNGA, 2015, p. 3)

These are the lines that make up the first paragraph of the subheading 'Our
Vision' in the outcome document of the summit, which was titled *Transforming
Our World: the 2030 Agenda for Sustainable Development*. Also found within this
document was the official announcement of the adoption of the 17 SDGs that
would be the focal points of the new agenda. Though this also was more a formal-
ity than anything else, the summit saw reiterations of the most salient points of
what had been partially re-baptised as the *2030 Agenda*. These included themes by
now familiar, such as strengthening global institutions, addressing climate change,
the interconnectedness of the various goals, and the importance of engaging all
stakeholders and ensuring a robust follow-up and review mechanism.

## Conclusion

The above-described ideational timeline's final instalment is *Transforming Our
World* – the outcome document to the summit that officially adopted the post-
2015 agenda, including the SDGs. The current development agenda and the
normative paradigm within which it has been constructed is a product of a long
process of organisational cultural change, affected by events, ideas and other factors of internal and external origins alike.

The purpose of this chapter has been to provide a brief genealogy of the UN
development agenda since its rearrangement around the start of the 1990s. It
started by providing a recounting of the summit and conference trajectory of
that decade as well as the contents of the annual HDRs. The summits and their
outcome documents acted as ideational *fora* and value statements. The global
context in which these large-scale meetings took place was also explored and
described as one in which the conventional assumptions relating to concepts such
as development and security were being questioned, allowing for new perspectives to inform various degrees of paradigmatic shifts. In large part, compounding
factors such as the end of the Cold War, the increasing rate and proportions of
intra-state conflicts, the rather calamitous development efforts of the 1980s, and
the various effects of accelerating globalisation acted together and formed ideationally fertile ground upon which other approaches could thrive. With regard to
the UN development agenda, this shift was represented by the introduction of the
human development paradigm. The normative and implementational prescriptions emanating from the HDRs amplified this ideational movement. (Chapter 4
covers the emergence and integration of the human development paradigm in
greater detail).

Human development, at its core, questions the links between economic growth and especially gross domestic product (GDP) as a measure of successful development. The new paradigm emphasises well-being and the expansion of the richness of human life and suggests that increasing people's opportunities and capabilities are the real *ends* of development and that economic growth is only one means by which to reach those ends. The implication is that development is contingent upon a number of interconnected aspects of the life of an individual, a family, a society, and a country. The focal point of the new agenda became poverty eradication, which became nearly synonymous with the general concept of development by the time the *Millennium Declaration* (UNGA, 2000b) was published. A more detailed account of the effect that this shift had on the direction of ensuing health development policies – specifically those included in the two sets of global development goals – through the trajectories of health norms, is provided in Chapters 5 and 6.

The chapter further recounts the period of practical implementation of the MDGs and provides an account of the mixed results that ended up characterising the framework as a whole. This time period (2001–2015) also featured a range of global trends and contingencies, such as the threats of terrorism, the disease scares – best exemplified by the 2002–2003 severe acute respiratory syndrome (SARS) outbreak – and the 2008 GFC. With failure looming, 2010 saw the initiation of the process to devise a successor agenda to the MDGs.

The build-up to the creation of this new framework, in the end embodied by the SDGs, was different from the summitry period that had characterised the precedent-setting 1990s that resulted in the MDGs. Although the MDGs had not been perfect, the core value system of the human development paradigm would not be challenged. The post-2015 preparatory process was widely publicised, transparent, and – above all – *inclusive* in terms of input from an array of stakeholders. Inclusivity was also a central component of the contents of the new agenda, second only to *sustainable development* – the new overarching imperative that the naming of the SDGs derives from. After an introductory consultation period, the process was further catalysed by the *Rio + 20* summit, which delegated tasks of creating the new framework, most notably through the work of the OWG, represented by member states. Alongside the already multifaceted endeavours of poverty eradication, further complexity was added by the explicitly holistic concepts of sustainability and inclusivity, resulting in goals that aimed to facilitate intersectoral improvements that would improve the lives of people in the present without compromising the ability of future generations to also lead fulfilling lives. Health remained central to this process, but was treated more holistically, aiming for sustainably healthy populations rather than focusing on the largely poverty-related illnesses addressed in the MDGs.

In the chapters that follow, the context in which these processes transpire are assessed from political and normative angles, particularly in Chapters 4, 5, and 6. The following chapter presents the literature on, and reflects upon, the connections between health, development, and IR, further contextualising the study and providing conceptual clarity.

## Notes

1  The OAU, established in 1963, was disbanded in 2002 and replaced by the newly founded African Union (AU).

2  Not all ideas included in the outcome documents of various conferences and summits over the course of the 1990s were truly agreed upon by consensus. Some summits were even boycotted by certain states because of the subject matter discussed. One example, which is further discussed in a subsequent chapter, is the 1994 ICPD and its associated focus on reproductive health. Shrewd diplomacy saved the conference from being boycotted by a large number of member states. Iraq, Lebanon, Saudi Arabia, and Sudan did boycott (McIntosh & Finkle, 1995). This particular conference is discussed further in Chapter 5. In another example, George W. Bush famously decided not to attend the highly publicised 2002 World Summit for Sustainable Development in Johannesburg, South Africa. This was attributed to disagreements between the White House and the summit attendees at large with regard to private business interests in relation to sustainable development.

3  As presented in the World Food Summit's *Plan of Action*, "Food security exists when all people, at all times, have physical and economic access to sufficient, safe and nutritious food that meets their dietary needs and food preferences for an active and healthy life" (Food and Agriculture Organisation, 1996, para. 1).

4  Super-norms are discussed in greater detail in subsequent chapters. For the time being, it is sufficient to state that a super-norm is "a framework that attempts to incorporate several different norms into a coherent structure. A super-norm seeks to achieve more than the sum of its parts because of the positive feedback interactions between each norm" (Fukuda-Parr & Hulme, 2009, p. 5). In their line of argument, poverty eradication binds together all the MDGs (which are also large norms in and of themselves, made up of smaller norms) and the entire development project.

5  More specifically, faith in the UN's role and capability in global peacekeeping had waned significantly; the disasters of Srebrenica – and the conflict in former Yugoslavia generally – and Rwanda in the early to mid-part of the decade had been particularly damaging. In terms of development discourse, the UN – led by a renewed UNDP – was more secure in its position as normative hegemon and practical arbiter.

6  PRSPs, as part of an approach, to poverty reduction were introduced in 1999 by the IFIs. Essentially, preparing PRSPs and annual progress reports were requirements for heavily indebted poor countries receiving debt relief and other funds. In theory, the PRSP approach would necessarily involve civil society and take a long-term approach (much unlike the Millennium Project's approach).

7  At the annual meeting of the Group of Eight (G8) in 2005, the leaders met at the Gleneagles Hotel in Auchterarder, Scotland. On the agenda were Africa and climate change, and the outcome was to double aid for Africa and to eliminate unpaid debts for the poorest countries. Aid was to be increased by $50 billion per year by 2010, half of which would go to countries in Africa. Additional funds would be earmarked towards specific problem areas, most notably the fight against malaria on the continent. All these efforts were explicitly inspired by the call for and directed towards acceleration of the processes that would ensure the success of the MDGs by 2015. In 2005, the G8 consisted of the U.K. (the holder of the presidency for that year), France, Germany, Italy, Japan, Canada, the EU, and Russia. The G8 is currently the G7, after the suspension of Russia following the annexation of Crimea in 2014.

8  MDG number 8 is 'Develop a global partnership for development'. This is a complex goal that involves making international agreements that are conducive to the progress of underdeveloped states. This includes working towards a more favourable global trading system for LDCs, to provide affordable medicines, and to make sure benefits of new technologies, such as the Internet, are available to as many people as possible.

9 The three dimensions of sustainable development are (1) social, (2) environmental, and (3) economic. The interdependent and cohesive elements constitute the foundation on which the post-2015 development agenda builds, as is made explicit in several documents. Additionally, the UN has attempted to integrate these dimensions system-wide with the goal of permeating the organisation. This process has been identified as '*Mainstreaming of the three dimensions of sustainable development throughout the United Nations system*', and the work towards it has produced several UNGA resolutions.

10 "Because of the great number of questions it is called upon to consider, . . . the UN General Assembly allocates items relevant to its work among its six Main Committees, which discuss them, seeking where possible to harmonize the various approaches of States, and then present to a plenary meeting of the Assembly draft resolutions and decisions for consideration" (UNGA, n.d., para. 1). The second committee is more specifically referred to as the economic and financial committee.

# 3 Development, health, and international relations

This chapter explores the links between three distinct but interlinked spheres: health, development, and IR. Our main focus is the nexus between health and IR, particularly the concepts of global health and global health governance (GHG). We begin by exploring the links between *health* and *development* historically and – in more detail – in contemporary settings. The main feature of this first section is its exploration of the expanding array of actors involved in global health efforts, where the main actor continues to be the World Health Organization (WHO). The relationship between health and IR is then examined in detail, with a particular focus on the inherent bi-directionality of global health, illustrated by its uneasy relationship with security. More specifically, this relates to the two dichotomous modes of approaching this relationship: namely, *state security* and *human security*. The discussion continues with a short history of HIV/AIDS and its relationship with security, before the chapter closes with a section on the inclusion of health in foreign policy and in the practice of health diplomacy.

In the opening pages of this book we mention of Bellamy's *Looking Backward: 2000–1887*, the futuristic book in which the author envisions a socialist utopia by the turn of the millennium. In a similar fashion, another writer, Thomas, laments what she views as the nonsensical absence of health issues in IR in *On the health of International Relations and the International Relations of Health* (Thomas, 1989). The final paragraph is titled *Looking to the year 2000*, and Thomas, seemingly inspired by ideas similar to those informing the nascent human development paradigm, suggests that the integration of health in both policy and research in IR is not only a normative necessity but a future inevitability:

> Changes in attitudes to health at local, national and international levels, albeit on a small scale, suggest the beginning of a revolutionary new path to tackling the problem of health, based on a new recognition of fundamental human rights, a conception of development which challenges the conventional orthodoxy, and a new political commitment to social mobilization, education and popular participation. . . . The consequences of the adoption of social mobilization as a vehicle to the fulfilment of the right to freedom from disease will have far-reaching effects on national politics and international

relations if they gather momentum. For the health of our subject, we ignore them at our peril.

(Thomas, 1989, p. 279)

Thomas's vision of the future was closer to reality than that of Bellamy's, although Thomas had the advantage of writing 102 years closer to the relevant date, as well as from the perspective of her professorship in global politics. Almost three decades after Thomas's article, many of the normative ambitions she mentions are in the process of being recognised and realised; connection points between health and IR are also gaining increased attention in the field. Exploring the processes that occur at the nexus of health, development, and IR can illuminate the processes that produced the circumstances in which the health norms of the MDGs and the SDGs evolved.

## Health and development: the evolution of a symbiotic relationship

When the SDGs were officially presented at *the UN Summit for the Adoption of the post-2015 Development Agenda* in September 2015, health retained its position as one of the cornerstones of the global development effort. While the explicit mention of health had been reduced from three of the eight MDGs to only one of the 17 SDGs, its role remained central to the endeavour as a whole. The single SDG health goal is, in fact, more comprehensive and holistic than the three health-related MDGs combined (Smith, Buse, & Gordon, 2016). Development and health have, directly or indirectly, been interconnected since the beginning of the global development effort. With the exception of the exalted *super-norm* of poverty eradication, specified and unspecified targets in fighting disease and minimising, for instance, child and maternal mortality rates, have always been top priorities of the development agenda. Health and development form a mutually beneficial symbiosis. Developmental efforts towards the improvement of health are inherently beneficial and contribute to the fulfilment of a human right. In addition, a healthy population is better equipped to accelerate further improvements in all aspects of development (Strauss & Thomas, 1998). Furthermore, health provides multiple non-controversial measuring sticks for development, as many indicators of health-related progress or regress are quantifiable – the health variable that makes up one-third of the HDI is perhaps the most salient example.

## Global health and health in development: a story of concentricity

For some, the origins of the relationship between health and development have roots that precede any formalised effort towards the mitigation of global inequality or alleviation of suffering. In one vein, some publications (Anderson, 1995; Palmer, 2010) describe how far less benevolent imperial practices can be viewed as important antecedents to the effort. They explore how Western ideas of health, hygiene, and medicine were introduced and imposed, with various degrees of force, on what was viewed as the primitive and unclean inhabitants of the colonies.

Historian of science Anderson narrates how American colonists in the Philippines, for example, found it necessary to purify all aspects of their surroundings:

> American colonial health officers in the early twentieth century turned their new tropical frontier into a desolate human-waste land, imagining everything "brownwashed" with a thin film of germs. Thus constituted, the tropical environment called for massive, ceaseless disinfection; the Filipino bodies that polluted it required control and medical reformation; and the vulnerable, formalized bodies of the American colonialists demanded sanitary quarantine.
>
> (Anderson, 1995, p. 641)

As all colonial powers, the Americans were not simply concerned with health problems associated with physical contamination. Disease, whether among colonisers or colonised, among its own citizens or the citizens of trade-partner countries, is detrimental to the economic profitability of the colony.

> Global health began in late 1913 when the newly chartered Rockefeller Foundation launched the International Health Commission to treat hookworm disease in a tropical band encompassing half the world's population that was of growing interest to the young imperial United States.
>
> (Palmer, 2010, p. 1)

There were, therefore, many reasons to introduce a degree of health care to the colonies. While intentions may have been explicitly selfish, whether from economic or medical self-interest or more crudely, from disgust for the unclean other – the idea was that a problem was being fixed. Fuelled by much of the same discourse as later modernisation theory, the assumption was that the introduction of medicine and hygiene was a step towards a more modern society and was considered a mutually beneficial process for the colonisers and the colonised alike. The emphasis of these efforts, however, seems to have been a largely self-serving one (Arnold, 1993; Wilmshurst, 1997).

Currently, the position of health in development is part of a larger discourse that also pertains to international health cooperation and coordination – namely, *global health*. Global health can be defined in various ways, but it generally refers to a coordinated reaction to worldwide health challenges. These challenges can be located anywhere and be responded to by local and international actors, or a combination of the two. The underlying assumptions that motivate these efforts are (1) the intrinsic values and beneficial by-products of healthy populations (Jamison et al., 2013) and (2) the recognition that health problems directly and indirectly transcend man-made borders. It is therefore – in the spirit of what IR refers to as *Liberal Institutionalism* – in everyone's interest that sovereign states cooperate in mitigating these health problems, often coordinated by IOs in which states are represented. It is an effort built not only on this sense of enlightened self-interest, but also on values based in human rights and global justice (see Pogge, 2001), which emphasises global health equity. *Health equity* is defined as:

> the absence of systematic disparities in health (or in the major social determinants of health) between social groups who have different levels of underlying social advantage/disadvantage – that is, different positions in a social hierarchy. Inequities in health systematically put groups of people who are already socially disadvantaged (for example, by virtue of being poor, female, and/or members of a disenfranchised racial, ethnic, or religious group) at further disadvantage with respect to their health; health is essential to wellbeing and to overcoming other effects of social disadvantage.
>
> (Braveman & Gruskin, 2003, p. 254).

This endeavour ranges from concerted efforts of treating acute pandemics such as cholera or Ebola; coordinated research, studying the array of aspects that pertain to health and disease, and distributing medicine and medical personnel as well as organising various forms of relevant training:

> Global health emphasises transnational health issues, determinants and solutions, involves many disciplines within and beyond the health sciences, and promotes interdisciplinary collaboration; and is a synthesis of population based prevention with individual-level clinical care.
>
> (Koplan et al., 2009, 1995)

While this alone is a formidable task, the scope of global health is even larger. As Koplan et al. (2009) suggest, global health does not only concern itself with diseases that literally cross the borders of states and continents, though these make up the most obvious area of concern. The increasing problem of antimicrobial resistance (Davies & Verde, 2013) is one example of a problem that is of increasingly acute interest to global health and is one of the top priorities identified by a Lancet Commission on Global Health (Hoffman, Cole, & Pearcey, 2015; Jamison et al., 2013). Further, "the global in global health refers to the scope of problems, not their location" (Koplan et al., 2009, p. 1994), and problems with a global scope are on the increase. For example, another major and growing aspect of global health is the multitude of health problems associated with global climate change, a problem recognised by the post-2015 development agenda and addressed within SDG 3. While this subject is explored in more detail in Chapter 6, the core issue is noted here: potential consequences of climate change can negatively affect all aspects of development, and health is certainly no exception (Ford, 2012; McMichael & Woodruff, 2005; McMichael, 2013; Patz, Campbell-Lendrum, Holloway, & Foley, 2005).

To add to this, non-communicable diseases (NCDs) are increasingly relevant to global health. There have been some notable success stories with regard to some of the efforts to curb the annual death toll attributable to NCDs, but problems persist and grow, particularly in developing countries (Patterson, 2018). These include issues such as alcohol intake and obesity associated with unhealthy diets and physical inactivity and their various consequences for the health of the individual; cancer, diabetes, and chronic respiratory disease are all major killers on a global scale and act as direct or indirect inhibitors of all aspects of human development (Beaglehole et al., 2011). In aggregate, these myriad challenges of global health are addressed by a vast and complex network of different types of local, regional, and international organisations worldwide, including health development.

The evolution of the place of health within the larger framework of the UN-led global development project is the main focus of Chapters 5 and 6, in which the subject undergoes closer scrutiny. For the purpose of the current chapter, it is sufficient to note that health has been – and continues to be – generally viewed as integral to development. This is true of earlier theories of development based upon the idea of modernisation, and it is also true of the contemporary rights-based frameworks within the human development paradigm and the related contemporary *leitmotif* of sustainable development. Furthermore, it is an essential component both for the MDGs and the SDGs. However, while health seems to have cemented a perennial position within development, much of the global discourse around health has changed both within the academic world and in policy, particularly since the end of the Cold War. This book is interested in the factors that have led to changes in norms, values, and cultural institutions for health in development, as explained by IR. The sections given later begin to explore the political nature of health in global governance and in foreign policy, emphasising in particular the continuous dialogue of material and ideational factors that combine to shape the present landscape in which politics and health meet.

### The actors and actions of global health

Although the precise definition of GHG lacks clarity and consensus (Lee & Kamradt-Scott, 2014), it generally refers to the way in which various global health efforts are organised and coordinated. "Broadly understood, [GHG] involves multiple actors, disciplines, and levels, recognises the effects of globalisation on disease, acknowledges societal responses to health and health solutions, and understands the linkages between health and economics, security, and the environment" (Patterson, 2018, p. 5). To an extent, these concerted and coordinated efforts include the early efforts of the major states that organised the international sanitary conferences in the late 19th century, although it is more accurate to refer to these conferences as part of *international* rather than *global* health governance. These efforts were far more explicitly self-interested responses to the adverse effects that epidemics – particularly cholera – had on important trade routes. The outcomes of these early conferences were largely agreements on quarantine and on limiting and monitoring population mobility across state borders. Early governing bodies such as the International Commission on Epidemics, founded in 1903, or the International Office of Public Hygiene of 1907 were mainly concerned with this kind of containment measure. In 1920, the League of Nations established its own health office, which was assisted financially and technically by the Rockefeller Foundation. In addition to disease containment and supervision, emphasis was also placed on "the provision of global standards for drugs and vaccines, and selected technical advice to countries on key health matters, including medical education" (Skolnik, 2012, p. 350).

GHG is a specified sub-type of the larger structure of *global governance*, a term which attempts to describe a set of behaviours by organisations and institutions that, in lieu of a central global government, aims to fulfil some of the work that national governments do domestically, but on a global scale. However, the direct analogy with government is limited:

> Both refer to purposive behaviour, to goal-orientated activities, to systems of rule; but government suggests activities that are backed by formal authority, by police powers to insure the implementation of duly constituted policies, whereas governance refers to activities backed by shared goals that may or may not derive from legal and formally prescribed responsibilities and that do not necessarily rely on police powers to overcome defiance and attain compliance.
>
> (Rosenau, 1992, p. 4)

Global governance implies the lack of a central authority; it is more appropriate to describe global governance as coordinated responses to an array of challenges and issues that go beyond the capacities of the individual state to mitigate and to challenges and issues that affect more than an individual state. Though there is some debate concerning defining characteristics of GHG (Lee & Kamradt-Scott, 2014), the concept – in short – refers to those global governance efforts that pertain to health. Importantly, GHG is not a value-neutral, rational enterprise in which the objectively best solutions always find their way into policy and practice. As some suggest,

> GHG is inherently political because it raises fundamental questions regarding where power and authority does and should lie in governing to protect and promote human health, and whose interests should be served or not served by the distribution of costs and benefits arising from such authority.
>
> (McInnes et al., 2015, p. 4)

GHG is a normatively contested space, in which meanings and interests are pitted against each other and in which framing becomes an important political tool. As with other forms of global governance, GHG was for a long time the responsibility of the UN and its specialised agencies. Shortly after the creation of the UN came the establishment of the WHO in 1948. The WHO's endeavours are often separated into the two respective categories of facilitating normative and technical cooperation in global health matters (WHO, 2017a). Effectively, the WHO acted as the closest semblance of a global health authority for decades, during which time it orchestrated a number of successful and significant global projects.

However, with increasing globalisation, the field has become more populated and more complex: "forces of global change, in various forms, have intensified cross-border activity to such an extent as to undermine the capacity of states to control them" (Dodgson, Lee, & Drager, 2002, p. 18). Indeed, as with health governance in general, the first decades of the WHO's efforts are more accurately characterised as *international* health governance. The *global* nature of these efforts only appeared later, with globalisation. Fidler defines GHG as a concept used "when thinking about how globalization affects the national and international pursuit of public health" (Fidler, 2002, p. 6). He further describes GHG as referring to:

> the use of formal and informal institutions, rules, and processes by states, intergovernmental organizations, and nonstate actors to deal with challenges to health that require cross-border collective action to address effectively. This definition's relative simplicity should not obscure the breadth and complexity of this concept.
>
> (Fidler, 2010, p. 3)

The WHO's stated objective is "the attainment by all people of the highest possible level of health" (WHO, 1948, p. 3). This aspiration has yielded several ambitious efforts over the decades, laying the foundation for how global health is coordinated today by, among other things, cementing countless good practices and norms in terms of ethical considerations, practical implementation, and in mobilising global cooperation. Projects such as the eradication of specific communicable diseases are often seen as the WHO's most successful endeavours. A global immunisation campaign with the goal of eradicating smallpox was started in 1966 and successfully concluded in 1980. A similar programme to eradicate polio was started in 1988 and has, at the time of writing, taken great strides toward succeeding, with less than 50 cases worldwide per year (and decreasing). The WHO has also been at the forefront of battling HIV/AIDS, malaria, and tuberculosis in various capacities, thereby greatly reducing deaths and limiting spread.

The WHO has also put considerable resources into reducing the negative effects of NCDs. Obesity, the abuse of narcotics and alcohol, diabetes, various cancers, and smoking of tobacco are examples of some of the major problem areas within the category of NCDs. According to the WHO, these various health challenges kill around 38 million people per year, almost three quarters of which take place in low- and middle-income countries. The organisation, in cooperation with other global health actors, puts in place a variety of measures to reduce these numbers, including, for example, cancer prevention through more available screening and limiting the advertising of alcohol and tobacco. Perhaps most famously, the World Health Assembly, the forum through which the WHO is governed by its 194 member states, adopted the *WHO Framework Convention for Tobacco Control* (FCTC) in 2003. The FCTC, legally binding in 180 ratifying countries, requires all tobacco products to be clearly marked with the health risks associated with its use. For many, the FCTC is an early example of a formal multilateral treaty directly prioritising health concerns over economic interests. It was the first multilateral and binding treaty regarding a chronic, non-communicable global health issue and stands as a milestone in global cooperation towards the mitigation of NCDs.

In a sense, the WHO has long acted as the normative hegemon of global health. As some suggest, the organisation was, from the time it was established, "a normative agency endowed with unprecedented constitutional powers" (Gostin, Sridhar, & Hougendobler, 2015, p. 1). However, with the increasing pluralisation of health governance, the WHO currently finds itself alongside a number of other major actors:

> Also important to the system are other United Nations and multilateral agencies that have health components (e.g., [UNICEF], the World Bank, and the regional development banks), along with a diverse set of civil society organizations, multinational corporations, foundations, and academic institutions. This pluralistic landscape has been enriched by a set of innovative and influential hybrid organizations, such as the GAVI Alliance (formerly the Global Alliance for Vaccines and Immunization), UNITAID (which works to improve the functioning of global markets for commodities for the acquired immunodeficiency syndrome [AIDS], tuberculosis, and malaria), and the Global Fund to Fight AIDS, Tuberculosis, and Malaria, which are governed by representatives both from within and from outside national governments.
> (Frenk & Moon, 2013, p. 937)

The 2014 Ebola outbreak of West Africa was symptomatic of the waning status of the WHO's role as "the directing and co-ordinating authority on international health work" (WHO, 1948, p. 3). In dealing with the crisis, the World Bank and the African Union (AU) were able to allocate far more funds than the increasingly financially restricted WHO. Coupled with a response to the crisis that was considered to be slow and which drew criticisms from organisations such as Médecins Sans Frontières (MSF), the Ebola epidemic contributed to the questioning of the WHO's capacity for fulfilling its role as a leader in responding to global health crises, a role that had already been called into question prior to the outbreak: "[t]he current trajectory suggests that WHO and powerful donors will continue their slow dance of death, with the organization becoming increasingly irrelevant and sidelined by other institutional players" (Lee & Pang, 2014, p. 7). However, the WHO does remain at the core of GHG and global disease control, particularly because of the role of its *International Health Regulations* (IHRs), which provide global guidelines for the minimisation of the spread of disease (Davies et al., 2015).

In general, although the WHO has seen many successes in its time as the virtually undisputed leader of GHG and global health security, and while the organisation and its norms and institutions retain a significant position in these spheres – particularly through the IHRs – its power has declined over the last two to three decades (Youde, 2012). Hoffman (2010) describes this ongoing atrophying process by applying regime theory's[1] *hegemonic transition framework*. The organisation ascended to a position of hegemon of its speciality almost immediately upon its formation in 1948 and has, since then, originated and integrated much of the *ethos* that continue to characterise GHG and global health security in stated purpose and in practice. Newer actors in the field – for instance, large NGOs like MSF or the Bill & Melinda Gates Foundation – largely base their beliefs on many of the same principles but have different approaches that have enabled them to become influential actors in a previously solitary playing field. This, in combination with the increased prevalence of new associations of states with specialised health security interests (such as the G7's Global Health Security Initiative) have resulted in a decreased dependence on the WHO as the sole legitimate leading figure in GHG. The timing of this hegemonic decline is likely not arbitrary. Hoffman (2010) suggests that as the volume and density of the field increases, so does the likeliness of hegemonic decline and transition. This coincides with the material growth of the field that happened in the beginning of the 1990s. Singular events such as the organisation's inadequate response to the most recent major outbreak of Ebola in West Africa have also contributed to this hegemonic decline (Gostin et al., 2015).

One aspect that is often referenced and subsequently characterised as an increasingly significant part of global governance in general – including the endeavours of global development and GHG – is the emergence of powerful, well-resourced NGOs, and philanthropic foundations. This is thought to be significant primarily because of the new interests and identities these bring to the arena, which tend to contrast with, or at least are less ambiguous than, the identities and interests of the average state actor, and by extension, IOs. Another facet that separates NGOs from states is their inability to make and enforce law, as they lack any form of rational-legal authority.

Often, the motivations and interests of NGOs within general and health-specific development tend to approximate the sentiments of globalist, cosmopolitan frameworks such as the human development paradigm and the concept of human security. Global health (and general health) NGOs exist in different sizes and formats. For example, there are those focused on specific diseases, such as the many that concentrate on HIV/AIDS, or malaria; others focus on specific cancers, others still on reproductive health. Multipurpose organisations such as the Bill & Melinda Gates Foundation target a slew of different areas connected to what they perceive as threats to health. Another category constitutes alliances that are made up of sometimes hundreds of specific organisations in order to unite for a larger, common denominator – such as the NCD Alliance. More multipurpose still are entities such as the Rockefeller Foundation – a foundation that aims to generally promote human well-being through avenues such as health, food security and sustainable agriculture, and technological innovation, among others. These actors all have in common that they work towards improved prevention, education and awareness, treatment, research, and access to care and/or medicines.

The lack of self-interest in terms of security is what most strikingly sets non-state actors apart from the traditional state actor. Non-state actors have no territorial integrity to protect; they are – in the realm of global health – truly global actors created and moulded by, and therefore inherently adapted to, a globalised world. The state actor and its interests, by contrast, face the numerous consequences of globalisation with varying degrees of ambiguity. The lack of ambiguity displayed by variables such as the statements, fund allocations, policies, and actions of NGOs make them less complicated than states and IOs, whose corresponding variables can be contradictory, fleeting, inconsistent, and opaque.

## Plurality, squared

To complicate the matter further, various global health issues are affected by organisations, actors, and forces that are ostensibly not associated with matters pertaining to health. Increasingly, decisions made regarding areas like migration, trade, and climate change are continuously changing and complicating what is considered to be indirect determinants of health. Major policymaking actors in *these* spheres are therefore also significant for the general global health situation. The cross-sectionalism of these spheres of influence is a clear and recurring theme of global health when considering the vast range of health's potential determinants. The MDGs, for example, have three discrete goals dedicated directly to health issues, while the five remaining goals are all relevant to *social determinants of health* in one or several different ways to one extent or another.

The notion of social determinants of health refers to variables that *indirectly* affect the health of an individual. This includes the circumstances in which people live and work, where they are born, and where they grow old. It is dependent on a set of indirect forces and systemic specificities that shape the conditions in which people live their lives. Social norms, political and economic systems, and poverty as well as any type of structural violence are all considered integral social determinants of health. In the words of the WHO's Commission on Social Determinants of Health (CSDH), these factors have massive consequences for the health of individuals and populations:

> The poor health of the poor, the social gradient in health within countries, and the marked health inequities between countries are caused by the unequal distribution of power, income, goods, and services, globally and nationally, the consequent unfairness in the immediate, visible circumstances of peoples lives – their access to health care, schools, and education, their conditions of work and leisure, their homes, communities, towns, or cities – and their chances of leading a flourishing life. This unequal distribution of health-damaging experiences is not in any sense a 'natural' phenomenon but is the result of a toxic combination of poor social policies and programmes, unfair economic arrangements, and bad politics. Together, the structural determinants and conditions of daily life constitute the social determinants of health and are responsible for a major part of health inequities between and within countries.
>
> (CSDH, 2008, p. 1)

One of the most recognised social determinants of health is local social status, which often goes hand in hand with higher income and better education. Racial discrimination is also a common causal factor; gender norms and taboos affect health in various ways, a topic explored more closely in Chapter 5. Even less tangible factors such as support from family, friends and local communities are also rightly included in this category, as is the notoriously labyrinthine concept of culture. Defining these indirect and often fluid determinants of health is among the more challenging obstacles of global health actors, particularly because of specific cultural or economic contexts.

As a result of this plurality of determining variables, a number of dynamics attributable to globalisation compound this already complicated picture, and major global policy decisions in seemingly separate areas tend to be crosscutting as well. For example, the WTO's 2001 *Doha Declaration on the TRIPS Agreement and Public Health* (henceforth referred to as the *Doha Declaration*) and its 2005 amendment concerning pharmaceuticals – discussed further in Chapter 6 – came about as a global health response to increase the availability of affordable medicines (Frenk & Moon, 2013). On a more local level, access to, for example, better roads can mean access to better health services. This serves as a reminder of the symbiotic and interdependent relationship between health and development and the occasionally counter-intuitive causal trajectories that can act as determinants of health. This "hyper-pluralism" (Ruger, 2013, p. 267) of variables, determinants, and actors contributes to a number of complications for the coherence of GHG. As identified by Ruger (2013), these include, among others, a lack of accountability (the other side of the coin of a corresponding lack of legitimacy), a lack of a coherent global strategy, and a lack of dispute resolution mechanisms.

### Health in development versus global health

The endeavour of health-specific global development as organised and implemented by the UN is an integral part of the larger body that comprises GHG. However, there are certain attributes that set health development apart from many of the other practices of GHG. The notion of global health "suggests issues that people face in common, such as the impact of a growing and aging worldwide population on health or the potential risks of climate change to health" (Skolnik, 2012, p. 7). While the latter point concerning the looming threat of climate change is indeed central to the post-2015 development agenda, health's place in development did not initially emanate from the recognition or concern of the global nature of certain health problems. It was rather merely one part, albeit an integral one, of the process of attempting to mitigate global inequality, as briefly described in Chapter 1.

Global health and GHG only truly manifested decades after the start of the development agenda in the 1950s, although it has roots stemming from at least the mentioned international sanitary conferences of the late 19th century, both in terms of motivation and in terms of organisation. Today, partly owing to its plurality of relevant actors, GHG is driven by the motivations that inspired both these respective efforts. From this perspective, global health is simultaneously altruistic and self-interested, reflecting a self-proclaimed cosmopolitan ideology of connection, directed at addressing shared challenges and finding solutions, while also emphasising a level of shared threat that alludes to existential vulnerabilities. The transformation from the explicit approach of the pure self-interest of the sanitary conferences to the current more humanitarian-framed endeavour is emblematic of an international norm change in which explicit references to human rights have begun to supersede the concern for a state's interests. These bi-directional but not mutually exclusive motivations for global health cooperation are recurring themes in the study of nearly all aspects of GHG and global health in general. Although humanitarian norms tend to be more publicised, there is little doubt that there is a large degree of self-interest involved in the way that states engage in the rules and activities that make up GHG. *Disease Diplomacy: International Norms and Global Health Security* (Davies et al., 2015) explores how the most recent revision of the IHRs (WHO, 2005b) was a culmination of a number of international norm changes that came about through the interaction of material changes and ideational innovation. These included the increasing securitisation[2] of health that occurred in the early 1990s, built on the oft-repeated narrative that increasing globalisation leads to more frequent and faster travel by people and therefore the diseases that they carry. Another security concern, which became more salient after 2001, was the possibility of pathogens being weaponised for the purposes of bioterrorists, most infamously exemplified by the American anthrax attacks of that year. This aspect of global health, *global health security*, is discussed in more detail later.

Development, on the other hand, has traditionally had little to do with security and self-interest and more with altruism, with an underlying sense of a global divide between *haves* and *have-nots* included in its foundation. Indeed, the dichotomous binary of developed and developing (or underdeveloped) states and regions as vocalised by Harry S. Truman in his 1949 Four Point speech, refers to a sentiment that is at its core far more interested in helping those who find themselves in the latter category rather than ensuring the safety of those in the former, which was seen as an altogether separate enterprise. While intentions may have originated in different sentiments, the lines separating global health and health development are currently not easily identifiable – particularly since the advent of GHG and the globalisation of health that heralded its emergence. Health-based development is now inextricably linked with global health efforts generally, as the two spheres are affected by many of the same variables. This link also exists in terms of security and securitisation in relation to global health, through what some refer to as the *security-development nexus* (Hettne, 2010; Keukeleire & Raube, 2013). The points of contact between security, health, and development have developed over time as responses to material and ideational transformations. The manner in which norms pertaining to these interconnected spheres have evolved in relation to the UN's development agenda form a prominent subject of analysis in Chapters 5 and 6.

## Health and international relations

The increasing number of actors and determinants of global health in a globalising world has generated a corresponding plurality in the scholarly and practical fields to which global health has become relevant. Its infiltration into the realm of IR, a multidisciplinary field concerned with matters of global significance, is not exactly controversial. Two decades into the new millennium, the points of concentricity between the two spheres are becoming increasingly numerous, both in the realms of academic research in both fields and in the policies of states and organisations. Novel areas towards which IR and health both tend to gravitate have been, and are still being, identified, opening up a number of nascent areas of research.

Several of these areas of intersection have been, to one extent or another, explored over the last 10–15 years. Price-Smith's work *The Health of Nations: Infectious Disease, Environmental Change, and Their Effects on National Security and Development* (2002) shows that increased disease often has direct negative effects on economic and political stability and, overall, reduces state capacity. The Department of International Politics at Aberystwyth University has a Centre for Health and International Relations (CHAIR) dedicated to the study of the link between the two fields. CHAIR also has links to a number of academic and institutions globally as well as links with organisations such as the United Nations Educational, Scientific and Cultural Organisation (UNESCO).

A 2014 special issue of the *Review of International Studies* was dedicated to the subject of global health in IR, in which a wide range of topics was covered, and in which a wide range of theoretical and methodological approaches were applied. The featured articles discuss, among others, matters of health diplomacy[3] and soft power, health in and post-conflict contexts, the political role of pharmaceutical companies in GHG, and the links between health and security. Other recent publications include *Global Politics of Health* by Davies (2010a); *Global Health and International Relations* (2012) by McInnes & Lee, and *Global Health Governance* (2012) by Youde. More specifically focused, a 2016 special issue of *Third World Quarterly* was titled *The international politics of Ebola*.

In spite of their increasingly clear common areas of interest, the association of these two fields has traditionally been far from straightforward, a fact nearly invariably mentioned by all these publications. Importantly, IR scholarship has also become more varied in its areas of concern due to parallel and complementary developments, both in ideational terms within the field and in terms of material developments within areas of concern in the field: the relationships between global actors and the emergence of new actors. Twenty or 30 years ago, health did not have a place in IR in the way that it does today (Thomas, 1989). However, both IR and global health are fields in flux. As their subject matter has gone through significant changes, the disciplines have necessarily found ways to adapt:

> Both, as multidisciplinary fields, continue to struggle with questions of identity, of what they are – and are not – concerned with. Both, in practice, also struggle with a world of ever greater complexity and interconnectedness. Two distinct fields have thus been brought together in the early twenty-first century by the development of shared concerns, of uncertain disciplinary

boundaries, and of a mutual need for more effective policies in a changed and changing world.

(McInnes & Lee, 2012, pp. 1–2)

The increasingly eclectic spheres of relevance to both fields have led to the realisation that they share large and complex swathes of common ground. For global health experts and practitioners, areas of knowledge that fall under IR's expertise such as global political economy, trade, foreign policy, and global security are increasingly apropos. Additionally,

> [t]he linkage also challenges those studying national security to consider issues, such as the relationship of public health to a state's material capabilities, previously alien to national security debates. The different perspectives on the meaning of security further relate to larger theoretical concepts concerning the structure and dynamics of international relations. The linking of public health and national security thus raises deeper theoretical issues and controversies about world politics in the global era.
>
> (Fidler, 2003, pp. 788–789)

One major reason for the previous separation of the two is an obstacle presented by one of the major tenets of traditional IR thinking. In IR (a field for decades concerned mostly with conflict, power, and national security), health concerns have often been considered – if considered at all – as part of the second tier of the field's binary hierarchy of *high* and *low* politics: "[m]atched against other foreign policy crises and priorities, . . . global health problems stay part of the low politics of foreign policy, where health issues historically tend to reside" (Fidler, 2009, p. 22). In IR, *high politics* refers to what is viewed as ever-present concerns of a state's foreign policy. In essence, the matters that are imperative for the survival of the state belong in this category. Currently, military security is the only consensually defined aspect of a given state's concern that can truly be said to possess this quality. In diplomatic terms, it refers to "a state's security relationship to other states in the international system" (Barnett, 1990, p. 531). Low politics, on the other hand, is associated with concerns that are secondary, "economic and social affairs" (Keohane & Nye, 2011, p. 19). In the end, the implication is that low politics always plays second fiddle to high politics.

This distinction owes much to the traditional underlying assumption that low politics pertains more to domestic and national politics rather than having an influence on international affairs, which is the overarching unit of analysis of the field: "[i]n particular, health appeared to [IR] scholars as a domestic concern largely unrelated to matters of national security" (McInnes & Lee, 2012, p. 26). As Thomas writes,

> The subject has been overlooked because it does not fit neatly into the dominant state-centric approach of the discipline, and discussion of health might

be seen to contravene the aged principle of non-intervention in the internal affairs of other sovereign states. Also the discipline, rooted as it is in developed, and more particularly Western, states' experience and perceptions, has concerned itself with the more threatening scenarios of military security, the social dimensions being settled by way of the welfare state and falling within the realms of low politics. . . . A discussion of health draws on interdisciplinary debates about human rights, development, self-determination, the role of state and non-state actors in international affairs and many other issues. It challenges the conventional wisdom of the subject of International Relations, and forces us to look beyond the state-centric paradigm to understand social, economic and political linkages between local, national and international levels of activity.

(Thomas, 1989, p. 273)

For reasons already alluded to, the categorisation of health as part of low politics, as well as the validity of the binary categories themselves, is becoming less clear-cut. Indeed, decades after her article, the suggestions listed by Thomas were beginning to come to fruition:

this thriving growth in the study of health in IR responds to the heightened density of global health activity. There is a growing awareness that – like many international environmental issues – pressing global health challenges transcend national borders, and because of their centrality to human and societal well-being, they generate a sustained political demand for more concerted international responses.

(Davies et al., 2014, p. 2)

Many changes in global health over the past decade or so have seen an increase in these concerted international responses. The first shift was a renewed sense of crisis, as affluent states, long unconcerned with the disease problems experienced more typically closer to the equator, were faced with serious novel infectious diseases, as well as the increasing occurrences of drug-resistant strains of a number of diseases assumed permanently curbed, for example tuberculosis. The SARS crisis in 2003 made it abundantly clear that no state was immune to the travel of infection and that increased proactivity in global cooperation and coordination would be necessary in order to maintain stability and security both within and among states. This can be seen as a reaction to the direct security threat of disease physically entering the borders of states and thus presenting a risk to its citizens. These can be characterised as *state security health norms* and were central in the UNSC's *Resolution 1308*, which framed HIV/AIDS as a global security threat – a process returned to below, as well as in Chapter 5. A second shift was the realisation that health's increasingly global relevance also affects other areas of concern. For the same reasons that health is important for development, disease – wherever located – is a global economic issue (WHO, 2000). However, disease continues to disproportionately afflict the poor, despite the efforts of health development. For Davies et al. (2014), a sense of failure in terms of the endeavour to eradicate illness has acted as an additional motivation for more efficient cooperation in the global fight against disease. Both these factors suggest an ascendance of global health closer to a position in the category of high politics, which may act as a contributing factor regarding the success or failure of an emerging health norm.

In the same vein, state-actors have stepped up their work in global health coordination, in which state and non-state organisations pursue common goals in the spirit of liberal institutionalism. "This can be seen in the way that key international institutions – from the [UNSC], [UNGA], the World Bank and the [G8], through to the [WHO] – have converged on seeking to tackle many more global health issues" (Davies et al., 2014, p. 3). As suggested earlier, a number of increasingly powerful and resourceful NGOs have also grown to become significant actors in GHG as, for example, the H-8, mentioned in Chapter 1. From the view of IR, then, the range of threats relevant to the security of the traditional actor has changed. Non-state actors, with different interests and identities to those traditionally attributed to the traditional sovereign state actor, have come to the fore, and are taking up increasingly significant roles in the sphere of global health.

This, however, is not sufficient to explain the full range of reciprocal interest areas that exist between global health and IR. As suggested, specifically in relation to the binary of high and low politics, major changes in the empirical realities in the field have the potential to challenge its theoretical underpinnings. Or conversely, the theoretical underpinnings in the field must be open to the possibility of including non-traditional but relevant variables, a possibility that was not afforded by IR scholars for a long time. Indeed, the area that deals most directly with the health threats, and thus tightly connected with security, that of "infectious disease control, of whatever variety, was a neglected aspect of international relations" (Fidler, 2004, p. 800). Alongside material consequences attributed to the various trajectories of globalisation, new perspectives within the field started emerging as serious alternatives towards the end of the 1980s, particularly gaining traction and popularity after the end of the Cold War – and in part as *a result of* the end of the Cold War. These perspectives offered several challenges to the conventional wisdom of what famed constructivist scholar Alexander Wendt (1992) has called the *rationalist*[4] theories of IR. As some suggest, "[t]he emergence of feminist IR, critical security studies, constructivism and post-structuralist IR has been critical for the area of Global Health to be explored and, even, accepted in the discipline" (Davies et al., 2014, p. 6).

## Health and security

Whether naturally occurring or intentionally inflicted, microbial agents can cause illness, disability, and death in individuals while disrupting entire populations, economies, and governments. In the highly interconnected and readily traversed 'global village' of our time, one nation's problem soon becomes every nation's problem as geographical and political boundaries offer trivial impediments to such threats.

(Smolinski et al. in Lo Yuk-Ping & Thomas, 2010, p. 447)

One prominent link between IR and health is a shared emphasis on security. In the growing body of literature that bridges the two fields, security is a major point of connection as well as a major subject of debate. Indeed, there has been significant growth in literature in both policy and academia since the early 1990s, and particularly since the beginning of the millennium (Davies et al., 2015). For IR, any talk of security was long automatically prefixed with *national* or *state*; the discipline as a whole was under the impression that:

the referent object of security is the state; that the main concerns are direct threats, usually military in nature; that the context is one of an anarchic international states system where self-help is the order of the day; and that stability (both state and international) is privileged over issues such as rights and justice.

(McInnes, 2015, p. 8)

An emphasis on the state is, however, only one of the ways to view the linkage between health and security. The connection, which is often referred to as *global health security* (Rushton & Youde, 2015), has many meanings. It is a contested term with no clear definition or consensus with regard to what it entails, much like the term *security* is in its own right (Buzan, 1991; McDonald, 2008). This means that any view of what health security is, or should be, is a subject of debate, in which the various perspectives have meanings that

[are] constructed for a particular purpose including promoting a certain agenda and privileging certain interests over others. . . . The lack of an agreed definition is not due to the lack of effort but because in its different uses and terms it reflects different interests and agendas.

(McInnes, 2015, p. 7)

At the heart of this lies a conflict that seems innate in the relationship between health and security: "[m]any scholars have argued that there is an inherent tension between policies that prioritize state security interests and those that promote human health and wider health obligations, particularly when those obligations evoke duties of justice beyond national borders" (Brown & Stoeva, 2015, p. 304).

The dichotomy of self-interest and selflessness as motivating factors in pursuing endeavours in global health security correspond roughly to what Davies (2010a, 2010b) refers to as the *statist* and *globalist* perspectives. Davies's typology is often mentioned in discussions on the ambiguity of interests that characterise global health security (see Caballero-Anthony & Amul, 2015; Rushton, 2011). She has written extensively about the ways in which the field of IR engages with global health issues and emphasises that these perspectives are rather "modes of thinking and prioritization than cogent theories" (Davies, 2010b, p. 1170) and that most approaches are most appropriately placed somewhere in the middle of the two. Nevertheless, the typology is useful for categorising the divergent views on the dynamic between foreign policy and health. The *statist* perspective holds that the state is the referent object of security. In this sense, health issues are only salient when it affects the security of a state, be it political, economic, or military. In this view, health challenges, urgent or otherwise, become national security threats, the protection against which is the main goal of contributing to global health. For the *globalists* on the other hand, the referent object has shifted to the individual, and the state is only one of many actors responsible for ensuring its security. In fact, they argue, the state must adapt its own security needs to fit that of the global individual – and if it fails to do so, it must be held responsible. We refer to these two perspectives as *state security* and *human security*, respectively.

### State security

IR's traditional view of the connection between health and security was openly statist, mostly focused in terms of the effects of health concerns on the military, then focused later on general national security, as globalisation enabled the uninhibited travel of pathogens (McInnes, 2015). Indeed, the global health security discourse was originally situated in a statist paradigm. Several authors (Davies et al., 2015; Weir, 2015) refer to the U.S. Institute of Medicine's (IOM's) 1992 publication *Emerging Infections: Microbial Threats to Health in the United States* (Lederberg, Shope, & Oaks, 1992) as the point of inception for a security-based global health discourse, particularly through its emphasis on the novel concept of *emerging infectious diseases* (EIDs). As one observer notes, "*Emerging Infections* reframed contagious disease prevention and control through the invention of a new disease concept, EIDs, that was cast as the most significant problem for public health in the United States and, by extension, the world" (Weir, 2015, p. 19). In the report, infectious diseases were framed as a national threat, and it further suggested that the problem was global and subsequently that the U.S. government should "approach the WHO to implement a global surveillance system with the capacity to detect and respond to EID outbreaks" (Weir, 2015, p. 19). This was a significant step towards securitising health both domestically and, shortly after, globally. As Davies et al. (2015) suggest, the timing of this publication exploited a 'gap in the market' of national security in the immediate post-Cold War era, a context in which Washington's ears were open for suggestions. As the Copenhagen School suggests (Buzan, Wæver, & De Wilde, 1998; Lo Yuk-Ping & Thomas, 2010), the first step toward securitisation is the identification of an existential threat to an actor's existence. EIDs were soon identified as a threat within the context of U.S. security. This identification was thereafter exported to the WHO, which subsequently identified it as an existential *global* threat.

Indeed, the ideas of the IOM's report had, after a series of meetings, by 1996 been re-contextualised into global policy via the WHO. The WHO then established a new division called Emerging and Other Communicable Diseases (EMC), which would act as an identifying and responsive mechanism for limiting the spread of EIDs globally. The infiltration of the securitised status of disease into the WHO is illustrated in the *1996 World Health Report*, which describes a global crisis related to EIDs (WHO, 1996; Fidler, 1997). As Weir suggests, the U.S., along with Canada and the EU, went to great lengths to expand their perceived localised security threats into a frame of global security and global health. Many countries from the Global South were opposed to the idea, suggesting that the framework was primarily designed to protect the Global North from the diseases of the South, and not to prevent and treat disease in a truly global sense, a point which is discussed later.

Generally, the link between health and security is rather ambiguous. Much work has been done to assess the relevance of health concerns to foreign policy and whether these concerns warrant a classification within the category of *high politics*. The state security paradigm is built on the assumption that there are several causal links between global health problems and national – as well as international – security and stability. Though these are not agreed upon without controversy, they typically include the detrimental relationship between poor health and economic growth, the perceived inevitable migratory behaviour of poor people with poor health, the negative effects on militaries active in areas of high disease prevalence, and simply higher mortality and morbidity – though the empirical validity of these causal relations remain largely unsubstantiated or outdated (McInnes, 2015). From this perspective, increased globalisation means increased threat levels:

> With the complexities brought about by globalization and the emergence of new, more virulent pathogens, health challenges have increasingly been labelled as security issues or as exemplars of collective insecurity for sovereign states in particular. This frame presents effective health governance as a matter of national and international security that demands sophisticated surveillance, institutionalization and health policy prescriptions crafted at the multilateral level and then applied to the whole world. In so doing, public health challenges, which are usually discussed as 'low' politics, focusing on soft issues including social, justice, human rights, and the general delivery of services, are legitimized as security challenges, which are thus rendered exceptional, as 'high' politics.
>
> (Fourie, 2015, p. 105)

This state-centric approach has been criticised for being increasingly anachronistic and simplistic as well as unethical. Brown and Stoeva (2015), professing a more *cosmopolitan* view of the connection between health and security both in academia and in policy, argue that:

> The current literature also promotes an ethos of security over an ethic of care, simply because traditional understandings of security as 'security from' external threats inhibits an ethic of positive care. They are grounded in traditional theories of international relations, which assume a duality in the

moral standards that apply to individuals and to states. This is so, due to the assumed *raison d'être* of states, which authorizes the use of any means to achieve the overriding aim of the preservation of the state.

(Brown & Stoeva, 2015, p. 306)

As the authors point out, this tension is one of seemingly perpetual contestation, in a similar way to the theoretical debates within security studies as well as within IR in general. In practice, this tension is also reflected in the bi-directional frame of GHG, in which security – for states individually and collectively – as well as a normative message of global justice and human rights, are emphasised. In promoting a cosmopolitan perspective, Brown & Stoeva fully reject a state-centric health security paradigm and, with it, the assumption that the interests of a state and the interests of its citizens align. Rather, they emphasise individual health, human rights, and social justice, and "demand ethical duties for health beyond state border, and seek to draw attention to the structural causes of poor health versus simply focusing on the securitisation of existing symptoms" (2015, p. 310). This is both a normative and a practical argument: while demanding justice built on the idea that all human beings have universally equal status and rights that other states have a duty to fulfil; it also argues that states should not be the focus of something that they cannot individually control:

The idea being that if globalization has broadened the scope of health security relationships beyond state borders (as a statist position on global health admits), then the state loses its boundedness in favor of new political formulations that can better capture the interrelations that exist in a globalized world and their impacts on human health.

(Brown & Stoeva, 2015, p. 311)

Many of the sentiments found in this *cosmopolitan* view, in particular the emphasis on the human rights of all people (including the right to health) and the subsequent duty and necessity to combat disease in order to ensure these rights, are central tenets of the WHO, as seen both in its constitution and in the most recent revision of the organisation's IHRs (WHO, 2005b). The second principle of the constitution proclaims that the organisation should strive for "the enjoyment of the highest attainable standard of health [which] is one of the fundamental rights of every human being without distinction of race, religion, political belief, economic or social condition" (WHO, 1948, p. 1).

Global health practitioners are typically associated with a perspective termed *global public health security*. While the WHO is no longer the unquestioned hegemon of GHG, it is strongly associated with global public health security, and the explicit ideational underpinnings of the organisation reflect much of what this perspective entails. In its 2007 *World Health Report* (WHO, 2007), the WHO defines health security risks in a much wider context than territorial integrity: it includes infectious diseases, new and old, as well as disasters concerning the environment, natural or otherwise. It also somewhat uniquely includes food security and generally shifts the emphasis from the state to the general public and its vulnerable position in the face of globalisation.

However, framing global health concerns in a security discourse, rather than one in which human rights were emphasised, was an important method for the secretariat of the WHO to garner support for its new IHRs in 2005 (Davies et al., 2015). The regulations are not presented in a traditional state-centric security frame but rather in a frame that focuses on *collective* security, rationalised to a significant extent by the examples of the 2003 SARS outbreak and the threatened spread of the H5N1 pandemic in Asia. As is evident in the 2007 *World Health Report*, the WHO emphasises the impacts that global health threats can have "on economic or political stability, trade, tourism, access to goods and services and, if they occur repeatedly, on demographic stability" (WHO, 2007, p. 5). As Rushton (2011) suggests, the state remained the referent object of security in this paradigm, although the focus had shifted more toward goals that are common for all states and that behoves cooperation between all states, as well as with non-state actors. Writing at the time, Fidler (2005) articulated that

> [t]he world of global health security is one in which governments, intergovernmental organizations and non-State actors collaborate in a 'new way of working' by contributing toward a common goal through science, technology and law rather than through anarchical competition for power.
>
> (Fidler, 2005, p. 392).

Like the WHO in general and the realm of GHG at large, the IHRs have a nuanced and less than straightforward history, affected by various events and developments. Utilising Finnemore & Sikkink's norm life cycle, Davies et al. (2015) trace the evolution of the newest edition of the *IHR* (WHO, 2005b). The now familiar narrative of globalisation and its subsequent mobility of infectious diseases and risks of bioterrorism, which at least partly securitised certain communicable diseases, hastened the 2005 revision process. The authors identify norm entrepreneurs present within U.S. policy circles – including the authors of the IOM report – as well as individuals within the WHO's secretariat who worked towards the spread and reinforcement of these ideas. Contemporaneous outbreaks such as the 1994 plague outbreak in India and the emergence of new technologies that enabled the WHO to gain knowledge of outbreaks without the help of the affected governments, contributed toward initiating a revision process. A confluence of changes in circumstances and ideas, interests and values were the necessary precursors to this revision. The authors, wary of the narrative that links security, health, and globalisation, emphasised that every piece of this confluence is interdependent on the other and that the ideational and political factors of this process were essential:

> It is clear, for example, that pathogens are 'material facts' that cause disease within the human body and which (in some cases) have the potential to kill millions of people. Likewise, some of the capacities that countries need to

respond, such as laboratories to diagnose illnesses and medical facilities to treat them, are also material. Yet how we respond to disease outbreaks and whether or not we decide as societies to invest in such items as laboratories and medical facilities, is a product of ideas about the nature and scale of the threat posed by pathogens, what we should collectively do to address that threat, and how those measures should be ranked in relation to other priorities we have as societies. The idea that pathogens are a global threat requiring international cooperation rests on a similar set of ideas and beliefs, ideas and beliefs that are socially constructed.

(Davies et al., 2015, p. 10)

The IHR revision process lasted a decade, from 1995 until 2005. From a normative perspective, the process was a dialogue between material and ideational developments. During protracted negotiations, the SARS crisis in 2003 was particularly significant, as it largely resonated with what had been depicted within the securitised frame of global health described earlier. In fact, SARS was a nearly perfect exemplar that illustrated many of the arguments that had spurred the revision and that set off a norm cascade that significantly sped up the process toward internalisation: "the adoption of the revised IHRs only two years later would not have been possible without the fear and panic that SARS induced" (Davies et al., 2015, p. 139).

### Human security

Human security is a paradigm of security most famously advocated by the UNDP, most particularly their 1994 HDR. The main catalysts for the emergence of this paradigm were the end of the Cold War and increasing intra-state conflict. There was also "an improved understanding of socio-economic development [which shone] light on the neglected everyday insecurities faced by the world's poor and excluded" (Chen & Narasimhan, 2003, p. 182). Globalisation also played a major part, as it continues to erode the primacy of state sovereignty and territorial integrity. Together, these factors spurred a re-examination of the traditional concept of security. Human security draws the attention away from the state and directs it toward the individual; it argues that the assessment of security should rely on whether individuals are *free from want* and *free from fear* – regardless whether the source of fear is external or internal.

The concept of *human security* has been accused of being 'airy-fairy' and too wide in scope, rendering it less useful:

everyone is for it, but few people have a clear idea of what it means. Existing definitions of human security tend to be extraordinarily expansive and vague, encompassing everything from physical security to psychological well-being, which provides policymakers with little guidance in the prioritization of competing policy goals and academics little sense of what, exactly, is to be studied.

(Paris, 2001, p. 88)

Indeed, human security "has not had the impact in both policy and academic circles which its proponents had hoped for" (McInnes & Lee, 2012, p. 146). However, the width of influential variables *on* and referent objects *of* security are seminal ideas in their own right that have contributed to alternative modes of thought among both scholars and policymakers. From some points of view, the human security paradigm reflects far better the complex security threats faced by individuals:

> for most people in the world, the much greater threats to security come from disease, hunger, environmental contamination, street crime, or even domestic violence. And for others, a greater threat may come from their own state itself, rather than from an 'external' adversary . . . international security defined – territorial integrity – does not necessarily correlate with human security, and [an] overemphasis upon statist security can be to the detriment of human welfare needs.
>
> (Newman, 2001, p. 240)

This a far cry from the traditional idea that the state represents the individuals who comprise the population within its borders; if a state is secure, so are its people – simply by default. For human security adherents, a view focusing solely on state military security from external threats is oblivious to the realities of citizens in the 21st century. Caballero-Anthony and Amul (2015), using Davies' (2010a) typology, draw parallels between the *statist* and *globalist* perspectives on global health with state security versus human security to point out the limitations of the former approach: "[s]tatist perspectives result in narrowly focused policies that are not able to adequately address the complexities of the health security issues seen today or the cross-linkages between poverty, health, and development" (Caballero-Anthony & Amul, 2015, p. 36).

The human security paradigm does not exclude state security from the equation; it merely removes it from its traditional pedestal and includes it among a range of other variables. In IR, as in development – illustrated by the sentiments featured in the 1994 HDR – the conception of human security is deeply normative, as it suggests a strong ethical responsibility in ensuring the individual's human rights, while simultaneously questioning the state's ability and potentially even its willingness to do so in certain circumstances. It also questions the primacy of the state as the primary actor in the international arena, as regional and IOs, NGOs, and local communities are all relevant to human security.

In the rationalist tradition, the inherently anarchic nature of global relations unavoidably leads actors to be self-interested. The view holds that regardless of any amount of interaction between actors, the axiom of self-interest is not subject to change. In fact, self-interest sets the terms for interaction as a whole; actors are exogenously constituted and cannot fundamentally change their identities and interests. Critical theorists and constructivists are unconvinced of this inevitability, as well as of the causal powers of the anarchic structure of international affairs:

"[d]espite important differences, cognitivists, poststructuralists, standpoint and postmodern feminists, rule theorists, and structuralists share a concern with the basic 'sociological' issue bracketed by rationalists namely, the issue of identity and interest-formation" (Wendt, 1992, p. 393). As suggested earlier, the emergence of these alternative perspectives took place alongside global material developments. The rationalist *modus operandi* of brushing aside changes as inconsequential side effects of the unchangeable identities and interests of state actors either vying for or working together to maximise power and ensure interests, was becoming increasingly unconvincing as the 1990s progressed. This coincided with the burgeoning critical and postmodern branch of IR theory that had started to gain a significant foothold in the late 1980s (see, for example, Der Derian & Shapiro, 1989). Scholars favouring varieties of non-materialist schools of thought allowed for a wider and more plural set of variables to come into play when defining the identities and interests of actors – and indeed defining what constitutes an actor at all. An international scene that evolves in terms of an increasing plurality not only with regard to actors, but also in terms of interests and motivations and, significantly, in threats to security, all but demanded alternative explanatory narratives. "Clearly structural realism would not be sympathetic to the concept of human security, which relies upon the significance of agent-oriented processes, the emergence of nonstate forces, and the impact of ideas and values" (Newman, 2001, p. 247).

One health norm favoured by adherents of the human security paradigm is the aforementioned *right to health*. Connecting health with human rights, the right to health is ensured, in various conceptualisations, by a number of international agreements – including the *Universal Declaration of Human Rights* (UDHR), the *Constitution* of the WHO, the *International Covenant on Economic, Social and Cultural Rights*, and the *Convention on the Rights of Persons with Disabilities*, "and in more than 120 constitutions worldwide" (Amon, 2015, p. 293). It was further elaborated upon in ECOSOC's *General Comment No. 14*, published in 2000, which expands on the mentioned covenant. In these agreements, health is defined in terms encompassing freedom from physical and mental disease and includes considerations of various social determinants of health, including the relationship between the right to health and other human rights. The *Constitution* of the WHO emphasises the obligations of the state to uphold these rights. In *General Comment No. 14*, ECOSOC augmented this idea and suggested that states and IOs have various responsibilities to *respect, protect, and fulfil* the right to health both directly and indirectly, with an emphasis rooted in *health equity*. Among others, these include preventing any manner of discrimination in care-delivery, providing proper guidelines, and avoiding the implementation of embargoes on medical goods and services. Essentially, the state should not interfere in any way with people's treatment or prevention of any type of illness; it should explicitly plan and implement public health programmes and ensure and expand access to health care. More indirectly, the duty of states includes ensuring that social determinants of health are also protected, such as housing, access to water, and freedom from violence.

The 1994 HDR defines health security in a holistic manner, including both communicable and NCDs, global health inequities as well as environmental and social determinants of health. A 2003 report by the Commission of Human Security expanded on this and emphasised the central role of health in the fulfilment of human security. Specifically, it identified the main threats that negatively affect human security as global infectious diseases, poverty-related health problems as well as ill-health as a consequence of various forms of violence (Caballero-Anthony & Amul, 2015; Commission on Human Security, 2003). Some authors (Aldis, 2008; Caballero-Anthony & Amul, 2015) explicitly link human security with global health security, suggesting a high degree of compatibility between the two.

### Health norms, bi-directionality, and the WHO

Though not mutually exclusive in practice, the ambivalent narratives of the WHO and of GHG generally – that is, those of rights-based duty and altruism and those of self-preservation through cooperation, have very different angles in a normative sense. Lakoff (2010) describes this divide as

> two contemporary regimes for envisioning and intervening in the field of global health: *global health security* and *humanitarian biomedicine*. Each of these regimes combines normative and technical elements to provide a rationale for managing infectious disease on a global scale. . . . While these two regimes by no means exhaust the expansive field of global health, their juxtaposition usefully highlights some of the tensions inherent in many contemporary global health initiatives.
>
> (Lakoff, 2010, p. 59, original emphasis)

For the purposes of this book, this divide is broadly referred to as the described categories of state *security* and *human security*, respectively (see Table 3.1). While

*Table 3.1* Motives and rationales underlying health norms: state versus human security

|  | State security | Human security |
| --- | --- | --- |
| **Referent object** | Sovereign states | Individuals within and among states |
| **Emphasis** | Limiting spread of disease across borders, ensuring territorial integrity, guarding *instrumental* benefits of health | Limiting and preventing disease outright; human rights, guarding *inherent benefits* of health |
| **Identity** | National/regional | Cosmopolitan, global |
| **Interest** | Self-protection | Communal protection |

(Source: The authors).

not exhaustive representatives of the field, this divide is helpful in categorising and juxtaposing two subtypes of *health norms*.

Norms associated with state security in health are associated with protecting the security of the state from infections and from the subsequent consequences affecting the populace within its borders. The norms within this category there-fore appeal to the self-interest of states to protect themselves, as exemplified most clearly by the early sanitary conferences and their resulting policy of quarantining the infected. Implied in this perspective is the fact that diseases and other vari-ables that negatively affect health are exogenous and malevolent and that they need to be restricted or prevented and their effects minimised. In such a view, health is part of the larger concern of state security, and it becomes more analo-gous and adjacent to an aspect that can be attacked by an enemy – the chief one being infectious and travelling disease. The rationale used to securitise diseases, for example, is based on this same logic, and health norms that inspire securitisa-tion are framed as security threats, such as the EIDs described earlier.

Health norms associated with human security, on the other hand, deprioritise the integrity of states and their borders and place their emphasis on the individual, global citizen. While this also includes preventing the spread of disease across borders, the underlying rationale is to protect the interests and health of the peo-ple, viewing these as more inherently important than the consequences border-crossing diseases may have on the state.

> It focuses on a broad understanding of security that encompasses not only the security of states against external or internal armed threats, but also the secu-rity of people living within states against non-military threats, such as disease, environmental degradation, economic and social instability etc.
>
> (Vieira, 2007, p. 144)

In this view, the state can be held responsible for not protecting its populace from new health problems or threats or adequately addressing existing ones. The right to health, for example, is an overarching health norm assumed within the viewpoint of human security. This approach is concerned with targeting diseases that afflict the most vulnerable demographics, such as the poverty-related issues targeted in one of the health MDGs: namely, malaria, tuberculosis, and HIV/AIDS (Lakoff, 2010). Further, because threats can be internal as well as exter-nal, infectious diseases are not the only concern relevant to security. Underlying health systems, such as access to health care and affordability of medicine, are also of prime concern – as are other social determinants of health. A similar norm is 'health for all', a norm that is integral to the WHO's constitution, and which is at the foundation of the *Declaration of Alma-Ata* (WHO, 1978) and reaffirmed by the World Health Assembly (WHA) in 1998 (WHO, 1998). This norm, explicitly defined by Halfdan Mahler, director-general at the time, posits that *everyone*, each person in the world, should attain a state of health that enables that person to lead a socially and economically productive life (Mahler, 1981). While the WHO's actions towards realising this ambitious norm have been irregular and inadequate, parts of its content and spirit were reinvigorated in the early 1990s within the WHO by individuals such as Jonathan Mann. Subsequently, these norms were successfully invoked by NGOs in the early- to mid-2000s, in a global campaign for access to essential medicines, particularly antiretrovirals (ARVs) for people afflicted with HIV/AIDS. This normative victory, which was also able to merge human and state security (Hein & Kohlmorgen, 2009), is explored in greater detail later.

The way GHG is *practised* by the WHO does not fully embrace the normative and practical implications of human security, nor does it represent an approach inspired entirely by state security. While explicitly referring to ideas attributed to a view closer to the human security, human development, or cosmopolitan paradigms, the main goal of the organisation remains preventing the spread of disease across the borders of the member states comprising it (Rushton, 2011). The 2007 *World Health Report*, for example, frames disease control as reducing the vulnerability of populations with regard to border-crossing disease (WHO, 2007), a frame that puts human security first, but simultaneously appeals to state security. This bi-directionality may be caused by fundamental institutional tensions that complicate the WHO's identity and that ultimately impair its functioning (Gostin et al., 2015).[5] Others argue that the fact that the WHO has, for the last decade and a half, been authorised to collect data and gather information from independent non-state actors and not just member states, has effectively pushed the WHO's focus away from norms of sovereignty and towards those of human security (Fidler, 2005). This pattern of ambiguity from the main actor of global health and disease control illustrates the divide between selflessness and self-interest, or that between the globalist and statist, so prevalent in the health security discourse. Elbe (2011) suggests that this is rooted in the relatively sudden association of the two different policy communities of foreign and security policy and that of public health policy – leading to what he refers to as the *securitisation of health* and the *medicalisation of insecurity*.

Fourie (2015) suggests that the origins of this tension, or bi-directionality, may be found in two major historical modes of thought, each culminating in events that were seminal for the intellectual and ideological architecture of the modern world. The first is the *Treaty of Westphalia* of 1648, which established the modern state system and the idea of state sovereignty. Westphalian sovereignty, now an integral part of international law, emphasises the territorial integrity of a state – that is, to say, its geographical territory and domestic affairs, codified in law by the principle of non-interference:

> No State or group of States has the right to intervene, directly or indirectly, for any reason whatever, in the internal or external affairs of any other State. Consequently, armed intervention and all other forms of interference or attempted threats against the personality of the State or against its political, economic and cultural elements, are in violation of international law.
>
> (UNGA, 1970, p. 123)

Westphalian sovereignty, however, is challenged by the ideas that culminated in the French Revolution of 1789, which emphasise the rights of individuals and the responsibilities of states towards their people. These ideas are also well represented within international law and international conventions and declarations. Furthermore, Fourie submits, this latter idea later inspired Marxist modes of thought, in which the focus was less on the rights of individuals and more on the plights of economic classes of people "resulting from material inequalities and structural deficiencies at the national and global levels" (2015, p. 110). These three ideologies, particularly the first two, directly inspired the formation of the UN after the end of the Second World War – a process which saw the codification of the convictions that constituted them:

> The ideal thus became a rather interesting hybrid of Realist and Liberal discourses applied within the multilateral organization, with members of especially the new second and third worlds emphasizing (discursively at least) notions of greater global class equity and fairness.
>
> (Fourie, 2015, p. 111)

Today, the tension between these ideologies is part and parcel of the global health dialogue, and while they can work together in mutually beneficial ways in some instances, other circumstances put them at odds with each other (see Michaud & Kates, 2013).

Another characteristic resulting from this ambiguity is the plethora of meanings attached to the concept of *global health security* (McInnes, 2015), with the result that this concept tends to remain as contested as other topics pertaining to security (Buzan, 1991). Aldis (2008), for example, explicitly laments the fact that the many meanings of health security in literature and in policy are confusing and that the plethora of definitions not only allow for contestation but also risk rendering the concept hollow. Another concern for Aldis is the favouring of the Global North in the current global health security discourse. Indeed, as Rushton (2011) points out, academic literature on global health security is, with very few exceptions, "written in the West and focuses either upon Western policy communities or the major multilateral institutions" (Rushton, 2011, p. 782).

Rushton disagrees with the sentiment that the paucity of definitional clarity is the main issue. In fact, he argues, there is broad consensus over the core meanings of the term. They are identified as (1) the familiar fact that disease travels with people with increasing frequency in a globalised world; (2) a concern about the weaponisation of pathogens, also known as bioterrorism; and (3) that serious specific disease burdens can potentially have detrimental effects on the social, economic, political, and military stability of states and regions. These three points also tend to dominate relevant policy documents, the IHRs being the most common and salient example. McInnes (2015), more of a believer in the inherent contestation of any security discussion, suggests that the prevalence of some aspects of global health security over others is the result of *one* narrative or understanding being promoted over another:

> That much of the discussion over health and security focuses on a similar range of issues – usually severe and acute epidemic infectious diseases, HIV/ AIDS, and bioterrorism – has helped to create the sense that this is a coherent picture where there is agreement over the landscape. What differences do emerge are therefore deemed second-order issues concerning how to respond to such risks, rather than the first-order scene-setting issues of what is being discussed within the realm of health security in the first place. . . . Health security is essentially contested with a number of identifiable terms each reflecting a particular perspective and with its own narrative of health security. Crucially these narratives, which attempt to explain the social world, are not objective accounts of observed phenomena, but help to construct social reality by promoting particular understandings.
>
> (McInnes, 2015, p. 14)

Illustrative of this sentiment is the fact that not all infectious diseases are equal in the eyes of the typical health security researcher or policymaker and that biases exist in the global health security discourse. One such bias emphasises (and securitises) certain diseases that are perceived as being the most acute for populations, although they are not necessarily the most lethal. Generally, global health security is mainly concerned with the containment of pathogens that are highly publicised: "[t]his seems to be borne out in practice where the focus of attention in terms of naturally occurring threats has overwhelmingly been on pandemic influenza, emerging and re-emerging infectious diseases (SARS is an oft-cited example) and HIV/AIDS" (Rushton, 2011, p. 783). As Rushton and others (McInnes & Lee, 2006; Stevenson & Moran, 2015) point out, these emphases generally do not reflect disease prevalence or mortality rates. NCDs and other, more indirect determinants of health are traditionally rarely mentioned, though they are responsible for increasingly significant proportions of the global health burden (Figure 3.1).

The omittance of NCDs is particularly striking and may be partly explained by certain aspects that set them apart from communicable infections. Benson and Glasgow (2015) explore how and why NCDs have been neglected in global health security: a sphere where the most topical diseases have been HIV/AIDS and the more temporary outbreaks of SARS, H1N1, and Ebola. The authors suggest three main reasons for the security pedestal these have attained while NCDs have been largely ignored in the health security discourse: "that sudden, violent, and widespread infectious disease epidemics can be a powerful catalyst for socio-political change; that the agents responsible for infectious disease can often be targeted and contained or eliminated; and that there is an immediacy to them that necessitates response" (Benson & Glasgow, 2015, p. 178). Some parallels can be drawn in relation to the similarly skewed priorities of the MDGs. Infectious diseases invoke images of suddenness and exogeny, as an attacker that has the potential to uproot society as a whole – bubonic plague being the most salient trope of this type of

# Disease burden by cause (2016)

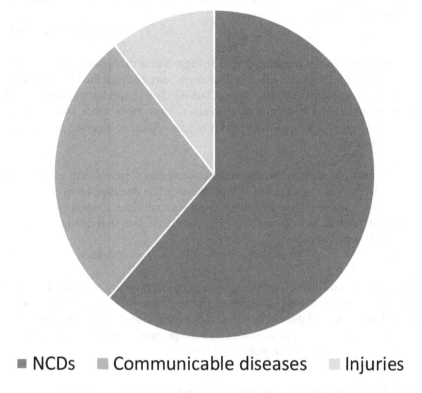

■ NCDs    ■ Communicable diseases    ▨ Injuries

*Figure 3.1* Global disease burden by cause, 2016. Measured in Disability-Adjusted Life Years (years of life lost and years lived with a disability)

(Source: Global Burden of Disease Collaborative Network [GBDN], 2017).

narrative. Second, infectious diseases are targets that can be cured and eradicated and, therefore, appear as clearer objectives towards which goals can strive. Last, the suddenness of infectious diseases conjures a sense of urgency, connotations that the slower, ambient presence of most NCDs do not provide.

The problem with this is twofold. First, the heavy focus on these few diseases obscures the dangers of de-prioritising these diseases or other causes of ill-health that have not been securitised. Second, the securitised diseases tend to be those that Western states and multilateral organisations fear the spread of from the Global South, highlighting a favouring of the interests of the few rather than of all:

> Global health security has effectively been (and will continue to be) defined through practice, not some separate process of definitional negotiation. Such

practice is inevitably fundamentally affected by the distribution of power in the international system. It should be no surprise that a global system designed to protect states from disease privileges the protection of the most powerful states in the international system.

(Rushton, 2011, p. 791)

In practice, Stevenson and Moran (2015) suggest that the strong focus on these highly publicised diseases and their containment have not benefited lower-income countries in terms of primary health care. Indeed, disease-specific emphasis rooted in sentiments related to securitisation tends to draw more funds and resources than broad-based improvement of health systems. Another observer, in the same vein, argues that

even though successful health securitization efforts have led to increases in absolute spending on global health issues, it has diverted funds away from critical, poverty-related health challenges as solutions towards single-securitized illnesses, most prominently HIV/AIDS, in ways that do not reflect the global burden of disease.

(DeLaet, 2015, p. 339)

The sentiment that this process has led to the neglect of health-infrastructure, and particularly of poverty-related health challenges that are – in fact – the leaders in global mortality and morbidity, supports the suggestion that high-income countries are the prime beneficiaries and indeed the primary referent object of security in the current architecture of global health security.

### HIV/AIDS, securitisation, and universal access to medicines

Surely, future generations will look back on the era of HIV/AIDS as one of the most remarkable periods in the history of human disease, in which civilization was challenged by a devastating pandemic EID and aggressively addressed it from a scientific and global health standpoint, leading to the real possibility of effective control in a relatively timely manner.

(Mourens & Fauci, 2015)

HIV/AIDS was one of the main disease threats specifically identified and placed within the category of EIDs by the IOM's 1992 report. Fourie (2015) assesses how the placement of HIV/AIDS in a security framework progressed and how it ended up doing a disservice to the endeavour to mitigate the pandemic and help those affected by it. This securitisation process, perhaps starting as early as 1987 – thus preceding the mentioned EID report – by a U.S. agency associated with government security, was further solidified by the Central Intelligence Agency (CIA) in 1990 (Fourie & Schönteich, 2001). Once the identity of HIV/AIDS as a security threat had been established, constructing a narrative with "martial overtones"

(Amon, 2015, p. 293) was the logical next step, similar to the response to other securitised objects such as terrorism or drugs. Statements relating to these are couched in language that declares a state of warfare between the specific threat, which is depicted as the enemy, and the referent object of security, which is depicted as the righteous victim of attack: "[b]y making appeals to *states'* security, and by crafting AIDS as an 'enemy' that needs to be 'battled' and 'defeated', a number of effects can be achieved" (Fourie, 2015, p. 108, original emphasis).

These effects include the elevation of the specific concern from low to high politics, an elevation that was made explicit in the case of HIV/AIDS (McInnes & Rushton, 2010). As with terrorism, an overarching sense of danger is created by the narrative and reified by the trademark over-exposure and perhaps disproportionate focus and allocation of resources on the specific subject of securitisation. Additionally, concerns still belonging to the category of low politics, such as human rights, may be de-emphasised in order to effectively combat the enemy, and laws and regulations interfering with this effectiveness can more easily be eschewed.

With this in mind, this process can be characterised as a powerful political tool that can breed unintentional and adverse side effects: for example, Fourie (2015) alludes to the rabbit hole comprising terrorism, the Patriot Act, and nationalist tendencies. More specifically related to HIV/AIDS, side effects included the further stigmatisation of homosexuals, intravenous drug users, and sex workers. However, the securitisation of HIV/AIDS was primarily fuelled by legitimate fears of a very real disease: by the end of 2016, an estimated 36.37 million individuals were living with the disease, and approximately one million people died as a result of their infection that same year (GBDN, 2017). Furthermore, it is a disease that is slow to detect, even by the person carrying it, and one that still does not have a known cure.

Global health response to the global HIV/AIDS pandemic is symptomatic of the bi-directionality inherent in global health security and GHG generally:

> Discursively, one of the ways in which this tension has been playing itself out has been through appeals to either a (hard) securitization agenda that make appeals to the dangers that AIDS implies for state survival, or an agenda that appeals more directly to a softer, human security approach that underlines the nefarious implications of the epidemic for individual human rights to health. The latter approach has been most closely associated with a developmental agenda. Either way, global AIDS governance has become supremely political.
>
> (Fourie, 2015, p. 109)

In practice, the securitisation of AIDS reached its zenith in 2000, and had, by some accounts "[become] a recognized international norm" (Vieira, 2007, p. 144). The UNSC – a "state-centric vehicle par excellence" (Fourie, 2015, p. 111) – debated the issue in early 2000, and the result was *Resolution 1308* (UNSC, 2000) of July that same year, a process explored in more detail in Chapter 5. While the wording of the resolution balanced rights-based and security-based reasoning, the discourse was not entirely cemented: "various AIDS watchers have been making claims and counter-claims regarding the link between the pandemic and its impacts. This discourse is constantly revised – a process that takes place in an increasingly political and particularly multilateral environment" (Fourie, 2015, p. 112). The amount of resources allocated to the global fight against HIV/AIDS grew quickly, reinforcing the idea of the disease as a security threat seemed to yield the biggest shares of these resources. However, the insistence upon the validity of this link was rarely properly substantiated with evidence and often exaggerated to unrealistic extents. One example used is the perceived causal and reciprocal relationship between HIV/AIDS and state fragility suggested, initially by the CIA, coupled with the topical link of fragile states as breeding grounds for terrorism.

Beginning around 2005, with HIV/AIDS as a security threat now seemingly a part of conventional wisdom, some scholars and professionals within the sphere of security policymaking and research started changing their views and questioned whether the connection with security is truly legitimate, particularly the one linking state fragility with HIV/AIDS. This was the result, Fourie (2015) suggests, of a hastened process to create the link in the first place, guided by ideological and normative motivations rather than by evidence. Securitisation is an enticing and, as suggested earlier, very powerful tool to mobilise resources and support, but is – at its core – a reactive rather than proactive method of addressing the problem. The latter requires a versatile, evidence-based approach that addresses systemic root causes and that does not compromise essential human rights. In sum, "the proactive, long-term changes required in gender relations, sustainable behaviour change, and cultural adaptation are not served by the knee-jerk reactivity and short-termism of recent AIDS securitization" (Fourie, 2015, p. 115).

On the other hand, contrasting aspects of the global response to the HIV/AIDS epidemic are often thought to have shifted the global health discourse toward adopting human security-related health norms. At the turn of the millennium, ARVs were estimated to cost the average patient around $10,000-$15,000 per year (Pérez-Casas, 2001) – an insurmountable amount for the vast majority of the infected global demographic. This growing problem had been recognised by a host of NGOs in various local settings since the late 1980s (Smith & Siplon, 2006) but made its first global headlines when a group of pharmaceutical companies sued the government of South Africa for its *Medicines Act* of1997. This legal action, popularly framed as 'Nelson Mandela vs. Big Pharma', was one of the catalysts that acted as a call to global action for activism on the principle of access to medicines (Ferreira, 2002; Hoen, Berger, Calmy, & Moon, 2011). The mobilisation included developing countries, as well as regional powers such as Brazil, which was the first country in the Global South to provide widespread access to ARVs for its citizens.

However, legal complications related to international patent agreements emanating from *The Agreement on Trade-Related Aspects of Intellectual Property Rights* (*TRIPS*) made it difficult for countries to provide affordable medicines without breaching the agreement. By 2001, the narrative that pitted pharmaceutical companies against those on the side of affordable treatment had deepened, and when the court case against South Africa was eventually dropped, the normative climate was ready for a significant shift, codified by the *Doha Declaration* of that year. The *Declaration* is an amendment to the *TRIPS* agreement and gives WTO member states flexibility in circumventing patent rights with regard to access to essential medicines in cases of "national emergency or other circumstances of extreme urgency" (WTO, 2001, p. 25). What constitutes a national emergency is up to each member state to determine. Though often couched in terms of its contribution to human security, the *Declaration* also acted as a further mechanism for connecting disease with state security. "This meant that, in a situation of threat to public health, governments could manufacture, buy and import generic copies of patented medicines. The Doha agreement of 2001 was an unprecedented move towards the securitisation of severe epidemic diseases" (Vieira, 2007, p. 152).

An important component of this hitherto unprecedented global campaign was the invocation of the health norm 'health for all' and of connecting universal access to ARVs with the universality of human rights. In what can be seen as a victory for human security, "AIDS activists embraced and further developed the global right to [a] health norm by advocating for a commitment to addressing health as a shared global responsibility, and not a responsibility confined solely to the borders and budget of a nation state" (Hammonds & Ooms, 2014, p. 12). The *Doha Declaration* further placed the onus on states to prove that public health crises were not taking place, clearly shifting the referent of security object to the individuals within and among states. State security, however, was also central to the process. While the explicit sentiments expressed were based on universal human rights, the subject matter also spoke to protecting the interests of states:

> They [NGOs] framed this conflict by addressing the scandal of the disaccord between high prices of drugs and the suffering and dying of millions of AIDS victims. Furthermore, this campaign fell on fertile ground as the governments of industrialized countries were more and more anxious about the transborder spread of infectious diseases and the consequences for international security.
> (Hein & Kohlmorgen, 2009, p. 101)

This dual accommodation, balancing rights-based altruism and self-interest, is symptomatic of how states interact with issues of global health, and health norms have a greater chance of cascading if they appeal to both categories, perhaps especially when the benevolent aspects can be highlighted while those relating to self-interest caveated as fortunate side effects. As Hein and Kohlmorgen (2009, p. 96) argue, in certain cases "the social and human rights interests of [NGOs] coincide with self-interests of industrialised countries like containing the risks of a global spread of infectious diseases and of political instability".

## Health in foreign policy and health diplomacy

Health issues as a foreign policy concern can be traced back to the mentioned sanitary conferences of the mid-19th century, but the last two decades have seen an increase and a more explicit consideration of the relationship. Alongside the expanded influence and place of health in global security discourse, health also experienced greater inclusion in the foreign policies of specific countries, in which the bi-directionality of altruism and self-interest is similarly reflected. Michaud (2015) suggests that the tendency of a gradually increasing incorporation of health in foreign policies owes its existence to many of the same reasons as those which precipitated a global health security discourse in general. This refers to the "now conventional wisdom among policy makers and political leaders that health issues can and do impact the traditional security and economic concerns that are the focus of foreign policy" (Michaud, 2015, p. 265). Relatedly, there is also a sense among the same policymakers and political leaders that globalisation, trade lib-eralisation, and the free flow of people – along with the infectious diseases they may carry – have made states both vulnerable to and wary of disease outbreaks in any geographical location. The reaction to these factors – that is, the inclusion of health in foreign policy – generally falls within two categories. The first category comprises those policies and foreign involvements that address specific perceived threats: for example, working towards limiting the possibilities of the spread of potential pandemics. Another example would be working towards an agreement such as the FCTC. The second category of the inclusion of health in foreign pol-icy is the realm of health diplomacy, in which states use various health-related resources as diplomatic tools with which to build relationships with other states or with NGOs. This can include medical personnel and equipment, medicines, earmarked resources, or technical assistance.

For some, particularly (global) health practitioners, the increased inclusion of health in foreign policy was a welcome, and perhaps transformative, addition. For example, in a much-cited comment published in the *Lancet* in 2007, the editor-in-chief, Richard Horton, suggested that "health moves foreign policy away from a debate about national interests to one about global altruism" (Horton, 2007, p. 807). This is reminiscent of the aforementioned meeting of health and security and the reciprocal influence of various fields' values and norms upon each other. Horton's assumption is that the *ethos* inherent in health care would be able to modify the cold, self-interested world of foreign policy and diplomacy to become a positive force that is guided by an assumption of interconnectedness and mutual benefits. However, this assumption suggests a one-way street of acquiescence that seems to largely ignore the other direction of this reciprocal relationship:

> While there is widespread recognition that health and foreign policy are increasingly linked, there is an ongoing debate about how and when (or even if) health shapes foreign policy and vice versa. Is foreign policy driven by *increased interest in achieving health goals* or is there increasing use of *health as an instrument to achieve traditional foreign policy goals* such as economic growth and national security?
>
> (Michaud, 2015, p. 267, original emphasis)

These questions may not have unambiguous answers. An illustrative example is the *Oslo Ministerial Declaration* (Amorim et al., 2007). In 2007, the foreign min-isters of Brazil, France, Indonesia, Norway, Senegal, South Africa, and Thailand signed the *Declaration* and its *Memorandum of Understanding* (MOU). It is worth noting that this selection of states is rather eclectic in terms of geography, culture, in economic stature, and in domestic circumstances, which may suggest a universal sentiment towards the cause. In short, the *declaration* repeatedly emphasises that health is a matter of fundamental human rights and that it is the duty of every state to ensure it. In addition to addressing this sense of duty, the rhetoric is based around ideas of interdependence and common interests among states. It argues that "health is deeply interconnected with the environment, trade, economic growth, social development, national security, and human rights and dignity" (Amorim et al., 2007, p. 1), thereby hinting at the crosscutting relevance of health in foreign policy. Indeed, it posits, global health and foreign policy are mutually beneficial and its coordination full of potential and that "powerful synergies arise when national interest coincides with the need for concerted regional and global effort" (2007, p. 1). The *Declaration* actually argues that health should be prioritised over all other interests and that it should be "a point of departure and defining lens" (2007, p. 1) in the foreign policies of its signatories. As such, it prioritises health as the primary goal of foreign policy, which is framed as a tool to achieve health goals rather than *vice versa*. For the ministers, it is the effects of globalisation that have pushed health issues to a point where common interests and the primacy of upholding basic human rights trump that of traditional national security characterised by self-help.

The message in the *Declaration* suggests a symbiosis between the pursuit of mutual – even universal – interests and the duty of upholding human rights. While the follow-up and actual implementation of this declaration has been mixed (Fidler, 2011), Norway is an example of a signatory that has at least begun to adopt these sentiments into actual policy. In a *White Paper* published by the Ministry of Foreign Affairs five years after the *Declaration* was signed (Norwegian Ministry of Foreign Affairs, 2012), this narrative of win-win situations is also reflected. In line with Norway's long-standing and successful line of soft power politics and humanitarian endeavours (de Carvalho & Neumann, 2014), this particular publication heavily emphasises the altruistic side of the relationship between foreign policy and global health, referring to and promoting the paradigm of human security on numerous occasions. Benefits for the world at large and specifically for the public health of Norwegians are repeatedly mentioned, while any rhetoric around state security is subdued and rather implicitly suggested.

While central to the sphere of global health security discussed earlier, the low versus high politics categorisation is perhaps even more directly salient in the related subject of global health in foreign policy. This is particularly true of the *Oslo Ministerial Declaration*, which presents global health as a point of departure of foreign policy, rather than simply an aspect of it. This implies not only the introduction of an element long considered to belong to the low politics category into the realm of high politics, but the elevation of this element to as high, or higher, than considerations of military security. However, this may be largely contextual to the state in question. South Africa, another signatory, has barely mentioned global health or the *Declaration* in any of its foreign policy documents in the decade since signing it. This is typically attributed to the severe domestic health problems of the country, making it difficult to legitimise external resource-spending on matters of health, though some (Fourie, 2013) have suggested that the country's dire health situation can be considered a resource in health diplomatic relations, particularly in a context of South-South multilateralism. The current lack of such efforts is further attributed to the lack of experience, and perhaps even motivation, for prioritising soft power capabilities in general by the most recent administrations.

Norway and South Africa are only two examples of a very mixed global picture of the relationship between health and foreign policy. The U.S. *President's Emergency Plan for AIDS Relief* (PEPFAR)[6] is another example that both helps countless people *and* is explicitly part of a strategy of helping the country's soft power capabilities and general image. There are other examples where altruism clearly trumps self-interest, and vice versa (Michaud & Kates, 2013). Indeed, examples of different approaches to the integration of health in foreign policy contribute more to confusion than to clarification: "[a]dherents to any branch of international relations theory would have some evidence to point to support their views in the area of health and foreign policy" (Michaud, 2015, p. 274).

## Conclusion

The global development effort is largely predicated upon being explicitly apolitical: it is based in science and goodwill, motivated by liberal sentiments such as justice and human rights that consider global inequality normatively incompatible and unacceptable. However, many aspects of development are inherently political in nature. This includes trade agreements and regimes, such as, for example, the General Agreement on Tariffs and trade agreements, or the neoliberal SAPs of the 1980s. It also includes the very politicised nature of the securitisation of health and the security-development nexus (Hettne, 2010; Keukeleire & Raube, 2013) described earlier as well as repeated acts of protest from religious groups and single-issue alliances to any allusion to family planning. These examples both make an appearance later in this book, particularly in Chapter 5. The endeavour also involves states or groups of states brandishing or expanding their capabilities in both soft and hard power. Large global development summits have been publicly boycotted or otherwise undermined, while some of the commitments from seemingly successful summits have been followed up in a decidedly underwhelming manner or even virtually forgotten following the reduction of publicity that typically takes place some weeks after such an event. One example is UNCED (1992) and its associated framework of sustainable development, which rather quickly lost its momentum, only to be reinvigorated after the quasi-cataclysmic GFC of 2008 (Dodds et al., 2014).

Several examples of the political variables and motivations that have affected the evolution of the global development agenda over the years are discussed or alluded to throughout this study. The relationship between politics and global development is complex, and includes numerous areas of specific macro and micro-level research open to study by numerous methodologies from the field of political science and IR. This book aims to contribute to such research and to provide insight into how the dynamics of IR and global health interact with global development, particularly with regard to questions of security.

The purpose of this chapter has been to give further context preceding the analysis in subsequent chapters and to elaborate on concepts and terms central to the research problem and research questions. While the previous chapters provided an account of the evolution of the UN development agenda from 1989 until the present, the focus of this chapter has been on how IR, health, and development connect in a myriad of different ways. Another purpose has been to situate this study in the IR-health nexus and to provide a short account of the state of this subfield.

The chapter opens with an introduction of the conceptual and practical relationship of health and development, exploring the origins, actors, and variables that constitute the mechanics of global health governance. The concentricities and divergences between global health governance and health in development are also explored. Next, the chapter focuses more closely on the links between health and IR, with particular emphasis on how different conceptions of security have significant implications for the way in which global health is approached by various actors. A related discussion of the bi-directionality of global health follows, and responses to HIV/AIDS provide an illustrative example. Further, the recent emergence of explicit references to health in foreign policy is discussed. Finally, a brief exploration of the somewhat meagre scholarship of the relationship between development and IR is presented.

The focal point of the chapter is the complex concept of *global health*. While global health refers to concerted efforts to ensure and improve the health of the global population, its complexity is derived from the plurality of actors involved in the endeavour – including states, IOs, and NGOs. The ambiguous intentions of states is one point of contention, and the balance between altruism and self-interest constantly remains a contested question, perhaps best reflected in the behaviours of relevant IOs, particularly the WHO. With this tension in mind, the chapter elaborates on the perspectives of statist security and human security and proposes the utilisation of these as a categorisation device for health norms, which depends on their underlying rationale and consequential emphasis.

## Notes

1 Regime theory is based within the liberalist belief that non-state actors such as international organisations and institutions, multinational companies and non-governmental organisations exert influence on global behaviour. Krasner defines international regimes as "sets of implicit or explicit principles, norms, rules, and decision-making procedures around which actors' expectations converge within a given area of international relations" (Krasner, 1982, p. 186).

2 Securitisation theory describes the process of subjects being identified as security threats by the relevant actor, traditionally the state. The theory was originated by the Copenhagen School (comprising, most famously, Buzan, Wæver and de Wilde). The threat can be towards the state itself or towards another referent object, such as, for example, the rain

forest (Buzan et al., 1998). One major point in securitisation theory is that the threat may not necessarily *really* be as serious as perceived and that a newly securitised subject is often granted an inordinate amount of attention and resources.

3 Health diplomacy "refers to both a system of organization and to communication and negotiation processes that shape the global policy environment in the sphere of health and its determinants" (Kickbusch & Kökény, 2013, p. 159). Health diplomatic negotiations can include, among others, health personnel and equipment, medicines, and political support relating to specific diseases or general health care.

4 *Rationalism* is the term utilised by Wendt (1992) and others when describing the common ontologies of neorealism and neoliberalism in IR theory. Rationalists, from Wendt's description, both treat the interests and identities of actors as exogenously given (by the anarchic structure). In this view, states are the dominant actors in the system, and they are always and unchangeably self-interested.

5 For Gostin et al. (2015), the WHO suffers from five such fundamental tensions: (1) it is a servant to its member states; (2) it has been struggling with a paucity of resources, and has a relatively low budget to work with; (3) the funding that it does receive is often earmarked; (4) the organisation lacks institutional structures; and (5) the autonomy of its regional branches hampers centralised and unequivocal leadership.

6 Since its establishment in 2003, PEPFAR's impact on the global response to HIV/AIDS has been significant. The efforts of the institution has, at points, equalled half of all global treatments of the disease. As of the end of 2017, PEPFAR had helped treat more than 13.3 million people in total, including providing nearly 1 million children with lifesaving ARV therapy (PEPFAR, 2018). As some suggest, these efforts have continued – and even increased – even as the direct bilateral leverage portion of the endeavour diminish over time: "[a]id that is so closely linked to individuals' survival cannot reasonably be curtailed, even if serious differences arise between the donors and the recipients" (Lyman & Wittels, 2010, pp. 75–76).

# 4 Normative foundations

## The human development paradigm

In the next three chapters we will trace the life cycles of the norms that informed the health-related MDGs and SDGs. The chapters will describe the trajectory by which health norms were conceived and subsequently framed and advertised by relevant norm entrepreneurs, the manner in which these norms cascaded, and, finally, whether or not they successfully internalised. Throughout Chapters 4, 5, and 6 emphasis is directed towards the *norm emergence* phase to a greater extent than the other two phases: *cascade* and *internalisation*. This is because the first phase is where meaning is created through content and context. Individuals, organisations, timing, framing – as well as the characteristics of the norm itself – are all aspects of this phase. *Norm cascades* are set off by more or less specific moments that are referred to as *tipping points*, and pan out in the time following it – this phase is described as a series of documented indications that 'everybody's doing it', over the course of which a majority of relevant actors acquiesce to the emergent norm. The main evidence of *norm internalisation* in the context of this study is the inclusion of norms in the MDGs and the SDGs, though other significant representations of internalisation are also included when appropriate.

The current chapter is the outlier of the three because it does not treat specific health norms directly. Rather, it traces the trajectory of the *human development paradigm* and illustrates how its internalisation into the UN's development *ethos* was essential for laying the normative foundations on which the MDGs – and later, the SDGs – were constructed. It suggests that the system of values associated with the human development paradigm acted as a normative prerequisite for the health development norms that would emerge during the 1990s, earning the paradigm a status as *meta-norm*, as we call it. The chapter acts as a primer for the following goal-specific chapters by way of relaying the normative context in which the goals were conceived. Because the normative contents and institutions affiliated with the human development paradigm are so relevant to the two case studies explored in Chapters 5 and 6, an understanding of this foundation is imperative.

The first section of the chapter sets out the normative and political conditions in which the human development paradigm was conceived, while also offering a reflection on the inherent problem of finding the true origins of emergent norms. The remainder of the chapter offers an account of the evolution and most relevant contents of the human development paradigm, including the professional and intellectual trajectory of its main norm entrepreneur, Mahbub ul Haq. It also discusses the framework in relation to the *capabilities approach* of Amartya Sen (which was also developed by Martha Nussbaum), while exploring its explicit and implicit connotations for health development and global health governance. The UNDP is another central component of this evolution and its position as an organisational platform is elaborated upon.

## Pre-existing conditions

We are interested in the timeframe between 1989 and 2015. As has been suggested, however, the ideational seeds that laid the foundation for the creation of the normative tapestry for the MDGs in the 1990s were sown in earlier decades. Emerging norms are not borne out of thin air, but are conceived as responses to existing normative structures. Because the relevance of these ideas is fundamental, this chapter opens by establishing an overview of this pre-existing normative landscape.

Within the paradigm of modernisation that directed early global development efforts, health was considered part and parcel of general modernity. The idea was that as societies, countries, and regions became more modernised, their populations would become healthier as an indirect consequence. In broad strokes, a similar rationale was implied during the years of the SAPs. Just as wealth would ostensibly 'trickle down' and wet the mouths of the general public if 'job-creators' were given free rein and favourable legislation so benefits generated by the infamous neoliberal policies prescribed by the IFIs would trickle down to all aspects of society, health included. In hindsight, neither approach succeeded, the latter arguably negatively affecting health care in developing countries (see Ekwempu, Maine, Olorukoba, Essien, & Kisseka, 1990; Van der Gaag & Barham, 1998; Loewenson, 1993; Peabody, 1996).

These policies, precipitated in part by the unfavourable economic aftermath that the 'oil shocks' of the 1970s left in their wake, contributed heavily to the 1980s becoming a 'lost decade' of development. As a reaction to these failed policies, the years that preceded the end of the Cold War saw the emergence of a new set of ideas. These featured a normative framework that blended both emerging and established values to propose a new plan of action, while rejecting many traditional notions – particularly those suggesting that economic growth or modernisation should be the *leitmotifs* of development. Spearheaded by the *human development paradigm*, the sentiments that comprised this new approach grew in influence and subsequently prevailed in directing UN policy towards the very beginning of the 1990s; they consisted of a set of norms that were partly inspired by previous value statements such as the ones made explicit in the various UN Development Decade resolutions, the UDHR, and the *Declaration of Alma-Ata*. They were also partly the result of the norm entrepreneurship of central figures within the UNDP, particularly Mahbub ul-Haq – an undertaking detailed over the course of this chapter.

Prior to investigating the emergence of the relevant normative ideas and their diffusion in this chapter, a note should be made about infinite regress and the originality of ideas in general:

> Wholly new ideas do not suddenly appear. Instead, people recombine familiar elements into a new structure or a new proposal. This is why it is possible to note, "There is no new thing under the sun," at the very same time change and innovation are being observed. Change turns out to be recombination more than mutation.
>
> (Kingdon, 2014, p. 124)

Most people who have spent some time with the average three-year-old are likely to have experienced the child's propensity to consecutively ask its nearest trusted authority-figure the increasingly tough-to-answer question 'Why?'. Indeed, the line of questions typically ends with the replier having to concede that he or she does not know the answer; or to answer, in conclusion, 'That is just the way it is'. In epistemological philosophy, this is known as *infinitism*. In relation to the topic of this book, this becomes relevant when asking where norm entrepreneurs obtained their ideas from and, subsequently, where that source found its inspiration, and so forth, *ad infinitum*. To what extent can it be stated that a person or a group *originate* a normative standpoint or claim? Where does the ideational chain start? These questions, while valid, are epistemologically similar to a chicken-and-egg situation in the sense that pinpointing an origin with certainty is difficult or impossible.

However, finding the deepest roots of emerging norms is neither the purpose nor the utility of this book – nor of the *norm life cycle* framework in general. Rather, tracing the path of *norm entrepreneurship* is more a case of identifying how and when a particular set of normative values are utilised by a norm entrepreneur in a specific context and who has the ability to convince a critical mass of global actors, including states and IOs. This context is often an extraordinary circumstance or simply a platform such as an organisation from which the entrepreneur can act. Lenin was a norm entrepreneur in the form of a revolutionary in tsarist Russia. Lenin was explicitly influenced by ideas that Karl Marx had originated but nevertheless qualifies as a *bona fide* norm entrepreneur.[1] Relatedly, selecting a date to identify where a narrative or life cycle begins will inevitably have some degree of arbitrariness to it. In this book, the year 1989 has special significance for a number of reasons which, in aggregate, compound into making it the most logical starting point for this particular context.

In the *Millennium Declaration* (UNGA, 2000b), the notion of *freedom* tops the list of the fundamental values that the UN envisioned as essential for the organisation's successful role – and for international relations in general – in the new millennium. As presented in Chapter 2, the development section of the *Declaration* is heavily focused on poverty alleviation,[2] and poverty is viewed as the determinant that envelops all aspects of development, including that of health. More directly, a few health targets are mentioned, some more quantifiable than others. Primarily, they are concerned with reducing maternal and child mortality, HIV/AIDS, malaria, and other major diseases. The three health MDGs would subsequently take these topics and craft specified goals and indicators by which progress would be measured.

Today, these fundamental development principles and goals seem virtually self-evident; they have become internalised, and therefore appropriate and common sense. In actuality, they were the result of a process of negotiation, design, and redesign – particularly over the course of the 1990s. In the *Declaration*, 'growth' is not mentioned once; any reference to *economic* development is invariably followed by a mention of *social* development. This type of caveating is symptomatic of the norms that permeated the UN development system at the time – including those related to health. Explicit references to the health goals of reducing maternal and child mortality, however, have no caveats; neither do the stated goals of combating HIV/AIDS and other diseases. These are considered to be *inherently beneficial*, and their instrumental dividends are framed – at least publicly – as more of an added bonus than an actual goal. These are value statements that emphasise the experience of the individual – the *human* aspect of development, of which an image of the abject poor, HIV-infected and starving child and/or villager-turned-refugee represents the utmost destitution. By addressing and mitigating the interconnected causes and consequences related to it, the prevalence of this extreme image is what the MDGs attempt to minimise as much as possible.

## The meta-norm: Mahbub ul Haq and the rise of the human development paradigm

As mentioned when discussing the creation of the OECD's International Development Goals in Chapter 2, and as will be elaborated upon further in Chapter 6, Fukuda-Parr and Hulme (2009) build their own particular analysis on the MDGs using the *norm life cycle*. They focus on the role of *poverty* and how this one aspect of development gained primacy to the extent that poverty eradication became nearly synonymous with development over the course of the latter half of the 1990s. To illustrate the power that poverty eradication derived in this period, they introduce the concept of the *super-norm*:

> A super-norm seeks to achieve more than the sum of its parts because of the positive feedback interactions between each norm. Although each MDG is important as an individual norm, they are strategic components of the broader super-norm that extreme, dehumanising poverty is morally unacceptable and should be eradicated.
>
> (Fukuda-Parr & Hulme, 2009, p. 5)

This is in line with what was briefly explored in the previous chapter: namely, the existence of different levels of norms within a given society, including global society.[3] Indeed, the normative tapestry of any society is necessarily hierarchical, as some large-scale norms – such as those that inform the social institution of anti-slavery – are more universal, and act as prerequisites for related norms that may be smaller or less ecumenical. An example of a lower-level, more localised normative change that resulted from the institutionalisation of anti-slavery in the U.S. specifically, was a move towards equal rights and liberties for the erstwhile enslaved population – a development that would have been unthinkable had it not been for the initial, higher-order normative change. Anti-slavery norms were themselves inspired by the contradictions between the higher-order, established normative belief that *all men are created equal*, and the practice of extremely unequal treatment of the African-American population.

This example is intended to illustrate the dynamics of norms of different magnitudes. In the specific context of this example, *universal equality* belongs to a suggested category referred to in this study as *meta-norms*. Meta-norms are, in essence, normative paradigms that are based on one core imperative, such as the inherent equality of all human beings. They can be viewed as a *branch* of an ideological tree on which *leaves* (norms) of different sizes and significance can grow. The important point is that the existence (and general internalisation) of the meta-norm is necessary for its associated norms to follow. Meta-norms are characterised by generality; they make explicit and implicit sweeping statements from which other – more specific – norms are borne, can latch onto, and evolve from. We place the human development paradigm within the category of meta-norm because it provided the UN development endeavour with a novel and reflective approach that successfully challenged traditional assumptions about the *what*, *why*, and *how* of development – thereby causing significant *institutional change*. The MDGs would not have existed, or would have had markedly different attributes, had it not been for this institutional change that started from the sweeping, core imperative of the approach: development should be people-centred. That is to say that the norms that were at the forefront of discussion – and ultimately prevailed – at the summits and conferences throughout the 1990s, as well as the *Millennium Declaration*, would have been far less likely to succeed had it not been for the prior paradigmatic shift that had introduced the meta-norm of the human development paradigm.

There is little reason to set meta-norms apart from other norms of lesser magnitude with regard to the utility of the *norm life cycle*. One intuitive difference is that because of its larger normative scope and scale, the quantity and significance of variables – particularly in the *norm emergence phase* – outweigh those of a smaller-scale norm. Another disparity, perhaps, is that the internalisation of meta-norms is a longer process that includes within it successful internalisations of its associate, less sweeping norms. Again, it can be helpful to think in terms of the analogy of the meta-norm as the branch of a tree and its less substantial norms as its fruits. The fruits could not have grown without the existence of the branch, and the branch has not reached its potential without bearing produce. Furthermore, a strong branch will continue to grow, allowing for higher yields as time goes on, enabling the emergence of associated norms in the long and medium terms as well as the short term. Some norms may fail to grow to their full size, are too weak to fully materialise, and finally fall out of contention; others are sabotaged or rot while still others are outcompeted by norms that are part of a different branch which, at least temporarily, has a more favourable spot in the tree.

Most observers (see Cruz, Stahel, & Max-Neef, 2009; Jolly, Emmerij, Ghai, & Lapeyre, 2004), and certainly the UN itself, agree that the human development paradigm played a prominent role in bringing about the shift in emphasis in global development, evidenced by the change in policies that commanded the development efforts in the period up to the end of the 1980s versus those espoused by the MDGs (see Table 4.1). Though other sources of influence helped build the normative structure that underlies the MDGs, the explicitly human focus that rejected purely economic indicators of progress within the UN system was largely pioneered by the minds behind the human development paradigm. This section explores the *norm life cycle* of how these ideas were initiated, and how the ideas gained the influence that rendered them *passim* throughout the UN development agenda.

> Several 'schools of thought' flourished in the 1990s that were alternatives to neo-liberal approaches: feminism, basic needs, participatory development, social development and the human development/capabilities approach. The common element in these schools of thought is the concern with people and their wellbeing and empowerment. For all of these schools, reducing poverty and inequality is a priority. For want of a better term, they could be characterised as 'people-centred' approaches. These ideas were intellectually underpinned by recent academic and applied policy research, the most prominent of which is Amartya Sen's work on capabilities. Publications, such as Adjustment with a Human Face, and the UNDP's Human Development Reports launched by Mahbub ul Haq, were particularly influential in bringing policy research and public advocacy or people-centred approaches together.
>
> (Fukuda-Parr & Hulme, 2009, p. 16)

As is suggested by Finnemore and Sikkink (1998), emergent norms do not appear in a vacuum – they are presented by norm entrepreneurs who carry strong notions about the correct behaviour or values that ought to be implemented in their particular community. Further, the normative context in which the norm entrepreneur presents his or her case must be contestable, in the sense of the existence of an established normative framework that can be challenged; these act as the frameworks against which the new norms can be contrasted. Furthermore, the context must also have some degree of openness to change and one in which a norm entrepreneur may be given a platform to present logical arguments. The particular context, in other words, must be 'primed' for a change. One such situation arose when the project of global development experienced severe disrepute towards the end of the 1980s. As Sen suggested, "[T]he idea of human development won because the world was ready for it. Mahbub [ul Haq] gave it what it had been demanding in diverse ways for some time" (Sen, 2000, pp. 21–22). Indeed, in *A Decade of Human Development* (2000), Sen attributes to his then deceased colleague Mahbub ul Haq the idea of creating the human development paradigm; a first step in identifying the Pakistani as a *norm entrepreneur*. At one point, Sen refers to the approach as Haq's "brainchild" (Sen, 2000, p. 17), and reminisces about the summer of 1989, over the course of which Haq induced him to become involved in the process of establishing the HDRs – Sen eventually accepted.

For Haq, however, the paradigmatic shift within the UNDP which reached its first milestone with the publication of the first HDR (UNDP, 1990) was actually a continuation and manifestation of a set of normative and practical ideas that he had been thinking about for decades and that he had attempted to diffuse since at least the early 1970s. After graduating from Yale and subsequently doing postdoctoral research at Harvard, Haq returned to his native Pakistan where he assumed the position of chief economist for the Pakistan Planning Commission. While Amartya Sen and Haq were studying at Cambridge in the early 1950s, the two had already been discussing ideas such as "life expectancy and literacy and other measurable things beyond money that might provide a better indication of whether people have been given a chance for a complete human life" (Murphy, 2006, p. 243). These ideas were to evolve as a direct result of Haq's subsequent experience. During his 13 years of working with economic planning in Pakistan in the 1960s, the country had experienced an impressive rate of economic growth coupled with a strong growth in agricultural production. However, the situation for most people in the country had not improved. In spite of growth, real wages had actually decreased. There was inequality between different parts of the country, and the majority of the industrial wealth that the economic growth *had* brought about was situated in the hands of 22 families from whom there was little or no downward trickle. At the end of his term in the planning commission, Haq had become disillusioned with the ability of economic growth to deliver what he had now come to consider the true goals of development. In 1970, he made public statements that confirmed his increasing dissatisfaction with the traditional economic growth model that he himself had been a believer in, as exemplified in his first book, *The Strategy of Economic Planning* (1963). The statements included phrases such as 'turning development theory on its head' and to 'stand GDP on its head, since a rising GDP is no guarantee against worsening poverty'. The idea he wanted to convey was that development theory needed to become at once more focused and more holistic. Haq had begun to realise the limits of trickle-down economics and the models in which he had been trained; he was now convinced that the current approach did little but maintain the unequal status quo.

His professional debut in the field of global governance and international development came in 1970, when he was appointed to the World Bank. While at the World Bank, Haq held several positions, the most significant of which was that of director of the bank's policy planning and programme review staff under the bank presidency of Robert McNamara. Early in his World Bank career,[4] Haq shared some of these concerns at the World Conference for International Development held in Ottawa in 1971. At the time, this was much to the chagrin of his employer:

> I recall the reaction in the World Bank at that stage. It was one of shock and disbelief. I recall my first encounters with McNamara at that time. They were extremely unhappy ones. He suggested to me that this kind of belligerent

questioning of growth, at a time that the World Bank was committed mostly to production projects, was totally uncalled for.

(Haq in Asher, 1982)

Haq later admitted that, following this incident, he had offered to go back to Pakistan rather than further pursue his career at the Bank. McNamara, however, rather than entrenching himself, opted to ask Haq to compile his arguments in a coherent manner, to explain why focus should be taken away from thinking about trickle-down economics and directed towards targeting poverty and other, more specific sectors. Not long after, Haq was tasked with writing speeches for McNamara, and the latter began to espouse many of the ideas he had once found uncomfortable – especially as they were increasingly backed by evidence in the form of 'facts and figures', which was what McNamara put his trust in above all. In their time together at the World Bank, Haq, McNamara, and several other key staff members were instrumental in influencing the economies of developing countries through policies that encouraged direct focus on helping the poor. These policies included the investment in primary health care, primary education, and devoting resources to small farmers. Towards the end of Haq's World Bank career, something resembling *human development* tentatively began surfacing, illustrated perhaps most significantly in the *1980 World Development Report*:

> Human resource development, here called human development to emphasize that it is an end as well as a means of economic progress. . . . The case for human development is not only, or even primarily, an economic one. Less hunger, fewer child deaths and a better chance of primary education are almost universally accepted as important ends in themselves.
>
> (World Bank, 1980, p. 32)

As it turned out, however, the World Bank in the 1970s and early 1980s was not the ideal time and place for Haq to diffuse his ideas effectively. The 1970s energy crises were detrimental to this alternative thinking; while Haq had many support- ers within the bank, there were also a fair number of colleagues who rejected his approach. All the while, McNamara's devotion to the idea of human development waxed and waned, and ideas emanating from the Washington Consensus and its SAPs began to dominate the lending policy of the IFIs. Approaches now neglected included the Basic Needs Approach promoted by Haq and colleagues such as Paul Streeten, which had also enjoyed brief moments of relevance for World Bank Policy. By 1981, McNamara had been replaced by Alden Clausen as president of the World Bank. According to Haq, Clausen's position was not one that prioritised the targeting of poverty. Clausen focused almost entirely on the bank's relation- ship with the U.S. and less toward its client countries in the developing world. Fur- thermore, he was explicitly set against individual staff members expressing their personal views on matters without taking them through the proper channels. Haq not only disagreed with this philosophy, but it also served to make his work more difficult. This overarching intellectual chasm with the new leadership, along with related incidents over the course of the initial months of the new presidency, led Haq to finally resign from the World Bank in 1982.[5]

In the wake of his resignation, he moved back to Pakistan, and, in 1985, Haq was appointed finance minister.[6] Although the Pakistani government had long attempted to convince him to repatriate and apply his experience and skills to help his own country, his tenure was to be short-lived:

> He produced a programme for the liberalisation, privatisation, deregulation, and globalisation of the economy. He called for the collection of revenues through taxation, a chronic problem that had hobbled Pakistan's effort to generate economic growth from within the country. His revolutionary policies precipitated protest from many entrenched sectors: the bureaucracy, the landowners, and the business class all felt threatened by the reforms.
>
> (Cohen, 2004, p. 250)

Pressure from the powerful elites of these sectors led to Haq being removed from the position of finance minister less than a year after he had been appointed. However, many of the policies he had introduced remained in effect for the time being (Cohen, 2004), including efforts directed at human development and poverty alleviation:

> Many studies showed that during the period economic growth went up, poverty went down, and resources were mobilized for education. . . . For the first time in Pakistan, there was a focus on women's development in the planning documents, thousands of villages got electricity, family planning was introduced and institutionalized.
>
> (Haq, 2017, p. 4)

The mid- to late 1980s was a volatile period for domestic Pakistani politics. Under a caretaker government, Haq would return for a second tenure as finance minister. He prescribed policies and reforms of the taxation system. These almost immediately became hugely unpopular: "[t]his time Haq's policies were met with protests on the street. Factories and shops were shut, traders raised a hue and cry, and a political crisis erupted. Since then most elected governments have been wary of significant economic reform" (Cohen, 2004, p. 251). Haq left Pakistan in 1988, and the governments that followed only partly and intermittently followed his ideas with scattered efforts.[7] While his ideas had made a significant impact on the lives of many people, Pakistan was, in the end, not the correct platform at the right time for Haq's views to flourish.

### Additional antecedents: the roundtables

In the same time period, Haq was also part of a group of dedicated intellectuals who together worked towards formulating a coherent vision of what would become the human development paradigm (see Figure 4.1). This was known as

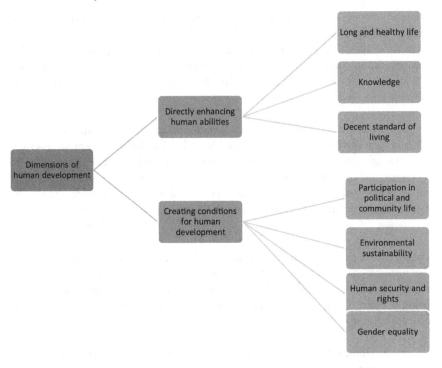

*Figure 4.1* Core attributes of the human development paradigm
(Source: UNDP, n.d.).

the North-South Roundtable (NSRT), which was part of the Society for International Development (SID).[8] The NSRT was spearheaded by four chairpersons: Mahbub ul Haq, his wife Khadija Haq, Barbara Ward – who had been one of Haq's teachers at Cambridge – and Maurice Strong, known for being both a self-made oil millionaire and the first executive director of the UN Environment Programme (UNEP). Over the course of the 1980s, three NSRT meetings in particular generated a coherent and explicit human development approach that would subsequently evolve into the foundation that underlies the HDRs. The roundtable meetings in question were those of 1985 (Istanbul), 1986 (Salzburg), and 1987 (Budapest), each of them addressing topics essential to the paradigm of human development. These are laid out in publications published after the meetings; many of the sentiments found in these publications are almost indistinguishable from those of the first HDR(s): "[t]he objective of development is people. The process of development may be measured in economic aggregates or technological and physical achievements. But the human dimension of development is the only dimension of intrinsic worth" (Haq & Kirdar, 1986, p. 7).

At the Istanbul Roundtable of 1985, health and nutrition are mentioned as one of the four main areas of action for the new paradigm. Alongside education, health had become deprioritised in the developing world following the economic challenges of the previous decade. Within the roundtable documents in general, health and education are often mentioned in the same sentence; aside from having intrinsic values in and of themselves, the two are paired together because they are both viewed as investments for development, a common theme for the double-edged sword that is health in development. The importance of health and the centrality of development are framed in the context of *capabilities* (Sen, 1999a), an approach returned to in more detail later. Relatedly, the indicators of health are presented as a central component in the measurement of the human dimension of development in a preliminary conception of what constitutes the HDI.

The generation and concretisation of ideas that occurred over the course of the NSRT initiative was crucial to the development of the ideas that would come to shape the UN's development efforts in the decades to come. However, Haq and his colleagues still did not have the prerequisite platform on which properly to influence the relevant actors in order to make their ideas effective, and there was still much work to be done. As Jolly comments,

> [N]o doubt some of the foundations of the HDR were laid. But it was no more than that. The major construction, the succession of annual HDRs, the HDI and other indices, the full flowering of the human development creation in the 1990s had to await the concentrated effort and full time commitment of Mahbub ul Haq, Amartya Sen and the other early members of the [Human Development Report Office], with the above members involved as consultants and Inge Kaul as chief of the UNDP team.
>
> (Jolly, 2007, p. 54)

The role of the UNDP as the appropriate organisational platform is explored in a subsequent section. In Finnemore & Sikkink's *norm life cycle*, such a platform is essential for the success of norm entrepreneurs in their effort to diffuse their ideas. For reasons explored earlier – that is, their rational-legal authority and position as global normative arbitrators in particular, IOs are in an especially potent position to act as platforms upon which individuals or groups can attempt to spread norms with a far larger probability of successfully reaching a tipping point and subsequent *norm cascade*.

### The influence and role of Amartya Sen and the capabilities approach

In the UN's official *Intellectual History Project*'s edition on the organisation's contribution to global development thinking, attention is directed more towards Amartya Sen than to Mahbub ul Haq when introducing the evolution and significance of human development: "the UNDP's [HDR] presents a subtle analysis of the relationship between human development and human rights, drawing directly on the work of Amartya Sen" (Jolly et al., 2004, p. 176). Today, Sen is indeed the more famous of the two. Perhaps this is caused by the fact that Sen is still alive while Haq passed away in 1998 (incidentally the year that Sen was awarded the Nobel Prize in Economic Sciences). However, Sen himself seems to shift more credit to Haq:

> The question with which I wish to begin is this: why has the Human Development Report received so much reflective attention with such speed in a world where new ideas often take decades, sometimes centuries, to receive the recognition they deserve? Why is the idea of human development such a success in the contemporary world? This is not a question about the profundity of Mahbub ul Haq's creative ideas, which is, of course, absolutely clear and not in any way in dispute.
>
> (Sen, 2000, p. 18)

His humble disposition aside, Sen's thinking and ideas had significant bearing on what would become the human development paradigm. When Sen was recruited by Haq during the summer of 1989, the two had already been friends for decades, and both were aware that their ideas about development were mutually inspired and significantly convergent. While Haq had spent much of his life working for government and in global governance, Sen's career had been confined within the world of academia. Most central in this context is Sen's *capability* approach, which reached the height of its popularity after the release of *Development as Freedom* (1999a). The idea had, in fact, first been articulated and presented 20 years earlier in Sen's chapter in an early edition of the *Tanner Lectures* (Sen, 1980).

The approach revolves around the concepts of *functionings* and *capabilities*, which refer to states and activities that a human being can experience. *Capabilities* relate to the opportunity for, say, achieving an education, while the corresponding *functioning* would be actually attending a place for learning and performing the various tasks that comprise the learning process. Without functionings, capabilities yield limited results; without capabilities, functioning is not even a viable option. Poverty, for example, is detrimental to a swathe of capabilities. What destitute or uneducated people in developing countries are actually in need of is not money or knowledge in and of itself, but the capabilities and subsequent functionings that these have the potential to allow. Human development and capabilities go so seamlessly together because while human development wants to direct development efforts towards human beings and factors contributing to the betterment of their lives, the capabilities approach provides one version of a road map that describes the dynamics that *constitute betterment* and therefore the ultimate end of development – the answer being to increase people's range of choices through capabilities.

> [The] human development approach developed a pioneering framework that integrated different development concerns and objectives. At the heart of this framework lay the notion of human capabilities, developed by Amartya Sen, which is in turn related to Sen's concept of [functionings] in different

domains of human life and action. The basic purpose of development is to enhance human choices and the human capabilities to undertake activities which people have reason to value. Thus, development policies, Sen argued, should be dedicated to enhancing people's capabilities through improved nutrition, better health, literacy, training, and civil and political rights. These ideas of welfare, choice, capabilities, and functionings introduced new and important theoretical foundations to many familiar development objectives and policies.

(Jolly et al., 2004, p. 179)

The connections between the human development paradigm and the capabilities approach are myriad and inextricable. While the capabilities approach was only fully presented in Sen's *Development as Freedom* (1999a), its ideas partly evolved alongside those of human development; one can hardly mention one without also mentioning the other. Phrases such as "human development is a process of enlarging people's choices" (UNDP, 1990, p. 10) exemplify the connection – the end goal of human development is increasing capabilities of the individual, allowing for the performance of an increased range of functionings (Fukuda-Parr, 2003); it is less about objective conceptualisations of well-being than about the opportunities available (Nussbaum, 2011). The manifold complexity of how choices are enlarged or diminished is also a point of mutual interest for the two approaches, as is the related intention to consider progress holistically. Both are fervent in rejecting economic growth as the *leitmotif* of progress and development, and both are keenly aware of the importance of social context – the list of concentricity goes on.[9]

One significant attribute of the normative nexus shared by human development and the capabilities approach is its connection with human rights – an example of an already established set of norms within the global community in general, and particularly within the UN. The norm entrepreneur can benefit from framing normative suggestions in a way that connects the proposed new norms to established ones, such as human rights. On a surface level, human rights and capabilities share many of the same attributes and creating a loose but convincing narrative equivalency was well within reach. In the introduction to the 2000 HDR, which deals specifically with the meeting point between human rights and human development, then administrator Mark Malloch Brown emphasises the common ground and interdependence between the two: "[w]hen adhered to in practice as well as in principle, the two concepts make up a self-reinforcing virtuous circle" (UNDP, 2000, p. iii).

Sen (2005) carefully explores the relationship between human rights and capabilities; he concludes that while there are significant overlaps, the two are not one and the same. For example, he asks, are human rights simply entitlements to capabilities – that is, the right to health?

It is possible to argue that human rights are best seen as rights to certain specific freedoms, and that the correlate obligation to consider the associated duties must also be centred around what others can do to safeguard and expand these freedoms. Since capabilities can be seen, broadly, as freedoms of particular kinds, this would seem to establish a basic connection between the two categories of ideas.

(Sen, 2005, p. 152)

When peeling back the layers,[10] Sen does uncover specific incompatibilities; the connection, however, and compatibility between the two generally remain congruent (Nussbaum, 1997, 2004; Vizard, Fukuda-Parr, & Elson, 2011). Indeed, from the perspective of the UNDP, human development and human rights are positively symbiotic. As the 2000 HDR suggests, the two enterprises both strive to ensure human freedoms. The fact that human development is so compatible with human rights has allowed the former a greater deal of moral legitimacy through the mechanics of norm-adjacency (see Table 4.1). On the other hand, human rights have benefited from the emphasis placed on long-term perspective and planning by human development: "[t]he concepts and tools of human development provide a systematic assessment of economic and institutional constraints to the realization of rights – as well as of the resources and policies available to overcome them. Human development thus contributes to building a long-run strategy for the realization of rights" (UNDP, 2000, p. 2).

### Health and capabilities in the human development paradigm

The introduction of the human development paradigm brought about a revolution with regard to how the UN considered and conducted its approach towards an internationally concerted global development effort. This process can be viewed as the emergence, cascade, and internalisation of a *meta-norm*, which was responsible for laying the foundations for the emergence of some of the subsequent norms that would inform the MDGs. This shift entailed a more holistic view of development and a reassessment of what constitutes its means and ends. The way of measuring progress would also be revamped with the intention of replacing the previously exalted position of economic growth[11] with a range of more nuanced indicators – among which economic growth would be considered but not necessarily prioritised. Instead, the concept of *capabilities*, itself a cluster of various considerations, became the core around which development progress would be evaluated. Importantly, the measurements also had to consider that the acquisition and formation of capabilities need to be supplanted by the ability to *use* these capabilities in order to realise their full potential, as conceptualised in Sen's *functionings*. Increasing and stimulating capabilities and functionings are thought to expand the range of choices and to increase the freedom of individuals, considered to be the true goals of development.

Health is at the core of the capabilities approach, and bodily health is one of the most tangible ways in which to measure capabilities and functionings: "health surely is substantially valued for itself: as a functioning or functionings. It may be taken as a proxy for many dependent capabilities, but this is not all: health is important in itself, not merely for its effects on other things (which could be compensated for by various means)" (Gasper, 2002, p. 25). It follows that ill-health is anathema to several of these integral capabilities and therefore to functionings. Sen's approach to health can be summed up as "the capability to live really long (without being cut off in one's prime) and to have a good life while alive (rather than a life of misery and unfreedom) – things that would be strongly valued and desired by nearly all of us" (Sen, 1999b, p. 619). Philosopher Martha Nussbaum, the 'other' renowned expert and champion of the capabilities approach, places *bodily health* second (topped only by *life*, and followed by the related *bodily integrity*) on her list of the 10 most central human capabilities (Nussbaum, 2000; Nussbaum, 2011). Sen has no such list, "although it is clear that he thinks some capabilities (for example, health and education) have a particular centrality" (Nussbaum, 2011, p. 20). For example, Sen writes that "health is among the most important conditions of human life and a critically significant constituent of human capabilities which we have reason to value" (Sen, 2002, p. 660).

From the perspective of the capabilities approach, health relates to development in several ways. In discussing the role of health within the approach, Sen tends to focus on the multidimensional sources – relating, to various extents, with other aspects of development – that have the potential to positively or negatively affect the health of individuals and groups. Emphasis tends to be on disaggregating the causal connection between economic growth and health improvement: "[w]hile there is a connection between opulence, on the one hand, and our health, longevity and other achievements, on the other, the linkage may or may not be very strong and may well be extremely contingent on other circumstances" (Sen, 1999a, p. 14). However, a consistent theme seems to be the focus on economic growth and health's *potential* for mutually beneficial symbiosis. Above all, he suggests that health is *integral* to development (as opposed to the more economically minded phrase *instrumental*, which he explicitly rejects), and that it is through coordinated and informed allocation of resources, and dissemination of knowledge for an informed public. Sen is candid in his assessment:

> Financial prudence is not the real enemy here. Indeed, what really should be threatened by financial conservatism is the use of public resources for purposes where the social benefits are very far from clear, such as the massive expenses that now go into the military in one poor country after another (often many times larger than the public expenditure on basic education or health care). It is an indication of the topsy-turvy world in which we live that the doctor, the schoolteacher or the nurse feels more threatened by financial conservatism than does the General and the Air Marshall. The rectification of this anomaly calls not for the chastising of financial prudence, but for a fuller accounting of the costs and benefits of the rival claims.
>
> (Sen, 1999b, p. 622)

Following the norms and logic embedded in the capabilities approach, human development introduced a momentous shift in terms of conceptualising what health is, as well as in terms of measuring progress towards it. The new paradigm also entrenched the role of health as one of the main aspects of development; the first HDR (UNDP, 1990) dedicates sizeable portions of text to discussing the importance of health, including the goals of increasing general life expectancy, of increasing and reducing unequal access to primary health care, and of emphasising preventive rather than curative treatment. There are also sections dedicated to children's and women's health, respectively. Nussbaum, in *Women and Human Development* (2001), suggests that reproductive health is an essential component of what she considers to be the *central capability* of bodily health; it is also part of a larger endeavour to minimise gender inequality and marginalisation in which it is implied that women stand the most to gain from a fully materialised human development campaign.

This adds to the point that the human development paradigm has a holistic view of health. This means that health is viewed not only as a state that enjoys the absence of any *physical* disease but includes the additional considerations of mental and social well-being. With this in mind, health is affected by a number of social and indirect determinants and is therefore dependent on the performance of several sectors and aspects of a given society. Reproductive health, which became a point of significant normative contention in the time leading up to the construction of the MDGs, is a case in point. The concept entails not only freedom from sexual ill-health but also the ability to exercise total control and freedom of choice over one's own reproductive system, including choices of whether to engage in sexual activity, whether or not to utilise contraception and whether or not to complete a pregnancy. These factors are highly contingent upon social context and its established norms, some of which are antithetical to freedom of choice in such decisions. The capabilities approach, particularly through Nussbaum, argues that any normative sensibilities that restrict freedom of choice and capabilities act as impediments to a universalistic sense of social justice. Such specific restrictions also contribute to the perpetuation of the pervasive problem of discrimination against women (Nussbaum, 2001). Indeed, any *normative* change that helps increase the capabilities and functionings, for example, related to managing one's own reproductive system, is part of the development process.[12] A further example is the tendency found by Osmani and Sen (2003) among certain South Asian communities in which gender bias is responsible for high levels of maternal under-nutrition, leading to intra-uterine growth retardation of the foetus, thereby complicating the future attainment of capabilities for the child. The approach implicitly and occasionally explicitly (especially through Nussbaum) critiques aspects of previous modes of development thinking and cultural and religious elements in the developing world alike, if deemed to be impediments towards the attainment of capabilities and to be contributors to marginalisation and discrimination (Nussbaum, 2011).

Furthermore, health is viewed as a human right and therefore it is the responsibility of states – individually as well as collectively – to ensure for its citizens a norm enshrined within the related concept of human security, as discussed in Chapter 3. These norms were not novelties brought about by the human development paradigm;[13] they were, however, augmented and brought to the forefront to a greater extent by the introduction of human development, particularly through the HDRs. With the explicit movement away from the previous paradigm, these considerations would now become central to measuring progress and success. Growth is not viewed as an end in and of itself but as a means that is helpful in order to reach the true ends of development, including that of health. Health has attributes that give it a superposition of both instrumentality and destination:

> A key analytical distinction in the capability approach is that between the means and the ends of well-being and development. Only the ends have intrinsic importance, whereas means are instrumental to reach the goal of increased well-being, justice and development. However, in concrete situations these distinctions often blur, since some ends are simultaneously also means to other ends (e.g. the capability of being in good health is an end in itself, but also a means to the capability to work).
>
> (Robeyns, 2005, p. 95)

While Sen tends to downplay the instrumentality of a healthy population while rather emphasising its intrinsic value, the power of this second-tier attribute is an important motivator for states in striving for and maintaining it. It can be seen as covering two different but related realms of interest for the state, related to ethical as well as to pragmatic considerations. While the former may (or may not) resonate with the social normative sensibilities of an actor such as a state, the latter is a clear benefit to the more economically focused side of behavioural determinants. Actors are more likely to comply with a norm if the norm also benefits their self-interest.

The WHO definition of health refers to more than the absence of disease. This sentiment is emphatically supported by the *capabilities approach*. Indeed, "health is a fundamental capability that is instrumental in the achievement of other capabilities. The unfair distribution of health capabilities may therefore affect social justice in several ways" (Ariana & Naveed, 2009, p. 238). Venkatapuram's book *Health Justice* (2011), in discussing the relationship between *health* and *capabilities*, explores and questions assumptions about the general conception of health. In his argument, he wishes to "break the mutuality between health and disease" (Venkatapuram, 2011, p. 41) in order to construct a perspective of health more in terms of people's ability to function and to "achieve or exercise a cluster of basic human activities" (2011, p. 42). These activities are relative to each individual's context. That is to say that personal biological specificities, extraneous physical conditions, and social circumstances all combine in interaction to create the extent to which health capability is fulfilled. More specifically related to social circumstances is *agency*, which refers to the ability of an individual actually to utilise her internal and external environs in order to *do* health functionings: "[m]aterial conditions such as availability of healthcare and adequate nutrition are determined by social arrangements, so material goods come under social conditions" (2011, p. 144). Again, reproductive health helps illustrate this point. Women and girls can be restricted from buying tools such as contraceptives even in situations where these may be technically available and legal, because they are not allowed to leave the house on their own, or because they have no access to money with which to independently make choices and purchase such products. Sen refers to these obstacles as social *conversion factors*,[14] which can nullify the influence that the presence of resources would have over someone's capabilities:

> It suggests that there are numerous factors influencing how different individuals convert resource inputs into valued functionings. These 'conversion factors' occur at the individual, social, institutional (formal or informal) and environmental level. Individual factors that determine how a given resource will be used include, for example, age, gender, metabolic rate, pregnancy, illness and knowledge. Social or family dynamics are also relevant in converting resource inputs to health outputs of value. Formal rules or informal regulations similarly intervene in our ability to use resource inputs to achieve desired functionings.
>
> (Ariana & Naveed, 2009, p. 235)

This is related to the *social determinants of health*, a concept in which the relationship between health and poverty is highly prominent. Poverty, enemy number one of the MDGs, gained prominence partly because of its interlinkages with almost every other aspect of development. In relation to health specifically, poverty has been shown to affect access to health care both in terms of quality and general availability (Feachem, 2000). A double-direction causality compounds this effect, as ill-health also tends to beget further poverty (Peters et al., 2008). The more indirect connection points are also plentiful, as poverty affects a number of aspects that are important for the capability conception of health, such as food, water, and sanitation. Education and knowledge about *what is healthy* is also statistically wanting in populations living in poverty (Arimah, 2004). Furthermore, as Ariana and Naveed (2009) suggest, health is among the capabilities that have the most lasting effect if it were to be compromised or stunted. People and societies can escape poverty and discrimination, even times and zones of war. However,

> deprivations in health may be irreversible. Once individuals have suffered from incurable diseases, they do not necessarily regain their health over a period of time. Such irreversible health losses may occur at any age. In the case of the elderly, irreversible dementia (the progressive decline in cognitive functions due to damage or disease), neural hearing loss and visual impairment are examples of irreversible health losses.
>
> (Ariana & Naveed, 2009, p. 242)

The importance of health in human development is evidenced by its inclusion as one of three component indicators of the HDI calculation. Choosing *life expectancy at birth* as the indicator that represents health was the result of considerations regarding which quantifiable statistic could best represent the health status of a country.

> The importance of life expectancy lies in the common belief that a long life is valuable in itself and in the fact that various indirect benefits (such as adequate nutrition and good health) are closely associated with higher life expectancy. This association makes life expectancy an important indicator of human development, especially in view of the present lack of comprehensive information about people's health and nutritional status.
>
> (UNDP, 1990, p. 12)

Life expectancy is seen to embody several aspects of a healthy life and is there-fore seen to fill the dual role of means *and* ends to the overarching goals of develop-ment. As Fukuda-Parr (2003) writes, Sen was initially against the idea of an HDI because he felt that the complexities that are involved in the quest for human development cannot be quantified in a single index. The myriad determinants of health, for example, represent one aspect of these complexities. However, Haq was able to persuade Sen to help develop the HDI for practical reasons; Haq was convinced that in order to catch the attention of policymakers, they would have to come up with a tangible form of measurement. The indicator of life expectancy at birth is considered to be the most representative single number regarding the health of an individual (UNDP, 1990).

### The UNDP as an organisational platform

> Development concepts cannot survive alone. They need to be framed and supported by organisational power. Organisations need, in turn, some sorts of shared ideas and values (including development concepts) for their existence in order to construct institutions.
>
> (Hirai, 2017, p. 22)

Emergent norms are more likely to be adopted on a large scale if they are supported and championed by an organisation, particularly an IO. Organisations can help an emerging set of norms by institutionalising, publicly endorsing, and actively dif-fusing its contents. This will often depend on whether or not the new normative suggestions dovetail with and incorporate already established norms within the given organisation. New norms can also replace antiquated ones or potentially fill void normative spaces that are discovered and subsequently deemed essential to the identity of the organisation.[15] An organisation's absorption of novel norms can have *constitutive* and *regulative* effects on its identity and behaviour (Katzen-stein, 1996). In the former instance, emergent norms can alter the identity and subsequent limits of appropriate behaviour of an actor. The latter – regulative – type of normative effect serves as providing new rules for behaviour that aims to supplement and optimise the organisation's rules of behaviour in order for its identity to remain cogent through changing circumstances.

Towards the end of the 1980s, the enterprise of global development was in crisis. The previous 10–15 years in particular had been catastrophically inadequate. Several prominent observers announced doom, gloom, and the end of development; the attempt had been made and had failed. For the UNDP specifically, the future was uncertain; in the early 1980s, they had chosen to support the SAP approach promoted and provided by the IFIs. As Hirai (2017) suggests, this support was probably caused by the UNDP's shrinking budget, leaving them little room to navigate independently. Indeed, governments had stopped funding them and were not listening to them as they had in the past – global development authority had increasingly shifted towards the pragmatic lending power of the IFIs. Pragmatic in their own way, the UNDP decided to align their views with the World Bank in particular in order to regain some of the influence that they had recently lost.

This state of affairs was, for several reasons, a temporary one. Human development, or ideas that in hindsight can be related to it, had been congruent with the nominal intentions and identity of the UNDP since the 1970s. In the mid-1980s, while still associating itself closely with the World Bank, the UNDP collaborated with the aforementioned NSRT in their early innovations in conceptualising and defining the purpose of human development.

When William Draper took over as administrator of the UNDP in 1986, several aspects of the organisation were due for evaluation and alteration:

> [I]n mid-1989, it was easy to believe that the Programmes' glory days were over. UNDP's engagements with revolutionary states and movements were unknown to me and most other observers (the engagements took place away from the public eye), and other organizations had begun to eclipse UNDP in its traditional fields. By then, most UN agencies carried out development projects funded from their regular budgets and many had their own representatives throughout the developing world. Moreover, compared with most of its competitors, UNDP had little focus – a complaint I later heard from scores of staffers. Hamid Ghaffarzadeh, who began working for UNDP in the mid-1980s, for example, says that he rarely contradicted his wife when she said that he 'worked for UNICEF; at least that made a picture in people's minds'.
> (Murphy, 2006, p. 232)

Draper was an outsider, an investment magnate and venture capitalist whom many perceived as possessing little or no relevant knowledge or experience related to development. He had been nominated to the position by Ronald Reagan – who features prominently among those who espoused a free-market, trickle-down economy approach. However, as Murphy (2006) argues, Draper was well versed in development and had strong motivations and particular convictions about how the UNDP could best fulfil their role.[16] One of these was belief that the UNDP needed to have a clearer identity, rather than be a passive facilitator for occasionally divergent paths of development. With this in mind, Draper wanted to unearth the values within the organisation and look for a way to synthesise these into policy:

> [M]ost were values shared by Draper . . . the desirability of democracy, the priority of improving the lives of the least advantaged, and, increasingly, the importance of raising the status and participation levels of women in society. Draper's embrace of 'advocacy' allowed those values to be put forward and made part of the staff's official remit.
>
> (Murphy, 2006, pp. 239–240)

Enter the human development paradigm. When Draper appointed Haq to the position of special adviser in 1988, the ideational climate within the organisation was ripe for a new focal point: one that corresponded to the value of the people who comprised it and one that could be effectively translated into policy. The points of connection that human development shared with those stated in the this quote were essential for the paradigm's relatively rapid diffusion within the UNDP *ethos*.

The institutional base of the UNDP at this point was a nearly ideal platform for Haq to diffuse his ideas. Importantly, the timing was also ideal in terms of the current climate of international politics. As 'softer' considerations slowly entered into the foreign policies of states previously encumbered with real and imagined fears of a war of unparalleled destruction, more nuanced approaches now had more room to manoeuvre. The extent to which Haq was granted free rein to pursue his convictions also played a significant role:

> When he joined the UNDP at the end of the 1980s, he insisted on a new division with editorial autonomy to run the [HDR] series and to bring the enlivening notion of human development to wide audiences. Thanks to Haq, the UNDP at last achieved important independent intellectual influence despite its pitifully small levels of research funding compared with those in the World Bank or [IMF]. Indeed, it came to set the agenda.
>
> (Gasper, 2005, p. 237)

Once the first HDR had been released, the shift in priority towards human development was immediately noticeable, and the UNDP experienced the largest budget surge in its history. This was the beginning of the *norm cascade* for the human development paradigm *meta-norm*. The concepts of human development, the HDI, and poverty had become the new buzzwords of development:

> It [the human development paradigm] has had an almost immediate impact on the allocation of development funds, especially donor funds, shifting them towards the priority concerns of poverty reduction and social welfare. In part, this was because the first reports coincided with the end of the Cold War, a moment when a shift from military spending was possible. It was also because the persuasiveness of the [human development] report's analysis convinced

a self-reinforcing cascade of development agencies to change their priorities. UNICEF's Jim Grant, for example, used it to pressure the Development Assistance Committee (the coordinating body of the major bilateral donors) to begin reporting the percentage of their aid allocations going to human development priority areas.

(Murphy, 2006, p. 245)

The first major UN-led summit of the 1990s, held only a few months after the publication of the first HDR, was symptomatic of this cascade. The optimism and buoyancy that followed after its publication created a favourable foundation on which the World Summit for Children would gain unparalleled traction, publicity, and participation. Not only did the summit set records in terms of high-level ministerial attendance, it also pioneered the practice of setting quantifiable objectives that member states could agree on, and to which they would commit. While its resultant outcome documents still contain allusions to the importance of growth, this is done in a noticeably subdued and caveated manner. The summit can be seen as the first of many to shift the mood held in the larger part of the 1980s, one that viewed the global development situation as an ideational and practical *cul-de-sac*. Additionally, further signs can be found in the Fourth UN Decade of Development (UNGA, 1990), which espoused many of the ideas presented by the new paradigm.

As St. Clair (2004) points out, the rapid adoption of the human development paradigm through the HDRs within the UNDP was the result of several dynamics. The combination of analytical utility and normative moral unassailability produced an attractive package for an organisation that was looking for a new approach and – to some extent – a newfound identity. The fact that these 'softer' considerations that dealt with the somewhat ethereal human condition could now conceivably be quantified was an important key to its diffusion within the UNDP. St. Clair further suggests that the diffusion of the human development paradigm had effects beyond its immediate scope, and that it fundamentally changed the operational structure of the UNDP:

[T]he effort to conceptualize the implementation of human development has forced the UNDP to re-assess the means used until now for this purpose. Many of the means now proposed by UNDP are also viewed as having intrinsic as well as instrumental value. In 1995, UNDP made poverty reduction one of its main objectives and created a division – the [Social Development and Poverty Elimination Division] – to work out ideas and strategies with enough holistic capacity to integrate the different dimensions of development and poverty. Capacity building, sustainable livelihoods, and the [Civil Society and Participation Programme], among others, are the result of UNDP's attempt to reach an understanding of the lives of the poor, and implement sustainable human development.

(St. Clair, 2004, p. 186)

"In most cases, for an emergent norm to reach a threshold and move toward the second stage, it must become institutionalised in specific sets of international rules and organisations" (Finnemore & Sikkink, 1998, p. 900). The main ideas of the human development paradigm had achieved just that – an infiltration into the institutional *fascia* of the UNDP. In addition, this infiltration precipitated a *constitutive* shift (Katzenstein, 1996) – a change in identity for the organisation, which saw its status lifted to one of increased authority with regard to setting the agenda for development policy. The significance of the imbuement of the *meta-norm* was therefore not limited to the generation of the conditions for which auxiliary norms could be advanced; at this moment in time, its particular content was so much in tune with global trends that it elevated its chief adopter's status – the UNDP – as a legitimate generator for frames and solutions for issues of global development.

## Haq, Sen, human development, and the UNDP

By 1989, Haq had been appointed as special adviser to the UNDP administrator, a job title created specifically for him by the recently appointed current administrator, Draper. He had been deeply impressed by Haq after having met him in Pakistan a few years earlier and put complete trust in his ability to discern for himself what his job would entail and the terms under which he would fulfil it.

Haq held several attributes that helped his eventual role as a norm entrepreneur. He brandished a combination of Western familiarity on account of his *alma maters* with a strong and credible attachment to the Global South, owing to his Pakistani credentials both as a native and as someone with significant experience working within the government of the country. "Haq's habitus as a development thinker and practitioner in and from the developing world therefore enabled him to criticize both countries of the South and the North more effectively" (Bode, 2015, p. 72). He enjoyed a dual citizenship of the North and of the South, which came with an implicit authority to speak on behalf of – or against – either. He was also known to be an exceptionally good storyteller, giving him a distinct advantage in terms of framing his cause to the intended audience. Bode (2015) emphasises this aspect:

> [A] second integral part in understanding Haq's empowerment in the UN development field of the early 1990s are his storytelling practices, performed on the basis of his constituted subjectivity. Haq constructed a story around the constitutive idea of human development through offering a chronological plot, including characters, and prominently featured himself as narrator. As Haq was a particularly 'present' narrator, the examination of his empowerment particularly showcases the analytical value of the story concept.
>
> (Bode, 2015, p. 79)

With his framing abilities, Haq was able to package the ideas of human development and subsequently the HDI in a way that was difficult to refute. There was little mistaking which group of ideas was the charitable protagonist and which was the malevolent antagonist. Tenets of the HDI were made to seem common sense, and the old way (i.e. a heavy reliance on observing the rise and fall of GDP) was made to seem foolish and inadequate. In this way he framed the normative context that he was contesting as – besides being less benevolent – actually making no practical sense. Evidence for the *norm internalisation* of these sentiments is found, mainly, in their permeation throughout the outcome documents issued in the wake of the various conferences and summits described in Chapter 2, and – as are discussed in Chapters 5 and 6 – throughout the value statements associated with the MDG and SDG frameworks.

Because Haq himself had converted from being an ardent believer in the reflexive relationship between an increase of GDP with a decrease in poverty levels, his own ideational evolution served as a microcosm for the larger ideational shift that he was now pursuing. His proof was simply to refer to the current state of affairs in the developing world and to point to countries in which the GDP was relatively low but other measurements for quality of life such as life expectancy and literacy were high – and vice versa. All the while, the aim was to drive home the claim that income growth does not necessarily equate to positive changes in the human experience of those who are supposed to be the target group. While such a positive causal link is plausible, so is an opposite effect. In the worst case, in fact, economic growth has the potential to deepen poverty within a country, depending on the related variables of institutions in place, political commitment, and levels of (in) equality; alternatively, its effects can be hardly noticeable in one direction or the other. The first HDR (UNDP, 1990) repeatedly pushes this point: "[l]ife does not begin at $11,000, the average per capita income in the industrial world. Sri Lanka managed a life expectancy of 71 years and an adult literacy rate of 87% with a per capita income of $400" (UNDP, 1990, p. 2).

This narrative created fertile ground for the ideas of human development to grow and replace the old and failing – perhaps even blighted – crops (see Table 4.1). In terms of the intrinsic characteristics of the human development meta-norm, there are two levels of conviction at work, introducing both *constitutive* and *regulative* change (Katzenstein, 1996) within the organisation of the UNDP. First, there is a sense of an overt moral and normative revolution with regard to the approach of global development policies; previous approaches were misinformed and wrong, while human development is thorough and intrinsically good and just. Second, there is a pragmatic argument in suggesting that the HDI is more effective than previous approaches in that it *actually* measures development progress in a way that is more plausible and realistic. The frame presented of human development (and the HDI) appeals to rational as well as to social norms, attaining a superposition that instils inspiration in both the economically minded and those more concerned with *doing the right thing*. "The normative value judgement is clear: the HDI is the 'better' way of measuring development, not least because of the policy optimism it conveys" (Bode, 2015, p. 82).

In Chapter 3, the health norm categories of human security and state security were introduced as devices with which to organise the various types and streams of interest that characterise them. By the description of the core tenets of human

*Table 4.1* Approaches in global development: the human development paradigm versus SAPs

|  | Pre-HDP (SAPs) | HDP |
|---|---|---|
| **Economic growth** | Top priority, the integral component that precipitates all other aspects of development. Best achieved by deregulation and privatisation. | One part of a holistic set of methods that can stimulate development. Emphatically a means, not an end. |
| **State role** | Limited. Supportive non-interference with the market. | State policies should be designed with the goal of maximising the capabilities of citizens. |
| **Human rights** | Not prioritised short term; expected to follow economic growth long term. | Essential means *and* ends, as well as of duty-bound inherent importance. |
| **End goal of development** | A higher standard of living brought about by economic integration, economic growth, and debt reduction. GDP the most common measure of success. | Expansion of freedom and range of choices through facilitating capabilities and functionings. Measured by the human development index. |

(Source: The authors).

development provided earlier, it is clear that the core assumptions that comprise its *ethos* are commensurate with those of human security. Indeed, human security is a conception of Haq's UNDP – specifically the 1994 HDR – and is intimately connected with the human development paradigm: "[i]t is proposed as a partner, rather than component, of human development; or sometimes even as its container, perhaps the biggest Russian doll of all (Gasper, 2005, p. 222). As has been suggested, the successful diffusion of the paradigm was partly dependent on post–Cold War circumstances, in which political neorealist and economic neoliberal assumptions were being questioned; globalisation was accelerated, and internal violent conflicts were on the rise. Human security, however, can benefit from statist security, in a similar way that human development can benefit from economic growth. The caveat is that these traditional ends, rather than being viewed as *panaceas*, are merely a single component of the whole.

The life (Figure 4.2) as a *meta-norm* is highlighted in such great detail in this chapter because the paradigm's position as a normative progenitor in the MDGs and the SDGs is considered ineluctable. As such, the paradigm successfully underwent the stages of *emergence*, *cascade*, and subsequent beginning phases of *internalisation*.

Several aspects of the process that facilitated the institutionalisation of the human development paradigm are recognisable. In the time leading up to the

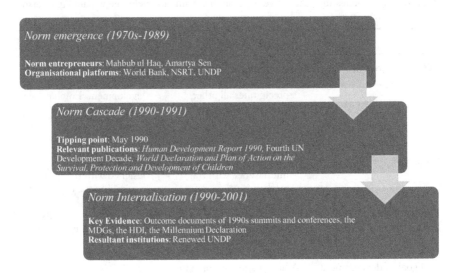

*Figure 4.2* The norm life cycle of the human development paradigm

emergence of the human development paradigm, global development discourse was dominated not by the UN, but by the IFIs and their associated SAPs (Jolly et al., 2004). A range of factors contributed to the challengeable nature of the normative space towards the end of the 1980s, allowing for Haq and his ideas to suffuse the *zeitgeist*. This situation fits the framework of the *norm life cycle* in a strikingly convenient manner. In its emergent phase, the normative context challenged by the human development paradigm *meta-norm* was in crisis and therefore highly contestable. Current wisdom was failing, and the neoliberal policy agenda had done little but stagnate or worsen conditions for most people in developing countries, and morale in the development community was low. Relatedly, the timing of Haq's UNDP employment was excellent, as it coincided with this general crisis as well as with the organisation's more specific identity crisis. More important, the ideas also resonated with the growing importance of political and broader cultural allusions to human rights, and the referent object of security shifting from the state to the individual (Vieira, 2007).

Added to this were the associated rise of explicit soft power politics and greater public awareness, the latter leading to connections between domestic elections and campaigning with allusions to *doing good* in the world (Finnemore & Sikkink, 1998; Kroenig, McAdam, & Weber, 2010). As a norm entrepreneur, Haq was ideationally committed and accomplished in the art of framing, as well as undeniably qualified in the field: he was as comfortable and as respected in the global North as he was in the South. Further, he found a nearly ideal organisational platform in the UNDP, an organisation with which his ideas entered into a mutually beneficial symbiosis – a relationship that would expand into the larger UN system and continue to produce more refined and specific norms. The meta-norm's cascade was initially swift following the publication of the first HDR, though its full manifestation would take the better part of the 1990s before it had (mostly) internalised. The mechanics of the latter process is what the next chapter concerns itself with. In part, it explores the *continued process* of internalisation of the *meta-norm* of the human development paradigm, while also narrating the full *norm life cycle* of health norms connected with the relevant MDGs.

Finnemore and Sikkink (1998) suggest that the variables *legitimisation, prominence*, and *world-time context* are important non-intrinsic variables that tend to play a role in whether or not an emerging norm will successfully diffuse. The implicit suggestion throughout this chapter has been that, for the initial normative incision of the human development paradigm, the most salient of these seems to be world-time context. Indeed, the fact that the UNDP embraced the paradigm at the time that it did – and that the normative contents of this paradigm *cascaded* soon after – reignited the organisation's prominence. Further, legitimacy was gained because the organisation's new stance stood in direct opposition to the recently deposed neoliberal development agenda, occupying the normative void with an *ethos* which, by emphasising human-focused policies, was explicitly contrary to the norms that it contested.

## Conclusion

This chapter describes and examines the ascendance of the human development paradigm; it also examines its contents in a more detailed fashion. The rationale behind this treatment is founded in the implications of its position as what is referred to throughout as a *meta-norm*. This term is introduced because its internalisation and normatively *constitutive* effect within the UN system, along with specific political conditions in the international arena, allowed for the emergence of new, *regulative* lower-order norms such as, for example, those concerning reproductive health. This example will be further examined in the next chapter. Aside from allowing new norms, the *meta-norm* also made it nearly impossible to oppose the now common-sense notion that health is worth pursuing in itself, thereby further solidifying its normative value as closely related to human rights and human security. The establishment of the paradigm further excluded notions not considered conducive or worthwhile, which meant that erstwhile imperatives of economic neoliberalism and a focus on GDP maximisation would no longer be abided by.

The chapter begins by analysing those challenges inherent in finding the roots of ideas in norm-based research, before the *meta-norm* concept is introduced. The rest of the chapter provides an account of the context in which human development emerged, with particular focus on the life of its main originator and norm entrepreneur, Mahbub ul Haq. Over the course of this narrative, the chapter elaborates on the *human development paradigm*, highlighting its connections with the *capabilities approach*, and more specifically with *health*. The UNDP is another main feature of the chapter, and its role is highlighted as the organisational platform from which the *meta-norm* could reach its stages of international *norm cascade* and subsequent *internalisation* into the UN development agenda, as evidenced by the permeation of its associated imperatives in the MDG framework.

A near-perfect storm of variables set the backdrop and came together to allow for this meta-normative shift. The human development paradigm's successful emergence resulted from a number of coincidental and favourable political conditions, coupled with a well-developed idea that was aptly framed by an ideationally committed norm entrepreneur who subsequently achieved the endorsement of the UNDP, an organisation in need of a new identity. Mahbub ul Haq's credentials, along with aspects of his personality, helped boost the paradigm's authority and legitimacy. Timing was a further important factor: an increasing emphasis on individuals as the referent object of security, along with the willingness of states to allocate resources to alternative spheres after the end of the Cold War, coincided with an urgent need for global development in general to reinvent itself.

In the following chapters, the influence of the human development paradigm will be re-examined in the context of investigating each specific health goal, along with other variables relevant to the *norm life cycle*.

## Notes

1  A norm entrepreneur does not necessarily originate a normative proposition. Indeed, this is rarely the case; he or she rather takes inspiration from ideas and modifies and adapts them to the relevant context.

2  As Hulme (2007) suggests, the terms of *development* and *combating poverty* were nearly synonymous by that time. Indeed, the subheading in the *Declaration* is *Development and Poverty Eradication*. As suggested, and as returned to below, poverty alleviation can be viewed as the *super-norm* – of the development agenda (Fukuda-Parr & Hulme, 2009).

3  As Buzan and Gonzalez-Pelaez (2005) point out, IR scholars and practitioners are notorious for using variations (i.e. global society/community, international society/community, or international system) of this rather loose concept, a tendency that has contributed to a sense of ambiguity regarding its meaning. For the English school, these terms are distinctly defined, each having a specific meaning. In the context of this book, *global society* is not meant to have any direct connection to the theoretically specific terms of the English School. Rather, it refers to the existence of a social arena of a global scope, where social rules apply, some by law. State sovereignty, self-determination, and territorial integrity are examples of such rules. As suggested, IOs serve an important function in global society, as they serve to define problems and solutions that are of common interest for every actor.

4  At this point in time, Haq was not yet a regular member of the World Bank staff. Rather, he was on leave from his work for the Pakistani government and was only beginning to be affiliated with the Bank.

5  Other reasons stated by Haq were that he felt that the field of international development was becoming so constrained that he would rather focus his energy on contributing to the domestic development of Pakistan, whose government had been inviting him to come back and work for them for quite some time.

6  In fact, Haq held several different governmental positions in the period after his return to Pakistan. His title as finance minister is highlighted for its special prominence.

7  As Cohen (2004) argues, the exception here may be Nawaz Sharif's government, which shared Haq's vision of liberalisation and which recognised the importance of globalisation.

8  The SID is a network of people and organisations dedicated to improving the develop-ment effort through several avenues of action. With values based in social justice and with an affinity for good research, the SID has since its establishment in 1957 been central in pushing for several of the values now integrated in the global development agenda. In terms of influence, "SID enjoys the highest consultative status, Category I, with the United Nations Economic and Social Council (ECOSOC). SID in addition, maintains consultative status with [other relevant UN sub-organisations]" (SID, n.d., para. 2).

9  The *Journal of Human Development and Capabilities*, for example, is testament to the plethora of concentric circles shared by the human development paradigm and the capabilities approach. The journal was founded in 2000, initially as the *Journal of Human Development* by the Human Development Report Office. After the establish-ment of the Human Development and Capabilities Association, the two entities co-operated more closely and eventually created a joint publication of the journal under the new name.

10  Sen (2005) goes into some detail to point out that capabilities and human rights are *not the same* but can be exceedingly helpful to each other's fulfilment.

11  Often, early development efforts are somewhat unfairly accused of being blind to factors other than economic growth with regard to what constituted development. Though economic growth was indeed the favoured metric for measuring the progress of development, the nuances of development were not entirely lost on those involved in the initial decades of the endeavour. As Streeten wrote as early as 1981: "[a]t this early stage [the late 1950s and early 1960s] we were quite clear (in spite of what is now often said in a caricature of past thinking) that growth is not an end in itself, but a performance test of development" (Streeten, 1981, p. 323).

12  As several authors (Alkire, 2005; Robeyns, 2005, 2006, Venkatapuram, 2011) note, Sen and Nussbaum are not in complete agreement with regard to what constitutes the totality of the capability approach. "The simplest distinction between Sen and Nuss-baum's approaches is to consider the Senian version as a descriptive framework while viewing Nussbaum's conception as a normative framework. Sen's approach has been described as providing an analytical device in contrast to Nussbaum's account of sub-stantive entitlements" (Venkatapuram, 2011, pp. 129–130). This distinction is largely false, as Sen *does* take normative stances varying from the opaque to the conspicuous in his writings; Nussbaum's approach is considered to be more direct.

13  Most notably, the *Declaration of Alma-Ata* (WHO, 1978) includes these norms. How-ever, the contents of the *Declaration* were soon deprioritised during the neoliberal developmental agenda of the 1980s, in which focus on primary health care particularly declined. The importance of social aspects as determinants of health were refined and reaffirmed in the *Ottawa Charter for Health Promotion* (WHO, 1986) – though they made a somewhat spectacular return in the early 2000s and a subsequent, more exten-sive return in the health SDG, as is explored more closely in Chapter 6.

14  Other classifications of conversion factors are *personal* (physical condition, intelligence, gender) and *environmental* (physical surroundings) (Robeyns, 2005; Sen, 1992, 1999a, 2009).

15  In the wake of numerous allegations of sexual assault and harassment during the sec-ond half of 2017, exemplified by the *#metoo* movement, companies and people within the American entertainment industry found it necessary to take a clear and strong normative stance against such behaviour. Though these normative values may have been previously present and/or nascent, the highly charged context demanded they be expressed or risk accusations of complicity.

16  Aside from being an ardent supporter of the core ideas of human development, Draper considered it essential to emphasise and strengthen the role of women in developed as well as in developing countries. He was responsible, in the end, for elevating women within his own organisation to higher positions on a whole different scale than had ever

been done previously (Murphy, 2006). In an interview years later, Draper stated that the two things he was most proud of from his time as administrator were (1) the conception of an organisation named Women in Development and of generally changing the culture of how women were viewed within the UNDP (which, he adds, was rather sexist at the time he arrived there) and (2) of helping to consolidate the HDR along with Mahbub ul Haq (UNDP, 2016).

# 5  The health norms of the Millennium Development Goals

The purpose of the previous chapter was to establish the importance and significance of the human development paradigm as a normative antecedent to the norms that are the focus of this chapter. The current chapter continues to utilise the norm life cycle by taking a closer look at the three MDGs specific to health. This will be done to identify and analyse their constituent health norms. Aside from the influence of the human development paradigm, influences emanating from the various political (and medical) ebbs and flows reflected in Chapter 3 are taken into account, keeping in mind the respective health norm categories of *state security and human security*. Considered together and in context, these considerations aim to illustrate the mechanisms operating in the contended normative spaces present within the spheres of influence connected to the global development agenda as set out by the UN during the 1990s, which in turn resulted in the creation of the MDGs.

In this chapter the life cycle of the health norms that embody the three distinct health MDGs will be investigated. Specifically, these include MDG 4 on reducing child mortality; MDG 5 on improving maternal health; and MDG 6, which focuses on combatting HIV/AIDS, malaria, and other diseases. Its main purpose is to apply Finnemore & Sikkink's *norm life cycle framework* in an attempt to identify and explain the normative and related political mechanisms that were decisive in the process that created the health MDGs. The anchor points of this analysis are the circumstances and documentation related to the time before, during, and after conferences and summits that took place during the 1990s, where much of the normative and practical policy groundwork for the MDGs was laid. The chapter opens with a short discussion of normative characteristics of global conferences and summits that typified the evolution of development discourse in the 1990s. The rest of the chapter treats the health MDGs listed earlier in numerical order.

## The role of conferences and summits in normative negotiation

The impetus, according to Jolly et al. (2004), for convening the various conferences held by the UN and its various specialised sub-organisations over the course of the 1990s, was the need to rethink and reframe global development thinking. Again, the motivational spur appears to have come from the crisis global development had found itself in after the relative failure of the efforts conducted in the 1970s and particularly in the 1980s. Some of the topics covered over the course of these conferences were as old as the global development endeavour itself and included hunger, unemployment, and shelter; some were new, such as a more pervasive focus on the environment and an added emphasis on various challenges unique to women. Issue areas such as the environment, gender equality, and women's rights had become increasingly pressing, topical, and mainstream over the previous decade or so but had yet to feature significantly in development discourse and policy up until that point.

These conferences were explored in broad strokes in Chapter 2. Many of them were specific to a certain cause, such as the UN Conference on Human Settlements in Istanbul; others, such as the World Summit for Social Development in Copenhagen, addressed more general terms about development at large. This chapter, utilising the insights from the *norm life cycle* and building on previous reflections regarding the nexus at which politics, norms, globalisation, and health converge, expands on those earlier reflections of the UN conferences of the 1990s that are most relevant to the subject matter – this describes the evolution of the health norms that informed the content of the health MDGs.

In terms of the mechanics of the *norm life cycle framework*, these conferences presented norm entrepreneurs with an organisational platform upon which to diffuse their emergent normative suggestions. Typically, norm entrepreneurs in such a setting express themselves and lobby on behalf of an invited organisation. The relevant organisation works as the platform for the individual, while a conference is a secondary, larger-scale platform for organisations to act as norm entrepreneurs. A simple way of assessing whether or not a norm has been successfully integrated into the value system is to check for its prominence in the outcome documents after a conference. A further test of the extent of their internalisation is to test for resilience – in terms of longevity and robustness – and to assess the ability to give rise to accessory norm emergence. A related indication can be found in its success rate when evoked as adjacent by a norm entrepreneur in the emergence phase. In this case, this is tested by the norm's inclusion or absence in the *core value statements* of the *Millennium Declaration* and, in particular, in the subsequent actual policy objectives found in the MDGs. This resilience is further tested in the next chapter, in which the health norms that constitute the SDGs will be examined.

### The MDGs and the primacy of poverty eradication

The gravity of the *super-norm* of poverty eradication (Fukuda-Parr & Hulme, 2009) as the core component towards which all the goals of the MDG framework gravitate is of major significance in the effort to understand which health issues were included in the framework – and which ones were not. While the human development paradigm is holistic and could accommodate a broader spectrum of areas to address, the MDG health goals all focus on ailments that disproportionately affect the poor. This suggests a framework mostly informed by human security, which is unsurprising when considering the underlying normative structure of the human development paradigm.

Fukuda-Parr and Hulme (2009) provide an account of the ascent of poverty eradication to the position of *super-norm* within the MDG framework. They argue that the "specificity and concreteness" (2009, p. 4), presented by a focus on mitigating the multidimensional causes and effects of poverty, was key to its internalisation and subsequent manifestation as the overarching imperative of global development. They identify norm entrepreneurs from several different stakeholders, such as NGOs, various UN officials, DAC representatives, and ministers within the donor community. Amartya Sen and his increasingly widespread *capabilities approach* – particularly in the wake of the publication of *Development as Freedom* (Sen, 1999a) – is also mentioned, as is the UNDP in general. The norm entrepreneurs diffused their normative convictions throughout several of the conferences held in the 1990s and in the negotiations surrounding the contents of *We the Peoples* (Annan, 2000), the *Millennium Declaration* (UNGA, 2000b), and the MDGs. These processes were all detailed in Chapter 2 and are to some extent discussed in this chapter, which deals with the MDG health norms.

As a result of this internalisation, all other MDGs – including those related to health – were framed within the unifying pursuit of poverty eradication. As the meta-norm of human development set the normative context for the renewed development agenda, which started taking shape after the release of the first HDR, the super-norm of poverty eradication set the more specific subtext for the MDGs. At first glance, such a subtext seems normatively rooted in human security and has little to do with state security. However, in the goals described later, health norms from the latter category came significantly to influence one of the three health goals.

## MDG 4: reducing child mortality

The 1990 World Summit for Children is remembered for putting global summits 'on the map' and for pioneering time-bound quantifiable goals that all member states could agree upon over the scope of a few days (Hulme, 2007), as well as being one of the early attempts at operationalisation of the human development paradigm. (In Chapter 4, it was mentioned as part of the *norm cascade* and as an early part of the *norm internalisation* of the *meta-norm* (Figure 4.2)). More pertinent, however, the summit and its outcome document *World Declaration on the Survival, Protection and Development of Children* (UN, 1990a) also acted as progenitors in highlighting the children's health issues that were to comprise the rationale behind MDG 4. Indeed, enhancing health and nutrition for children is identified as the *first duty* of the *Declaration*. This duty takes place in a predefined context described in the *Declaration* as one where children, being victims of their circumstances, are affected by several types of negative impacts – that is, violence, drought, malnutrition, illiteracy, disease, and poor living conditions – all inconducive to the development of a child's capabilities, or even more cruel still, to the child's survival. The goals agreed upon in the programme for action include the reduction of the mortality of children under the age of five "by one third or to a level of 70 per 1,000 live births, whichever is the greater reduction" (UN, 1990b, para. 2). This particular target is also stated in the first HDR which was published a few months prior, as well as in the document for the UN's Fourth Decade of Development, which was passed by the UNGA approximately a year after the Children's Summit. Given the many potential causes for child mortality, such a goal can be broadly interpreted to mean the amelioration of all the negative situational examples given earlier, plus potentially unlisted ones. A related and explicit goal was the elimination of children's malnutrition by one half of the 1990 levels by the year 2000, and more detailed emphasis was placed on this at the 1992 International Conference on Nutrition. The importance of protecting every part of a child's life, including health, is also reaffirmed in the documents that followed the World Conference on Human Rights.

The content of the children's health goal seems to be the least normatively controversial of all the health norms comprising the MDGs. The goal is positioned at the nexus between the right to health (as mentioned in Chapter 3) and the *rights of the child*,[1] both of which were relatively well-established normative constructs at the time. Reaffirming and refining these norms and subsequently concretising and further operationalising the contents of required policies with which to address challenges pertaining to them was therefore rather straightforward. It was a matter of *how*, rather than *whether*. The main change was a departure from approaches characteristic of the SAP approach (Table 4.1). A 1987 UN Children's Fund (UNICEF) publication, titled *Adjustment with a Human Face* (Cornia, Jolly, & Stewart, 1987) had argued for a modification of the SAPs by suggesting that it focus more on investing in *human capital*[2] and social safety nets. In other words, while lending more attention to the importance of capabilities in development, the emphasis is on their instrumental benefits: "it is growth, and technical prescriptions for attaining it through macroeconomic stability, privatization and liberalization, that dominates the discourse" (Cornwall & Brock, 2005, p. 1045).

UNICEF is mandated by the UNGA to protect and advocate for children's rights and to work towards the fulfilment of their basic needs and opportunities, and it constitutes the most authoritative institution in safeguarding children's health on a global basis. This value system is entirely commensurate with the goals of the human development paradigm and did not require a significant shift in terms of its imperatives after the emergence of the new *meta-norm*. However, the path towards attaining these imperatives had been shifted towards enhancing abilities and creating conditions conducive to these rights. On the basis of this observation, there is no natural room for a *norm life cycle* analysis of this particular MDG, at least within the specified timeframe.

Even if there is no clear point at which a previous norm was contested or any clear norm entrepreneurs who argued a normative case against a would-be established child-neglect developmental approach, children's health norms contain several of the properties and characteristics listed by Finnemore and Sikkink (1998) as tending to contribute to the success and robustness of a norm. First, children's health is universalistic. Nearly all people everywhere have children and are, to one extent or another, protective of the well-being of children, particularly of their own offspring – and especially of infants. Second, children constitute a group that is innocent and vulnerable – they cannot provide for themselves the necessities that they need to live a full life, or even to survive. Third, describing the health plight of children directly refers to bodily harm and, by extension, to the fragility, mortality, and survival of the human species. Fourth, there are explicit links with the more general normative framework of the UDHR, further strengthening the children's health norms through its *adjacency* to the established norms constituting the most exalted declaration of all (at large, but particularly within the UN system). States may adhere to emerging norms if by doing so it is considered to improve domestic legitimacy. In the case of children's health, its universal appeal creates a situation in which any government that would reject reducing children's mortality rates would quickly be considered illegitimate – even malevolent – in the eyes of the vast majority of their own population. Another sign of the internalisation of this norm across cultures and continents is that any state *opposing* this norm would rapidly reach pariah-status – as would be the case with a state openly supporting the practice of slavery.

The second point of the *Millennium Declaration* explicitly reinforces these values in a statement that illustrates their pervasiveness and fundamentality:

> We recognize that, in addition to our separate responsibilities to our individual societies, we have a collective responsibility to uphold the principles of human dignity, equality and equity at the global level. As leaders we have a duty therefore to all the world's people, especially the most vulnerable and, in particular, the children of the world, to whom the future belongs.
>
> (UNGA, 2000b, p. 1)

What had changed since the end of the Cold War was the *world-time context*. The reality of the political landscape had shifted, and with it emerged the potential for a truly concerted effort to improve children's health. The importance of this had been bolstered by the underlying normative framework of the human development paradigm *meta-norm* and the associated ideas of human security. Particularly salient is the normative message within it that emphasises the individual over the state and the latter's responsibilities to ensure the rights and welfare of the former. While this may in reality be 'hot air' (Paris, 2001) in a still self-interested world, the political climate of the day – of which the UN conferences and summits were symptomatic – seem to have further established certain rules of understanding (or logics of appropriateness). That is to say that while actors may still have purely self-interested underlying motives for adhering to the rules, the fact that there is a set of rules 'out there' that actors feel compelled to at least *appear* to have internalised and adhere to, helps actualise the existence and net power of these social institutions. Another novelty was a newfound spirit of optimism that had been reinvigorated by the internalisation of the human development *meta-norm*. There was a sense that *this time*, with the new and better tools as well as new and better intentions, the concerted efforts of the development community had a far better chance of succeeding (Bode, 2015).

## MDG 5: improving maternal health

A significantly more complicated trajectory was faced by the normatively contested issue of maternal health and mortality. While partly related to child and infant mortality (McCaw-Binns & Hussein, 2012), the norms surrounding women's health are far more disputed, particularly when it comes to health associated with childrearing and maternity. While children have a relatively neutral status, women's sexual and reproductive health sparks controversy in a number of different cultural or faith-based normative structures. The more interesting part of the norm life cycle for MDG 5 is *what was omitted* from the goal (though supplemented years later) rather than what was included.

Indeed, what was initially included was relatively straightforward. *Reduce by three quarters, between 1990 and 2015, the maternal mortality ratio*, partially by improving the rate at which births are attended by skilled health personnel – the latter an indicator suggesting progress on the former. The target was originally formulated in the plan of action agreed upon at the 1995 UN Fourth World Conference on Women in Beijing. These concerns held little novelty in global development discourse, as maternal mortality in developing countries had been recognised as a challenge well before the 1990s. However, little progress had been made, and any agenda based on human development could not accept such high mortality rates. In the first HDR, it is stated that "the maternal mortality rate in the South is twelve times that in the North – the largest gap in any social indicator and a sad symbol of the deprived status of women in the Third World" (UNDP, 1990, p. 2). Indeed, the only gap that surpassed maternal mortality at that point was that of GDP, in spite of these rates declining in certain regions in the preceding decades (Ronsmans, Graham, & Lancet Maternal Survival Series Steering Group, 2006).

The main causes of maternal deaths included haemorrhage and postpartum bleeding, postpartum infections, and complications arising from unsafe abortions. The overwhelming majority of cases were considered avoidable had the appropriate health facilities and skills been present; hence, the policy emphasis on increasing the attendance of competent health personnel. These more acute and direct aspects of maternal mortality generally deal mostly with situations *during* or in the immediate aftermath of childbirth – contexts in which the mother is fragile and vulnerable. These characteristics are reminiscent of that of a child, and the normative sensibilities discussed regarding the previous goal become relevant. Indeed, the similarities are striking. The issue is universal, the victims are particularly vulnerable; the issue regards bodily harm, and many aspects of the situation can be connected to adjacent established norms such as those enshrined in the UDHR. Another cognate set of norms are those associated with the closely related position of the child who faces life, from infancy to adulthood – without a mother. These health norms are, quite clearly, motivated by attempts to ensure human security and have little to do with its state security counterpart. Squarely placed within the normative parameters of the human development paradigm and the all-encompassing MDG *super-norm* of poverty eradication, they aim to benefit individuals and societies afflicted by these poverty-related and highly preventable causes of mortality and morbidity.

As with the norms that support the children's health goal, the ones that constituted the original form of MDG 5 were not particularly contestable and therefore did not require – or allow for – the actions and admonishments of a norm entrepreneur within the timeframe of this study. The relevant 1990s conferences and subsequent materialisation of global development goals relating to maternal mortality were more of a process reaffirmation and of concretising the way in which these ends would be pursued. Influences from the human development paradigm are tangible in the documents that emanated from the relevant conferences. The most general of these – the 1995 Women's Conference in Beijing – heavily emphasises the related nature of gender equality and women's health, keeping a holistic view of what is necessary to ensure the latter. Indeed, the conference papers mention a frighteningly wide spectrum of manifestations of discrimination against women and girls that can, in various ways, threaten their health. For example, a family might give their male child prioritised access to scarce resources of nutrition or health care over that of a daughter. This phenomenon, also known as *son preference*, is just one symptom of a discriminatory gender bias that exists in different iterations worldwide and something that only a holistic approach could mitigate.

In spite of these myriad considerations and sentiments, MDG 5 was limited to the very basic (and perhaps most easily quantifiable) goal of preventing maternal mortality, rather than tackling the more complex problems head on. The *norm life cycle* narrative of this goal is incomplete without elaborating on what was excluded from the agenda and which would be retroactively added some years later. This concerns any mention of family planning,[3] reproductive health, and the controversy surrounding these subjects regarding their connection to maternal health and women's health more generally. As Sending (2004) suggests, policies related to family planning had originally – from its earlier conception in the 1950s – been about curbing excessive population growth, as its implications were thought to negatively affect socio-economic development. U.S. President Lyndon Johnson articulated this belief in a speech at the UN in 1965: "[l]et us act on the fact that less than five dollars invested in population control is worth a hundred dollars invested in economic growth" (Johnson in Sending, 2004, p. 62). In the 1970s, an increasingly vociferous environmental movement also appropriated the notion of family planning – the logic being that a smaller population equals a smaller burden on the climate.

An approach to family planning that emphasised women's and reproductive health (and choice) as meaningful ends in themselves only began to take shape in the late 1980s, when a handful of research and interest groups began presenting evidence for the health benefits of family planning. Of particular note in this regard is the Population Council, founded by John D. Rockefeller III. Rockefeller himself and particular staff members and researchers were important for introducing a more overtly feminist perspective into the debate on population control and what they saw as the related topic of reproductive health. Indeed, the organisation and some notable individuals within it – such as Rockefeller himself, Joan Dunlop, Adrienne Germain, and George Zeidenstein – served important roles in contesting the conventional wisdom of population control while simultaneously advancing and promoting the importance of this connection and of women's rights in relation to reproduction generally. The norms advocated by this movement were characterised by defending women's rights to determine, manage, and control their own reproductive systems. The most important factor is the ability to decide whether, how, and when to have children – a significant increase in freedom of choice, in the parlance of the *capabilities* approach. The normative basis is built on ideas of equality, non-coercion, and respect for the agency of individuals. This includes not only the right to make such decisions but also that these decisions be informed through adequate education and information provision. Knowledge about contraception is a key aspect of this education; availability of and access to contraceptives is also considered essential for these rights-bound capabilities to materialise. Furthermore, practices that act to limit these capabilities, such as female genital mutilation and other harmful medical procedures, are condemned.

Though this effort included many dedicated and passionate individuals and organisations, Germain and Dunlop, in particular, stand out as norm entrepreneurs in this context. They combined their efforts in the mid- to late 1980s while working together at the International Women's Health Coalition (IWHC), a period that yielded significant evidence for their cause, accumulating scientific data to solidify their normatively motivated argument – a combination very much compatible with the then nascent human development paradigm. This is to say that the frame the movement operated within was one containing arguments of normative and rational/instrumental character alike. While the normative arguments had significant strength in an isolated sense, the addition of tying the effort up with the more plainly 'practical' issues of population control was the equivalent of adding an extra metal to form a normative alloy, which became more difficult to challenge. Not only *should* women's reproductive health be safeguarded in a strict moral sense, it also has instrumental value in terms of minimising the negative consequences of overpopulation.

In the many obituaries written following Joan Dunlop's death in 2012, the recurring sentiment is that she undoubtedly made the world a better place for women. Particularly, praise is given to her important work with the IWHC in the mid- to late 1980s as well as in the 1990s – her efforts prior to and during the ICPD in 1994 are especially lauded. Indeed, IWHC was the organisational platform from which Dunlop, the norm entrepreneur, most effectively disseminated her ideas. In a nutshell, those ideas stated that population problems could be greatly reduced only if the condition of women was improved. Included in this improvement was the right to proper (particularly reproductive) health care, education, and employment – all conducive to an increase of capabilities. Described by a colleague as "incredibly imaginative and yet viciously practical" (Thomas in Bumiller, 1998, para. 9), Dunlop was the one to originate and coordinate the idea of a *Women's Declaration on Population Politics*[4] prior to the Cairo Conference. She managed to

place her colleague and partner-in-ideas Adrienne Germain on to the U.S. delegation to the UN and lobbied with carefully selected people within the organisation
to make sure that their message would be heard at the conference. During ICPD,
she was responsible for organising early-morning advocacy meetings that would
become infamous: "In Cairo, she and her colleagues held 6AM war room-like
meetings. 'Where's Nigeria on this?' they would say. 'Are the Swedes obdurate?'"
(Bumiller, 1998, para. 11). The IWHC through Dunlop's leadership was essential
in bringing reproductive health into the sphere of global development, as the topic
had been "largely ignored in global policies until 1994" (Germain, 2018, p. 78).

Adrienne Germain – Dunlop's successor as IWHC president – also played an
instrumental role in the process of architecting the very same advocacy movement. Germain was particularly effective in negotiating and communicating the
message of the norms that she, Dunlop, the IWHC, and the general international
Women's Rights movement were attempting to diffuse. As suggested, Germain
was part of the U.S. delegation to ICPD and the subsequent women's summit in
Beijing the following year. Germain was able to utilise the powerful position of the
state she represented in order to give her arguments more weight, something that
may have made a difference in the final negotiations, particularly regarding the
ICPD's programme of action. Germain has continued her work in the same field
throughout her career and was awarded the UN Population Award in 2012 for her
lifelong work for the cause.

Opposition to the idea of family planning has come in various forms over the
years. The practice of family planning began in earnest to be encouraged by
the UN the 1960s – a time where population growth truly started accelerating.
Leaders of developing countries also recognised the issue relatively early on, and
exceptionally, many representatives from the Global South attended the 1965
World Population Conference in Belgrade.[5] Dissenting voices surfaced during the
next population conference, held in Bucharest in 1974, at which representatives
from several developing countries argued that 'development is the best contra-
ceptive' (Sai, 1997). The conference outcome documents recognise and emphasise the connection between development and population and encourage states
to inform and encourage their citizens about family planning and to integrate
these policies with larger developmental goals. During this period, the U.S. was
a strong supporter of using fertility control for these purposes, while other states
adopted a wide spectrum of approaches: China's controversial and aggressive one-
child policy – initiated in 1979 – being the most extreme example. By the next
population conference in 1984, family planning, particularly abortion, had become
a taboo subject in the eyes of the U.S., the Holy See, and a number of other
countries – these states now worked together to understate the impact and importance of related policies. Meanwhile, a varied selection of developing countries
had become more positively inclined towards family planning and the benefits of
population control, though some of the more conservative and Western-sceptical
countries were less convinced. Proponents of reproductive rights recognised that
framing the issue as reproductive *health* rather than in terms of *rights* – a concept
associated with ideas emanating from the Global North – would help the issue

become less normative, more matter-of-fact, and less culturally objectionable. The approach of the IWHC, though based on strong normative convictions regarding women's equality and human rights as essential means to attain economic and social justice globally, (Germain, 2018), were also – importantly – backed by evidence in numbers that could sway population researchers and health researchers who were less normatively motivated.

These different strains of contention coalesced at the ICPD, held in Istanbul in 1994. As suggested in Chapter 2, the ICPD received much of its publicity from the presence of controversy and dissent regarding family planning, with the Holy See and its 'unholy alliance'[6] taking centre stage. However, the general frame around reproductive rights and family planning seemed to have changed in a direction more in tune with the human development paradigm and the feminist arguments of the IWHC and the population council. Rather than focusing on the instrumentality of having fewer children in the endeavour to control population growth, the focus was increasingly on women's role in development and on the inherent rights of women with regard to reproduction, with the supportive, more practical argument that a lack of such rights would be detrimental to maternal health in particular.

> The ICPD Programme of Action recognizes women's education, equality and empowerment as paramount, and the importance of providing family planning within the context of full sexual and reproductive health care is stressed. It applies basic human rights principles to population and family planning programmes, and rejects coercion, violence and discrimination. It recognizes the central role of sexuality and gender relations in women's health and rights; asserts that men must be fully involved, but without veto, in decisions involving fertility, sexual behaviour, sexually transmitted disease and the welfare of their partners and children; and recognizes unsafe abortion as a major public health issue.
>
> (Sai, 1997, p. 1)

The ICPD was the apparent tipping point that set off the *norm cascade* for the reproductive health norm. The ICPD's programme of action in relation to reproductive health is heavily laden with human rights associations and the elevation of women to equal partners in development. The right to reproductive health is broadly defined, and includes the more controversial topics of access to contraception and sexual education. The common thread is the expansion of people's (and especially women's) choices with regard to reproduction, with population control being an added and naturally occurring benefit of ensuring these capabilities. It discourages female genital mutilation and allows for abortion where legal – a near-verbatim continuation of the policy outlined in Mexico City in 1984.

In the section on reproductive health, an asterisk informs the reader that the Holy See has certain reservations with the content. As David Hulme writes, the Holy See "'square-bracketed' the term 'reproductive health' 112 times and bracketed around 10% of the full draft document, with little or no support from member-states" (Hulme, 2009, p. 13). The reservations, in the end, did not stand in the way of the above content making it into the final version of ICPD's programme of action. The normative logic that was applied in the end is captured in a statement made by Norwegian Prime Minister Gro Harlem Brundtland towards the end of the conference. From the logic of this statement, larger, more *universal* norms trump those that are limited to a certain and more *specific* set of norms such as those found, in this case, within Catholicism and Islam. This is essentially a defence of the cross-cultural relevance of certain norms (or universal values), in the spirit of Nussbaum's iteration of the *capability approach* (Nussbaum, 1999). Indeed, for Brundtland, the latter are irrational and harmful to the common-sense proposed norms of reproductive health in a situation where lives are at stake.

> Sometimes religion is a major obstacle. This happens when family planning is made a moral issue. But morality cannot only be a question of controlling sexuality and protecting unborn life. Morality is also a question of giving individuals the opportunity of choice, of suppressing coercion of all kinds and abolishing the criminalization of individual tragedy. Morality becomes hypocrisy if it means accepting mothers' suffering or dying in connection with unwanted pregnancies and illegal abortions, and unwanted children living in misery.
>
> (Brundtland, 1994, para. 19)

Perhaps the most significant policy goal was the stipulation to achieve global reproductive health services for *everyone in all countries* by 2015. The norms established at ICPD were reaffirmed the year after, during the women's conference in Beijing. As a UN report suggested in the wake of the latter conference, "the atmosphere in Beijing was infused with a strong resolve not to unravel any of the ICPD agreements, particularly those pertaining to reproductive health and rights" (UN, 1995b, para. 2). The outcome documents from Beijing confirm this by connecting reproductive rights to human rights: "[t]he human rights of women include their right to have control over and decide freely and responsibly on matters related to their sexuality, including sexual and reproductive health, free of coercion, discrimination and violence" (UN, 1995c, para. 96). The participants in the conference further attempted to push the envelope by suggesting the partial decriminalisation of abortion, though not promoting it as a viable method of family planning. Reproductive health is also mentioned several times in the official report released in the wake of the World Summit for Social Development in Copenhagen in 1995. Its importance is repeatedly reinforced as essential to (1) ensuring proper and holistic health care to all and (2) in order to further the cause of equality between men and women.

The UNDP/UNFPA/WHO/World Bank Special Programme of Research, Development and Research Training in Human Reproduction (HRP), originally created in 1972, expanded its scope as a direct result of the ICPD "to include other aspects of health dealing with sexuality and reproduction, adding a specific perspective on gender issues and human rights" (Benagiano et al., 2012, p. 190).

While the HRP was involved in influencing the content of the ICPD's state-ments and programme of action,[7] it was also affected by the mainstreaming of the reproductive health norm that occurred in the aftermath of the conference – subsequently becoming an institution that *inter alia* aims to coordinate, generate, and implement research agendas for improving reproductive health. By the end of 1995, reproductive health seemed destined to be involved in UN-led develop-ment policy for the foreseeable future. On the face of it, the tipping point seemed to have been reached at the ICPD, and the *norm cascade* was apparently all but ensured.

Indeed, with two major conferences reinforcing the sentiments of reproductive health, the norms associated with the notion seemed to have attained near inter-nalisation within the UN. Indeed, as Hulme (2009) suggests, this was the belief of many of those who had ensured its success through lobbying and research ahead and during the ICPD, some referring to the effort as a "watershed, in that it sealed a paradigm shift with respect to gender and reproductive rights" (Standing, 2004, p. 239). This belief was further reinforced in 1996, as reproductive health featured in the DAC's *International Development Goals* (IDGs), in many ways the template upon which the MDGs were based – a relationship briefly relayed in Chapter 2. The ICPD+5 meeting held in 1999 also reaffirmed the positions of member states, further strengthening the belief that reproductive health was now a staple of the UN's development agenda.

As it turned out, however, this seeming internalisation was a temporary illusion. In Hulme's (2009) retelling of the events that led to the exclusion of reproductive health from the MDGs, he suggests that while those who supported its inclusion in global development policy were resting on their laurels, the other side had begun to recognise the importance of the impending Millennium Summit. The latter group now consisted of the Holy See, a few conservative Islamic countries, as well as an increasingly influential section of conservative evangelical Christians in the U.S. (Amstutz, 2013). Together, these *antipreneurs* (Bloomfield, 2016) created an image of the issue that connected reproductive health with its most controversial aspect: namely, abortion. Further, the encouragement of sexual promiscuity and homosexuality were framed as being highly connected with the paradigm of those who supported reproductive health. Framing the issue in this way stirred support with several more developing countries to the extent that Kofi Annan started feeling the pressure. At the G77,[8] countries less invested and concerned with the matter opted to support the conservative voices and to make the official position of the association one that opposed reproductive health goals in general.

> This message was forcefully relayed to the Secretary-General. No Secretary-General, and particularly one from the developing world, could ignore the G77 message. The concerns of these conservatives, that 'reduced maternal mortality' was a covert means of promoting reproductive health, meant that even this goal was also excluded from We the Peoples. . . . His priority was to achieve a progressive package of goals in the final Millennium Declaration that would be acceptable to all member countries. Losing the reproductive

health goals was no big deal from this perspective. European countries and the World Bank argued strongly that reproductive health was an essential component of a strategy for poverty reduction and that other Declaration goals could not be achieved if reproductive health was omitted. But the Secretary-General and Secretariat were not going to risk producing a document that the G77, the majority of UN members, would not approve. To the chagrin of reproductive health proponents around the world – and most poverty reduction specialists – the April 2000 Report of the Secretary-General to frame the Millennium Summit, We the Peoples, avoided mention of the Cairo Agenda.

(Hulme, 2009, pp. 16–17)

The growing evangelist movement in the U.S. also forced Al Gore, who had previously been a supporter of the reproductive health agenda, to tone down his support for domestic political reasons while running for president in 2000. Under threat of not signing the agreement, these forces combined to make sure that reproductive health was omitted from the *Millennium Declaration* as well; in spite of the support for its inclusion by "most OECD countries, the majority of developing countries, the [IFIs], specialised UN agencies and vast civil society networks" (Hulme, 2009, p. 18). While central to the IDGs as well as to the human development paradigm, reproductive health ended up being excluded from the MDGs because a few countries (and perhaps, above all, a non-state observer actor in the Holy See) had reservations toward some aspects of its contents. With political shrewdness, the 'unholy alliance' was able to frame the issue in a way that effectively reversed the previously surpassed tipping point, revealing the fact that norms of reproductive health had not yet been fully internalised.

This example stands out as an interesting case concerning the linearity of the *norm life cycle*, as well as the universality of human security. <u>*Antipreneurs*</u> (Bloomfield, 2016) such as the 'unholy alliance', responsible for overturning the positive trajectory that reproductive health had enjoyed during the 1990s, have the power and ability through the usage of timing, framing, and relative political power, to push back against norms that are seemingly past the tipping point. Viewed within the frame of Symons and Altman's (2015) concept of *international norm polarisation*, this retrocession of a seemingly internalised norm illustrates some potential blind or weak spots present in the framework, particularly regarding its assumptions of unidirectionality (Hofferberth & Weber, 2015).

So far, *legitimation* has been viewed as a force that facilitates norm diffusion and internalisation, by government adopting international norms to gain legitimacy and recognition in a domestic context. However, it is also a variable that has the converse potential of delaying, interrupting, or smothering the process of a norm life cycle. As evidenced by the case of reproductive health, the proposed norm clashed with central cultural standards of certain countries. International norms tend to have more legitimacy if they coincide with – or mirror – already existing domestic normative structures (Moravcsik, 1995). Conversely, "international norms that are inconsistent with prevailing social beliefs and values, are unlikely to enjoy high levels of domestic salience because their prescriptions do not accord with national understandings regarding appropriate behaviour" (Cortell & Davis, 2005, p. 6). In countries where the majority of the population feels that a woman should always obey her husband (see Bell, 2013), agreeing to support the full extent of reproductive rights would be going against the sensibilities of the electorate.

Less powerful, developing states have the incentive to conform to and eventually internalise norms emanating from industrialised democracies (Cortell & Davis, 2005), whereas states with more weight – or normatively aligned conglomerates of states that muster strength in numbers – can more comfortably protest against and disturb norm diffusion in multilateral contexts such as within the UN. This is related to the aspect of *prominence*, specifically through the decisive reservations noted by the G77, plus the somewhat erratic on-the-fence behaviour displayed by the U.S. The impact of Finnemore and Sikkink's (1998) notion of *world-time context* is less clear-cut in this example. Without the meta-norm of human development being prominent in the global normative context, the mid-1990s conversation about reproductive health is far less likely to have taken place. However, this particular aspect of the normative package shifted the emphasis towards legitimisation, while the prominence of the G77 in particular contributed to the internalisation process being left suspended and incomplete – at least for the period of time relevant to the formation of the MDGs.

Ultimately deemed integral as part of accelerating progress towards the goals, reproductive health norms were revived, and their internalisation reinitiated at the 2005 World Summit.

> Achieving universal access to reproductive health by 2015, as set out at the [ICPD], integrating this goal in strategies to attain the internationally agreed development goals, including those contained in the Millennium Declaration, aimed at reducing maternal mortality, improving maternal health, reducing child mortality, promoting gender equality, combating HIV/AIDS and eradicating poverty.
>
> (UNGA, 2005, p. 16)

Reproductive health goals were quietly added to the MDGs in 2007, and any reference to their earlier omission is difficult to find in any current official source. This latter point is an indication of its present status of internalisation; an MDG 5 without reproductive health is one best left forgotten, its status further reinforced by its inclusion in the SDG framework. More recently, the 2010 UNGA resolution requested a follow-up operational review of the ICPD and the status of its implementation. In 2014, ECOSOC's Commission on Population and Development announced its report pursuant to this request in the form of the *Framework of Actions for the follow-up to the Programme of Action of the ICPD Beyond 2014* (United Nations Economic and Social Council, 2014a). The report suggests that the monitoring framework will serve to provide inputs for monitoring population and development in the post-2015 development agenda, including mechanisms for measuring the extent of – and assessing the quality of – reproductive health

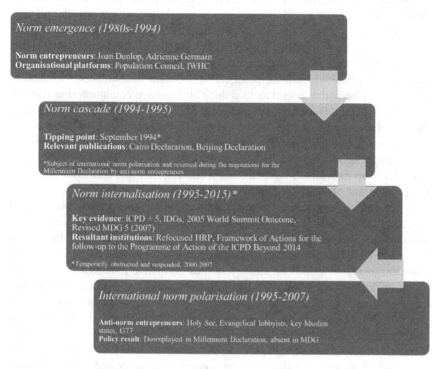

*Figure 5.1* The norm life cycle of reproductive health in the MDGs

care delivery. In conclusion, the *norm life cycle* of reproductive health within the MDG framework stands as an example of the potential non-linearity and political pliability that certain norms are subject to (Figure 5.1).

## MDG 6: combat HIV/AIDS, malaria, and other diseases

"To have, by then [2015], halted, and begun to reverse, the spread of HIV/AIDS, the scourge of malaria and other major diseases that afflict humanity" (UNGA, 2000b, p. 5). This is the wording for one of the main components constituting the normative and conceptual backbone of the health MDGs, namely the *Millennium Declaration*. Fighting disease has always been part of the development agenda of the UN. Indeed, the first UN Decade of Development document requests measures to be taken "to accelerate the elimination of illiteracy, hunger and disease, which seriously affect the productivity of the people of the less developed countries" (UNGA, 1961, p. 18). Later, the *Declaration of Alma-Ata* (WHO, 1978) connected disease eradication with *the right to health* – thereby elevating to the *end goal* the instrumental benefit of productivity that had been the focal point during the era of modernisation to the position of a beneficial side effect of ensuring the health of individuals.

As suggested in Chapter 1, these rights-based health norms took a backseat in development during the SAP era, as focus reverted to economic growth and market liberalisation. After these efforts were unsuccessful, the human development paradigm again de-emphasised concerns of productivity; statements painting disease as a hindrance to capabilities, choices, and social development in general, had become prominent talking points. The common denominator throughout, however, has been the intention to reduce and remove communicable diseases because of their universal negative effects. Though the emphasis has changed, the underlying premise is that disease has negative effects on instrumental as well as intrinsically valuable variables. At times these are separate considerations, but the overlap is significant. The inability to work and make a living, for example, are obstacles to an individual's capabilities and choices; they also constitute a liability for the economy of his or her family, community, and country.

In other words, targeting and directly treating disease has been a staple of global development efforts since the beginning, and so its amplification has never faced serious controversy or dissent. Indeed, the intention to rid the world of disease can be considered so commonsensical, so appropriate – or internalised – as to make any argument *against* it would constitute a serious normative transgression. In terms of the intrinsic characteristics of a strong norm as posited by the *norm life cycle* framework, such a position is to be expected. Disease represents a uniquely clear, tangible, and occasionally visually visceral threat of bodily harm; the vast majority of the victims of disease in developing countries are both innocent and particularly vulnerable because of circumstances such as poverty; a lack of access to health care, food, clean water; or the presence of conflict. As suggested, straightforward health norms that deal with *direct* suffering, misery, and death have favourable prerequisites in terms of successfully internalising, as do their connections with established, adjacent norms. Because of these intrinsic qualities, the formulation and frames of such norms do not play a very significant role, nor do the other variables discussed, such as domestic legitimisation and prominence of supporters. Indeed, the introduction of the human development paradigm and the subsequent creation of the MDGs served to strengthen these norms and the associated resolve with regard to combating disease, in large part by appealing to a common responsibility and emphasising issues of human security. This final point relates to the concept of *world-time context* (Finnemore & Sikkink, 1998), which suggests that large-scale global events such as the end of the Cold War can act as catalysts for norm change – a process from which the emergence of the human development paradigm meta-norm may have benefited.

Add to this the prevailing overarching theme of poverty eradication, and the MDGs' emphasis on diseases associated with poverty comes as no surprise. Malaria, the one disease aside from HIV/AIDS mentioned by name, had been the main scourge of the developing world for decades prior to the formulation of the goals. Emblematic of the dual relationship between health and development, malaria is not only far more prevalent in developing countries, it has also been shown to hinder progress towards various development indicators – particularly in terms of economic growth (Gollin & Zimmermann, 2007; Worrall, Basu, & Hanson,

2005). The less clear-cut facet of MDG 6 is the particular *exceptionalism* assigned to HIV/AIDS. For reasons similar to those mentioned earlier regarding malaria and development, the inclusion of HIV/AIDS is completely justified. However, concerns about the pandemic comprise two of the three sub-targets, while *all other diseases* are bunched together in the third sub-target.

One place to seek an explanation for this, as suggested by Rushton (2010), is not primarily in the *Millennium Declaration* but in *We the Peoples* (Annan, 2000) – the publication that somewhat infamously excluded any mention of maternal health. The health section of the document puts a rather extreme emphasis on HIV/AIDS – so much so that "a Martian reading the final chapter of *We the Peoples* could reasonably conclude that HIV/AIDS was the only health problem facing the Earth's poor people" (Hulme, 2007, p. 10). Indeed, while Annan does mention other scourges and their dire consequences, he disclaims further discussion of them before dedicating at least three quarters of the entire section solely to HIV/AIDS. The prevalent and relevant norm thus seems to be that this one disease merits more attention than other diseases (even combined). How did the norm of combatting HIV/AIDS ascend to this exalted position in the scope of disease in global development? Towards the end of their *UN Contributions to Development Thinking and Practice*, published as part of the *United Nations Intellectual History Project Series*, Jolly et al. (2004) have a section that mentions various 'omissions and missed opportunities'. The section includes major topics and areas that the authors feel had been neglected by the UN for too long. A short section on HIV/AIDS reveals that "all through the 1990s – while the number of infected persons multiplied rapidly – actions by the United Nations failed to rise to the scale of the challenge" (Jolly et al., 2004, p. 297). This observation amplifies the *sudden* nature of the rise within the organisation's development agenda of HIV/AIDS. Another observation further illustrates this suddenness: in resolutions, outcome documents, and declarations: it is customary within the UN to include a section that lists the previous commitments that the *current* commitment is meant to 'recall and reaffirm'. In the outcome document published in the wake of a UNGA Special Session on HIV/AIDS in June 2001, all 11 commitments that are referred to date back less than two years from the time of publication.[9]

The venture of raising awareness, understanding, destigmatising, treating, and attempting to cure HIV/AIDS has had no lack of dedicated individuals and organisations and, indeed, norm entrepreneurs. Countless *ideationally committed* people have contributed to the role that the disease has had in the world of health governance and development – for better or worse – since the mid-1980s (Smith & Whiteside, 2010). State actors such as South Africa have also played their parts, most notably by passing the mentioned *Medicines Act* in 1997. A plethora of small and large non-state actors were essential in providing scientific and normative weight that contributed to the attention and resources devoted to the efforts to mitigate the direct and indirect consequences of the pandemic (Vieira, 2007). Multiple books and countless articles have been written about several of these actors and their endeavours and deeds. In this book we limit ourselves to recounting an abridged version of the role of just a few.

One important individual whose efforts stand as significant precursors to the eventual focus on the pandemic is Jonathan Mann. Mann, a Harvard graduate epidemiologist, was tasked by the WHO in the mid-1980s to start the Special Programme on AIDS (SPA). His contribution to global responses to HIV/AIDS is substantial in at least two respects. First, he was one of the earliest global health professionals to recognise the scope and severity of the threat, particularly in regard to its potential negative effects on developing countries. Under Mann's leadership, SPA – later renamed the Global Programme on AIDS (GPA) – was able to generate significant funding, particularly from the U.S. government, and direct these funds towards mechanisms of surveillance and prevention in the developing world. One important aspect of this was to persuade developing countries to implement strategies and targeted campaigns that would combat the spread of the disease. This often took some convincing, as many governments were concerned that investors and tourists would be deterred if the country admitted that it had a problem. The GPA, however, was able to establish a vast network of national programmes that are likely to have saved countless lives: "[t]he emphasis was on risk reduction through information and education. People were encouraged to understand and change their behaviours. Condoms were distributed, testing and counselling made available, and occasionally, where appropriate, needle exchange programmes set up" (Whiteside, 2008, p. 106).

As he proved in his conference speeches and through his appeals to various institutions of the U.S. government, Mann was known for his ability to provoke inspiration, as well as his "intellectual acuity and magnetic presence" (Behrman, 2004, p. 41). Mann's efforts to make the world aware of the gravity of the situation, and to instil a sense of urgency in mitigating its present and future effects, were instrumental in the pandemic achieving a semblance of appropriate attention early on: "[h]e was able to shine the spotlight on the catastrophe as well as the deficiencies of the global response, yet frame the predicament as an opportunity, a chance to realize transcendent human aspirations" (Behrman, 2004, p. 49).

A second contribution attributable to Mann is that he recognised and advocated an approach that emphasised connections between human rights and disease. With regard to HIV/AIDS, he recognised that marginalised groups – the poor, homosexuals, prostitutes, drug users, and others – were those most vulnerable for infection, and that their diagnosis only contributed to their further marginalisation. He was an ardent champion of human rights and dignity and saw health care as integral to the fulfilment of these imperatives.

> Mann famously theorized that public health, ethics, and human rights are complementary fields motivated by the paramount value of human well-being. He felt that people could not be healthy if governments did not respect their rights and dignity as well as engage in health policies guided by sound ethical values. Nor could people have their rights and dignity if they were not healthy. Mann and his colleagues argued that public health and human rights are integrally connected: Human rights violations adversely affect the

community's health, coercive public health policies violate human rights, and advancement of human rights and public health reinforce one another.

(Gostin, 2001, p. 121)

Working with Halfdan Mahler – a well-known champion of *health for all* and the sentiments of the *Declaration of Alma-Ata* – in his time at the WHO, this underlying philosophy was the core motivation for Mann's work. A connection between human rights and health came to be salient in the MDG framework's approach to health, particularly through its connection with poverty eradication. The normative connection also comes into play in the health SDG, albeit from a different angle – this is further discussed in Chapter 6. Unfortunately for Mann, his career and influence would face a gradual atrophy after the appointment of Hiroshi Nakajima as Director-General of the WHO (Behrman, 2004), leading to Mann's eventual resignation in 1990. He would prematurely pass away in 1998, as one of the many unfortunate passengers – many of whom were top HIV/AIDS researchers – aboard the ill-fated Swissair flight 111.

Closer to the time of the MDG's formulation, two other individuals (and one organisation) stand out as particularly important norm entrepreneurs with regard to the position that HIV/AIDS finally attained with regard to the MDGs. The personal efforts of Richard Holbrooke, the U.S. Ambassador to the UN from 1999 to 2001, are considered to have been instrumental in connecting HIV/AIDS with security and with arranging the UNSC meeting about the matter in January of 2000 – a month in which the presidency of the UNSC lay with the U.S. Over the course of the 1990s, Holbrooke had seen the effects of the disease first-hand during trips to Asia and Africa. He held a general concern regarding the general conditions faced by many African citizens in particular, and he viewed HIV/AIDS not only as one of the most visceral aspects of these conditions but also as something that did *not* respect borders and would spread uncontrollably if left as is. The pandemic, in the eyes of Holbrooke, was already a humanitarian disaster, while having the potential to be a global security threat of unknown magnitude. The fruits of this January meeting would be the passing of *Resolution 1308* (UNESC, 2000) later that year. Holbrooke initially faced resistance in attempting to present his case. "A lot of people thought we couldn't make AIDS a security issue," Holbrooke said. "We needed the support of all the other members of the Security Council – all of them agreed, some more reluctantly than others." Holbrooke's use of the security frame was essential for this elevation of HIV/AIDS, as he managed to make the issue appear salient to – rather than far removed from – the security concerns of the most powerful states in the world (Shiffman, 2009). Holbrooke also had the support of his government, which itself "designated the global HIV/AIDS epidemic a threat to the security of the United States" (Vieira, 2007, p. 150).

A person with whom Holbrooke had consulted closely prior to the UNSC meeting, and one of the speakers at the event itself was Peter Piot, executive director of the Joint United Nations Programme on HIV/AIDS (UNAIDS) – the successor institution of the SPA and the GPA. With both an MD and a PhD in the medical sciences, Piot had had plenty of experience working with disease in the developing world.[10] As director of UNAIDS, Piot – much in the spirit of his self-proclaimed hero Jonathan Mann – encouraged and practised activism as a tool for bringing attention to the severity of the pandemic. In an almost self-referential norm-entrepreneurial manner, he once stated that activism "is the most potent force to get political leaders to overcome their unwillingness to act promptly on AIDS. . . . As so often in history, top leadership [is made up of] personal vision and responding to pressure from civil society" (Piot, 2005). Like Mann, Piot was convinced that the problem of HIV/AIDS was a problem of unique severity, both regarding health in isolation, but also as a major obstacle to development. Although difficult to imagine at present, few people in the Global North were sufficiently aware of the scope of the disaster for those in the developing world.

Piot was distraught at the lack of political interest and commitment toward the issue. Under his leadership, with limited staff and limited funding, "UNAIDS took on the challenge of combating such complacency in order to leverage a stronger and better-funded response from the developed world" (Joint United Nations Programme on HIV/AIDS, 2008, p. 74). This work included partnering with NGOs and afflicted individuals, by diffusing information through media awareness campaigns and supporting research related to learning more about how to ameliorate the effects of the disease. In 1998, Piot decided to shift his efforts more towards the UNSC and the UNGA and to finance ministers in powerful countries. He understood that a frame of the disease as a threat to *security and stability* was the most powerful tool with which to attract the interest of developed countries. In UNAIDS' own account, this was a defining moment. Piot approached his agenda with a flurry of meetings and events in different fora (from the Davos World Economic Forum, to the AU, to MTV), simply drawing attention to the harrowing facts of the pandemic. By 1999, finance ministers began discussing HIV/AIDS as an economic and developmental impediment. Kofi Annan had also begun espousing the message of UNAIDS and formed, along with Piot, a formidable team with a large measure of credibility:

> There has been a most fortunate synergy in having an African Secretary-General at a time when so much work was needed on AIDS – and [in having] his extraordinary leadership. . . . The Secretary-General's voice would just have been one voice without the back-up of UNAIDS and equally the reverse. They needed each other. I think it's been a very timely partnership.
>
> (Malloch Brown in Joint United Nations Programme on HIV/AIDS, 2008, p. 95)

One major event that helped put HIV/AIDS on the global agenda was the Durban International AIDS Conference in this very eventful month of July 2000. The speech by Nelson Mandela powerfully emphasised the problem, of which South Africa was at the core: "[t]his is, as I understand it, a gathering of human beings concerned about turning around one of the greatest threats humankind has faced, and certainly the greatest after the end of the great wars of the previous century"

(Mandela, 2000, para. 2). Commenting on the Durban event, a UNAIDS report later summarised:

> No one who attended the conference, and particularly the closing ceremony, had any doubts that a line had been crossed in the global response to the epidemic. The alliance of science, people living with AIDS, community groups, the UN, governments and civil society demonstrated just how potent a united stand against HIV/AIDS can be. The conference . . . recognized that AIDS is a crisis of governance. It also recognized that failure to apply the tools and resources available is a political issue. Leadership saves lives. . . . The Durban conference was critical in mapping out the need for an immensely increased resource flow.
>
> (Joint United Nations Programme on HIV/AIDS, 2008, p. 112)

Piot was exceedingly effective with UNAIDS as his organisational platform in talking to the right people, presenting the information about an existent problem that he viewed as neglected. In his speech given at the London School of Economics in 2005 titled *Why AIDS is exceptional*, Piot presented his view as one that sees HIV/AIDS as the ultimate nemesis of economic and social development. His frame was one in which the pandemic stands as one of the biggest major barriers that negatively affect the way in which countries can mitigate poverty. Finally, he added, the fact that the disease has stigma surrounding it by nature of it being sexually transmitted has complicated the matter to an unacceptable extent; if only prejudice, awkwardness, and discomfort were out of the picture, perhaps the matter would have been dealt with far sooner.

The descriptions of the Durban conference have the markings of a tipping point at which the *norm cascade* that precipitated the internalisation of the HIV/AIDS health norm began in earnest. There is, however, no objective point at which this tipping point can be identified. In the short paragraphs that comprise the UN's AIDS-specific sub-portal of its official website, the author refers to the MDGs and the *Declaration of Commitment on HIV/AIDS* (UNGA, 2001) as the beginning of the UN's mitigatory efforts specifically related to the disease. This declaration, along with the MDGs themselves – which represent the ultimate indicator for this assessment of the completion of the final stage of the *norm life cycle* – stand as the clearest signs of *internalisation* of the HIV/AIDS health norm:

> By this time, the securitization of the epidemic became a recognized international norm. This norm held a series of understandings, policy prescriptions and recommendations about the epidemic, which were internationally promoted as the panacea for efficient HIV/AIDS interventions.
>
> (Vieira, 2007, p. 168)

The commitments were reaffirmed at a 2006 high-level UN meeting, which also called for ambitious national targets on the road towards universal access to prevention and treatment of HIV/AIDS (UNGA, 2006).

As a regional punctuation to this process, African leaders made their own contribution. In April 2001, African heads of state met in Nigeria under the auspices of the OAU for "a Special Summit devoted specifically to address the exceptional challenges of HIV/AIDS, Tuberculosis and Other Related Infectious Diseases" (OAU, 2001, p. 1). In its outcome document, the *Abuja Declaration*, concerns of threats related to both human and state security are amplified:

> We recognise that the epidemic of HIV/AIDS, Tuberculosis and Other Related Infectious Diseases constitute not only a major health crisis, but also an exceptional threat to Africa's development, social cohesion, political stability, food security as well as the greatest global threat to the survival and life expectancy of African peoples. These diseases, which are themselves exacerbated by poverty and conflict situations in our Continent, also entail a devastating economic burden, through the loss of human capital, reduced productivity and the diversion of human and financial resources to care and treatment.
>
> (OAU, 2001, p. 3)

At the summit, the creation of what would become the Global Fund to Fight AIDS, TB and Malaria was suggested by Kofi Annan, who would personally make the first monetary contribution to its endowment. The creation of the fund was supported by all the summit participants in the *Abuja Declaration* and endorsed by the UNGA and the G8 that following summer; it established its first secretariat in January of 2002. Annan, along with Kingsley Amoako, was also a central figure in establishing the Commission on HIV/AIDS and Governance in Africa (CHGA) in 2003. CHGA was intended to oversee governance on HIV/AIDS in Africa, by (1) working to clarify the impact of the disease on economic and state structure on the continent and (2) working with governments to develop and implement various policies aimed towards minimising the adverse effects of these impacts.

Earlier signs include the fact that the pandemic is mentioned more than 30 times in the 1999 resolution which defines key actions for the fulfilment of the ICPD agreements (UNGA, 1999). The mentions include specific goals that focus on limiting infections through the diffusion of both contraceptives and information. A section of *We the Peoples* (Annan, 2000) also qualifies as an indicator of an ongoing cascade. As suggested, the report put most of the emphasis of its entire section on disease squarely on HIV/AIDS. As Rushton suggests,

> [c]rucially, it is the international development aspects of AIDS which are highlighted in this section of the text (which focuses strongly on Africa). In addition to noting that HIV/AIDS "threatens to reverse a generation of accomplishments in human development" the report explicitly links it with other development challenges such as education and nutrition.
>
> (Rushton, 2010, p. 9)

Over the course of these two or three relevant pages, Secretary-General Annan focuses largely on harrowing statistics regarding HIV/AIDS from the developing world in particular, particularly emphasising the plight and tragedy of children and those infected prenatally. The *Declaration of Commitment* that followed the 2001 UNGA Special Session covers a broad array of issues to which HIV/AIDS is related. The general argument is that the pandemic is responsible for exacerbating problems already present in developing countries: the points of connection run the gamut from negative effects on the practical attainment of human rights, capabilities, and the undermining of social and economic development. Particular concern is directed towards the most vulnerable demographic: namely, women, young adults, and children (particularly girls). Social cohesion and stigma are also included in the list, as are many other factors. In short, the pandemic is viewed as directly or indirectly detrimental to nearly all dimensions of development as well as to *political stability* in countries and potentially entire regions, with Sub-Saharan Africa being especially susceptible.

This type of frame connects the pandemic to countless other recognisable and negative realities within the sphere of development and is an effective way of creating and/or highlighting the emergent norm's adjacency to established ones. It creates a narrative in which, if one ignores HIV/AIDS, one also indirectly ignores the issues of poverty, inequality, health, marginalisation, and a slew of others. Indeed, the image created is that development at large is under threat by the pandemic. Add to this is the unfortunate fate of children and unborn infants contracting the disease, and the normative package becomes very difficult to ignore, let alone oppose. This effect was compounded by a growing global emphasis on the individual as the referent object of security – itself a normative package – that

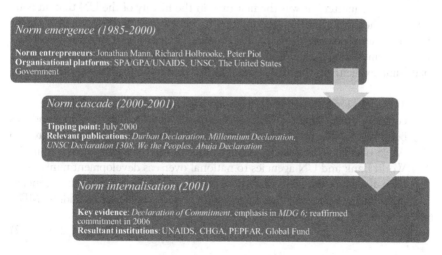

*Figure 5.2* The norm life cycle of HIV/AIDS in the MDGs

was growing in scope (and which had been explicitly espoused by the UNDP since the beginning of the 1990s. Though the relevance of HIV/AIDS to state security is salient – explored in its apparent securitisation considered later – the position of the pandemic as a human security issue made the effort adoptable by different categories of stakeholders: "HIV/AIDS clearly falls into this latter categorisation of [human] security, which led to the adoption of this broad perspective by a wide range of governments, multilateral agencies and academics" (Vieira, 2007, pp. 144–145).

The particular matter of HIV/AIDS differs from the other two health MDGs discussed earlier (and, indeed, the other half of MDG 6) in that it balances the line between high and low politics in a way that is quite unique for a pandemic, which disproportionately affects the poverty-stricken in developing countries. In Chapter 3, HIV/AIDS was presented in the context of securitisation. Notable in this context was *Security Council Resolution 1308* (UNESC, 2000), which is often regarded as the key moment of this process. There is some disagreement between observers regarding the extent to which this resolution *actually* securitised the pandemic (McInnes & Rushton, 2010; O'Manique, 2005; Vieira, 2007, 2011). Regardless, HIV/AIDS had by this time certainly cemented itself on the security agenda and could be viewed within a frame of state security as well as within a frame of human security: "HIV/AIDS has been framed as a public health problem, a development issue, a humanitarian crisis, a human rights issue and a threat to security" (Shiffman, 2009, p. 609). In the resolution, the characteristics of the pandemic are described as potentially having "a uniquely devastating impact on all sectors and levels of society . . . the HIV/AIDS pandemic, if unchecked, may pose a risk to stability and security" (UNESC, 2000, p. 1). The very fact that the UNSC – whose primary responsibility lies in ensuring the maintenance of international security and peace – would issue such a powerful statement, added weight to the matter: "it was the first time in the history of the UN that an issue related to health rather than the military had been considered a potential threat to international security" (Vieira, 2011, p. 4). The passing of this resolution may have informed the UN and Kofi Annan's decision not only to include the specific pandemic explicitly in the forthcoming MDGs, but to have it take centre stage.

> The inclusion of HIV and AIDS amongst the MDGs is perhaps the most concrete embodiment of the success of the development framing, and has been responsible for driving much of the increase in resources devoted to AIDS over the past decade. A huge range of international actors – from the World Bank and UN agencies to national overseas development ministries – formally align their goals with those set out in the MDGs, and new agencies, including the Global Fund, have been created specifically to address MDG targets.
>
> (Rushton, 2010, p. 7)

Inferential evidence suggests that the pandemic had become at least partially securitised in the way that it was prioritised in terms of resource allocation. "For instance, in the early 2000s HIV/AIDS received more than one-third of all major donor funding for health despite representing only around 5% of the mortality and morbidity burden in low and middle-income countries" (Shiffman, 2009, p. 608). Moreover, spending limited to within the scope of the disease has also not proven to be needs based. PEPFAR, an initiative that has saved the lives of a number in excess of 10 million people, initially prioritised providing assistance to countries whose numbers were far less severe than others. For example, Vietnam received funding while Malawi did not, in spite the latter having more than four times the number of infected individuals. The ability of the HIV/AIDS pandemic to accommodate concerns of altruism and self-interest at the same time may have contributed to the rapidity of its cascade and inclusion in the framework, as well as its exceptionalism. As the UN's fact sheet on *AIDS as a security issue* suggests, "[g]lobally, HIV/AIDS has emerged as a threat to *both human and national security* – so much so that it has become a concern for the [UNSC]" (UN, n.d.a, para.1). Indeed, this was the frame in which the mentioned norm entrepreneurs operated.

> *securitising actors/norm leaders* [sic] used both national and human security arguments to spread the idea that, because HIV/AIDS threatens the security/ survival of a referent object (either states or human beings), the epidemic should be treated as a special kind of emergency. As shown next, the new theorising about the security impact of the global HIV/AIDS epidemic, cou- pled with the growing acknowledgment of its multidimensional and destruc- tive impact, promoted a turn in the way the epidemic would be responded to.
> (Vieira, 2007, p. 146, original emphasis)

Whatever the proportions of the various motivations for combatting HIV/ AIDS, their aggregate effect resulted in an unparalleled prioritisation of the epi- demic within the scope of the health MDGs. The plurality of security concerns now facing states previously concerned primarily with the immediate threats of the Cold War, in combination with the related cluster of *softer* concerns such as human security, and the larger project of human development, created fer- tile ground in which an agenda focused on HIV/AIDS could take centre stage. Added to this was the effective framing of the disease's connection with virtually all other aspects of development. The heavy emphasis on this specific pandemic relied on its superposition of belonging to high and low politics alike, of relat- ing simultaneously to state and human security. While coordinating attempts to minimise the impact of the disease was normatively difficult to argue with in the first place, its skewed position in relation to other diseases in the MDGs can be attributed to the extra motivation brought about by its (real or perceived) secu- ritisation, orchestrated in part by individuals with organisational platforms such as Holbrooke and Piot.

The normative strengths discussed earlier regarding the abatement of general disease in global development efforts are equally valid for HIV/AIDS. Specific characteristics, however, amplified these norms and contributed to the excep- tionalism evidenced in the emphasis the pandemic received in MDG 6 and its preceding, ancillary documents. In terms of intrinsic characteristics, the goal is clear and specific; there is little doubt as to what the problem is and why it must be addressed. Though the bulk of the problems were located in developing countries, its status as a *pandemic* meant that HIV/AIDS – unlike malaria – had more universalistic properties which made it 'closer to home' for the Global North. Medically, HIV/AIDS has the unfortunate effect of being transmitted to unborn children: "it is a disease that attacks the young disproportionally [sic], its worst effects are concentrated in poor countries and it has a hideous potential to expand" (Annan, 2000, p. 26). In several sub-Saharan African countries, the disease directly contributed to significantly reduced life expectancies. A large number of mothers were affected, leading to higher rates of orphaning. In sum, the majority of the victims of this disease were the most vulnerable populations imaginable; in addition, the fact that the scope of the problem was growing rapidly added a sense of urgency to the matter. However, other diseases – particularly malaria – had similarly terrible and wide-reaching effects. Yet, being as atrocious as it is, the uniqueness of HIV/AIDS and its place in the MDGs cannot be reduced and attributed purely to its intrinsic characteristics.

Investigating the features that relate more to the *form* and framing of the issue helps generate a greater understanding of HIV/AIDS' augmented position. In terms of the variable of legitimisation, there was little doubt that many developing countries – especially in Africa – had populations with high infection rates. The pressure of a growing problem would make governments highly motivated to support a scaling up of the efforts to halt it. In developed countries, activism aimed towards increasing willingness to address the issue of HIV/AIDS had been present since the 1980s. In general, any policy stance attempting to minimise the extent of the problem would have been detrimental to the legitimacy of the transgressing government. Prioritising it at a level that may have been more elevated than was actually necessary (directly related to the efforts of Richard Holbrooke) was partly a result of the *prominence* of those initially responsible for this elevation. The authority of the endorsing actors involved in prioritising the issue, first with the U.S., and subsequently followed by the UNSC – perhaps the most prominent assemblage of states on the world stage with a global near-legislative authority (Talmon, 2005) – made general compliance practically unavoidable.

In the New Zealand comedy series *Flight of the Conchords*, one scene features the two struggling musician protagonists in a meeting with their manager. The conversation is centred on the band's intention to compose a song that raises awareness for canine epilepsy, in an attempt to win over a love interest whose dog is afflicted with the condition. Their manager expresses concern with the idea and argues that they may end up alienating the part of the target audience that are *for* canine epilepsy. He goes on to say that the same would be true if they were to write a song that was anti-HIV/AIDS; they risk losing potential fans that are pro-*HIV/AIDS*. The scene then continues to play on this theme, enhancing the absurdity of the manager's concerns. The absurdity, of course, stems from the intuitive and empirical observation that the existence of such a demographic is difficult to imagine. Therefore, there was little risk of a serious challenge by *antipreneurs*, or of an 'unholy alliance' pushing back on the idea of the inclusion of targets that would reduce the spread and impact of HIV/AIDS in the development agenda.

A relevant outlier is the failed *antipreneurship* of Thabo Mbeki, South Africa's second post-apartheid president from 1999 to 2008. While decidedly not *pro-HIV/AIDS*, Mbeki infamously rejected the notion that AIDS was caused by HIV, a connection held as being beyond dispute by the overwhelming majority of the global scientific community. ARVs were declared toxic, and alternative treatments including garlic, African potatoes, and beetroot were suggested. Resultant policies under Mbeki's rule saw hundreds of thousands of South Africans with HIV denied access to ARVs, leading to their premature and/or preventable deaths, including notable numbers of deaths resulting from prenatal mother-to-child transmission (Chigwedere, Seage, Gruskin, Lee, & Essex, 2008; Diethelm & McKee, 2009). The effects of the denialism, however, attracted little but disdain and ridicule outside of marginal scientific communities and fringe groups within the contemporary South African government. In the end, the South African Cabinet, enabled by the constitution, instigated a secret ballot that produced a policy that declared the connection between HIV and AIDS; in GHG and global development discourse, the matter was considered a tragic nuisance more than a serious contender in the policy space surrounding HIV/AIDS at the time. South Africa's reputation as a global health actor had been tarnished, and its clout diminished.

Relatedly, the concept of *world-time context* also comes into play. The aspects of globalisation and the end of the Cold War, the shift of the referent object of security migrating from state to individual, were central to the evolution of this norm, as it was for the emergence and subsequent internalisation of the human development paradigm. Medically, globalisation allows the virus to spread globally, creating the conditions in which the securitisation of HIV/AIDS could be carried out. Indeed, as discussed in Chapter 3, the 1990s was full of securitisation processes of health and infectious disease in general, with HIV/AIDS being the most exemplar. Faced with a concurrent normative wave of human rights and human security, the pandemic catered to concerns related to traditional notions of security as well as the softer side of health and politics that had recently begun to infiltrate the global normative establishment. The motives for states to endorse and adopt such an unbalanced prioritisation on HIV/AIDS therefore covered all the bases. The perceived threat to state security could work together with fulfilling the duties of taking responsibility for human security within and between borders, and helping to further the cause of global development.

## Conclusion

This chapter applies Finnemore & Sikkink's *norm life cycle* to analyse the emergence and diffusion of the prevailing health norms comprising the three MDGs specific to health development. The chapter identifies norm entrepreneurs and analyses narrated events in the light of the material presented in previous chapters. It begins with a brief reflection on the characteristics of UN-led summits and conferences in relation to mechanics of normative cementation and distribution. Next, the three health MDGs are treated in numerical order.

MDG 4 on reducing child mortality was a largely uncontroversial and uncomplicated normative package that required no norm entrepreneur to initiate a diffusion process. Though they became more explicit, clearly defined, placed within a human development context, and quantified in a set of goals at the 1990 *World Summit for Children*, norms related to child mortality were already relatively internalised within global development discourse. This may be related to the intrinsic normative characteristics related to the intention, as it aims to protect the vulnerable and innocent from physical discomfort, harm, and death. What had changed was the framing of this objective: the new approach inspired by the human development paradigm shifted the focus from the assumption that betterment of children's health would – among other benefits – come as a result of modernisation or of market liberalisation. The fact that high child mortality rates primarily affect poverty-stricken populations also put the goal in line with the overarching super-norm denominator of the general framework, further strengthening its chances of inclusion as an MDG.

Much of the same can be said about the components of maternal mortality that were included in the original edition of MDG 5. They aimed to reduce preventable suffering and deaths of a particularly vulnerable group, who in turn are responsible for another vulnerable group – namely infants – whose health is safeguarded in the previous goal. Omitting such a problem area would be considered inappropriate. On the other hand, the component of reproductive health, at least partly adopted by the UN at the ICPD of 1994, was only added to the goal nearly a decade after its original conception. The norms associated with this component, while universal in application and necessity, were not as viscerally connected to death and suffering as birth-related mortality rates. Crucially, they were not culturally value neutral, and faced significant opposition from untraditional religious case-specific coalitions who orchestrated shrewd political manoeuvring ahead of the *Millennium Declaration* – successful in part because of Kofi Annan's desire for full consensus, particularly from developing countries.

Reproductive health was also unable to appeal to health norms related to the category of statist security, something that HIV/AIDS managed to invoke to great effect. Again, there is a separation in the various components of MDG 6 that becomes salient in a discussion of its normative components. The inclusion of malaria 'and other (communicable) diseases', particularly and disproportionately affecting the poor are part and parcel of the human security-laden approach of the human development paradigm, while also consolidating the *super-norm* of poverty eradication that unifies all the MDGs. These mentioned diseases, however, are more accurately described as a side note of the goal that focuses most of its attention on reducing the spread and dire consequences of the HIV/AIDS pandemic. While addressing a real concern in the developing world as an inherent negative and as an inhibitor of development (such as the other diseases mentioned), HIV/AIDS was also a concern for developed countries, and the issue threatened human security and statist security alike, as explicitly stated by the UNGA itself.

Conclusions drawn from this analysis are somewhat of a mixed bag that – to an extent – question the linearity and variability of the *norm life cycle* framework, particularly in view of the reproductive health norms only retroactively included in MDG 5. In relation to the issue of HIV/AIDS, the implication is that health norms that cover simultaneous rationales from state security and human security are more likely to gain a prominent position in the development agenda; those that are limited to the frame of human security professed by the human development paradigm require nearly full congruence with the characteristics beneficial to the successful diffusion of an emerging norm.

## Notes

1 The most recent reinforcements of this had been the Convention on the Rights of the Child, a treaty adopted by the UNGA in November 1989. Previous iterations of similar value statements include, most notably, the 1924 Geneva Declaration of the Rights of the Child and the Declaration of the Rights of the Child adopted by the UNGA in 1959. There are also significant mentions in more specified sections of the UDHR; the International Covenant on Civil and Political Rights; and the International Covenant on Economic, Social and Cultural Rights. The rights of the child is also a central tenet in specialised agencies such as UNICEF.
2 Human capital refers to human attributes, such as skills, knowledge, and experience that can be quantified and assessed as being of cost or value to a particular business or country (see Becker, 1994).
3 A standard definition of family planning is the practice of controlling the number of children produced, as well as the temporal intervals between each offspring. Contraception of various types constitutes the main method in family planning, with the more momentous actions of sterilisation and abortion also belonging to this category.
4 The *Women's Declaration on Population Politics* was a document written and published by the IWCH in preparation for the ICPD. The *Declaration* essentially advocates a revision of how population policies are conceived and conducted and that the new approach should revolve around ensuring the empowerment of women, particularly through reproductive health. The *Declaration* was co-authored by Germain and two economists and women's rights activists, Geeta Sen and Lincoln Chen.
5 Illustrative of the growing scope of the problem is that the Belgrade Conference had more than twice the number of participants than a conference on the exact same topic that had taken place 11 years earlier.
6 An unholy alliance refers to an alliance or a coalition that is largely deemed undesirable and antagonistic. These alliances are typically made from parties that are not necessarily compatible in a general ideational sense, but whose interests may temporarily align, thus motivating the partnership.
7 The HRP provided a definition of reproductive health to be used at the ICPD – it was approved with only one amendment (Benagiano et al., 2012).
8 The Group of 77 at the UN is a coalition of nations in the developing world. Its purpose is to align collective economic interests and subsequently to provide a joint negotiating capacity from which these interests can be promoted.

9  Three of these are declarations for *further actions and initiatives* to implement the commitments made at the ICPD in 1994, the Beijing Women's Conference in 1995, and the Copenhagen Summit for Social Development in 1995, respectively. While HIV/AIDS is mentioned in the original outcome documents of these conferences, it is nearly exclusively mentioned in the same sentence as other diseases such as malaria and tuberculosis; it had not yet reached its elevated position.

10 Indeed, Piot is credited with co-discovering Ebola in 1976 while working at the London School of Hygiene and Tropical Medicine.

# 6    The health norms of the Sustainable Development Goals

This chapter identifies, describes, and explains the health norms that effectuated novelties in health development policy in the UN's post-2015 development agenda. The chapter is structured in a manner that incrementally narrows in on the health norms that are under investigation by means of the *norm life cycle*. The chapter is divided into three main sections. The opening section provides the most salient parts of the wider normative context in which the SDGs were formulated. It begins by focusing on lessons gleaned from the successes and the failures of the MDGs, before exploring the implications related to the continued realisation of the human development paradigm. Following this is an account of the new imperatives of the post-2015 development agenda – namely, *sustainability* and *inclusivity* – and how these normative concepts were introduced as primary and secondary *leitfmotifs* that together set the tone with which all the goals and targets aim to harmonise. *Sustainability* is the main focus throughout the section, which suggests that it arguably belongs in the category of *super-norm* in relation to the SDG framework, in the same way that *poverty eradication* did for the MDGs.

With this as a foundation, the next section introduces the single explicit health SDG. First, its features are represented and categorised into three groups: (1) targets that carry forward those that featured in the MDGs, (2) targets that are new to global development goal setting and form the focus of the subsequent health norm analysis, and (3) side-targets that are meant to improve and ensure implementation. Following this is an exploration of the specific connections between health and the imperatives of sustainability and inclusivity. These connection points are integral to the evolution of the final product that is the *health SDG*, because the aforementioned imperatives set the parameters for what is relevant in the pursuit towards the ultimate ends of development in the post-2015 framework.

With the general and health-specific normative context in place, the final section features two sets of health norms and their norm life cycles. The first norm life cycle relates to the inclusion of various non-communicable diseases (NCDs), while the second is concerned with universal health coverage (UHC). The analysis provides accounts of how the introduction and inclusion of these – through accommodating sentiments of both human and state security in parallel – came to constitute the most significant shifts associated with health development goals in the post-2015 global development agenda. Among other factors taken into account, specific effects of the omnipresent variable of globalisation and its contingencies are considered as is the increased number of actors in the realm of global health.

## The shortfalls of the MDGs

A section of Chapter 2 provided a condensed version of the process that generated the SDGs (see Figure 2.2): the set of goals that came to embody the post-2015 development agenda that was officially presented in September 2015. The goals were the result of a multifaceted procedure that had been conceived as early as 2010 and then expanded and carried out in the years following. Numbering 17 rather than 8 goals, the SDGs were part continuation of the MDGs, part innovation and improvement, and part significant expansion of what constitutes development.

As suggested in the previous recounting of the general process that resulted in the formulation of the SDG framework as the emblem of the post-2015 development agenda, the new framework is still both explicitly and implicitly devoted to the ideas of the human development paradigm. The imperative that *people* are at the centre of the development effort still reigned supreme, though a caveat had now been appended in the form of *sustainability*. The latter implies that today's progress must not detract from future human beings' ability also to lead fulfilling lives, free from want and fear, with their capabilities intact. While present as a component in the MDGs, *sustainability* had now become the new heading under which this next chapter of global development was to be written. The intensified influence of the norms of sustainability is one of the topics that will be analysed in this chapter, with special focus on its many connections with health. Generally, the new agenda is anchored in the essential components of the human development paradigm meta-norm. The goal is to increase people's capabilities and to ensure that their rights remain central to the ends of development. The timeframe, however, had moved: rather than focusing on present and short- to medium-term concerns of, say, the next 15 years, sustainability entails long-term reflection; it is concerned with guaranteeing the capabilities of future generations as well as of present ones. The scope had also changed, and emphases on indirect determinants, interrelatedness, and holism characterised the approach.

Unlike the 1990s, the decade succeeding it was not exceptionally active in terms of normatively ritualistic summits and conferences. With an understanding of the nature of the current *meta-norm*, this lull is to be expected. Because the human development paradigm had become internalised on such a large scale after the 1990s, a rather dramatic shift in global values would have to precipitate its displacement – such a shift had not occurred. The delayed integration of reproductive health targets for MDG 5 was indicative of a trend suggesting the opposite: rights and equality–based norms that largely resonate with human development experienced increasing traction on a global scale over the course of the MDG years (Besson, 2013; Fukuda-Parr, 2016). Rather than seminal summitry, it was the time for implementation, of 'waiting and seeing', and of observing the inputs and outputs of the MDG framework. What informed the options of approach for the post-2015 era was less a normative reckoning (*à la* the human development paradigm's reaction to the traditional notions of modernisation and the more recent Washington Consensus–inspired approach of the 1980s) and more a lesson in practical experience. The rules had not changed significantly with the SDGs, but the scope had widened, while the techniques of effectuation, implementation, and emphasis had – at least theoretically – improved.

As explained in Chapter 2, the initial period of the MDG framework amounted to a period of monitoring. The major impression from those first five or so years was that the project had experienced snags and drawbacks relatively quickly. For example, important donor states were not committing sufficient resources to ODA – the U.S. being the most prominent culprit. While efforts such as the *Millennium Campaign* and the *Millennium Project* were launched, and the *Monterrey Consensus* established, the enterprise, at large, continued to underperform, and projections after these first few years were already rather bleak. The 2005 *World Summit* was partly a rallying cry for member states to cease their business-as-usual attitudes and to magnify their efforts: developing countries needed to take more responsibility, and donor countries simply needed to give more of their resources, open up trade, and ease debt burdens. By 2008, however, even the most optimistic observers had begun to lose faith in the plausibility of reaching the set goals; newly appointed UN General-Secretary Ban Ki-moon went as far as assessing the situation as a potential "development emergency" (Ban, 2008, p. 2). By 2010 the attitude of many MDG-related publications had shifted from the optimism that had been slowly waning over the years towards a defensive narrative attempting to limit the extent to which the endeavour would eventually undershoot its objectives.

## The shift: from MDGs to SDGs

As suggested earlier, the SDGs are, in many ways, a continuation of the MDGs, altogether dependent on the existence of their predecessors. In attempting the second iteration, a person, society, or an organisation assesses what has succeeded and what has not. In the next version, the actor builds on successes and learns from mistakes, adjusting future actions accordingly in order to maximise the chances of positive results. In a personal setting, these adjustments are often subconsciously orchestrated, though particularly conscientious individuals may cultivate organised self-improvement schemes with professional systematism. In an organisational setting, conscientiousness is institutionalised and serves as a key mechanism in assessing the past, present, and future, in attempts to optimise on the basis of past experiences and present opportunities. IOs, in spite of all their exceptional qualities, are no exceptions. On the contrary, they do well to be as thorough as possible, as large-scale UN projects, for instance, face a significant – though justified – amount of public scrutiny from the watching eyes of laymen and expert observers alike. In its first decade, the MDG framework was the beneficiary of reviews ranging from scathing maledictions to felicitous praise, from opinion pieces to journal articles and conferences through to government policy reactions. For all its insufficiencies, the MDG project had a gravity about it that had made it the world's business. It is therefore unsurprising that an exceptionally elaborate process to find the optimal solutions to a post-2015 agenda was initiated as early as 2011. In normative terms, this was a process that partly further internalised the established norms of the MDGs and partly one in which large and small-scale emergent norms were coming to the fore and cascading into mainstream development thinking and practice. The ambition of the next step was clear: carry the momentum of the MDGs. While the essence of human development and quantifiable goals would be retained, other major aspects of the framework would require significant refurbishment through the elimination and replacement of the different levels of problems and complications that had become clear over time – in terms of conception, operationalisation, and implementation (Sachs, 2012).

First to be examined: the auspicious properties of *momentum*. The MDGs *had been* a success story in a number of different ways, and the aspirational actions towards their fulfilment are rather uncontroversially responsible for the improvement of millions of lives across the developing world. As the UN and its more specified sub-organisations like to emphasise, the MDGs had been instrumental in creating a truly global set of goals for development, which in turn orchestrated the largest coordinated and successful endeavour in the history of global development. Ban Ki-moon, in the foreword of the final MDG report, published in 2015, characterises the effort as a 'landmark commitment' and states that:

> [T]he MDGs helped to lift more than one billion people out of extreme poverty, to make inroads against hunger, to enable more girls to attend school than ever before and to protect our planet. They generated new and innovative partnerships, galvanized public opinion and showed the immense value of setting ambitious goals. By putting people and their immediate needs at the forefront, the MDGs reshaped decision-making in developed and developing countries alike.
>
> (Ban in UN, 2015, p. 3)

Indeed, the strides taken toward improving those metrics that had come to define what constituted development had been unprecedented in the period 2000–2015. These metrics were, of course, defined in the creation of the MDG framework, and each of them experienced progress in absolute numbers. During the last five or so years of the framework's timeframe, most observers agreed with the general sentiment that the MDGs had been a laudable attempt, an important call to arms that had changed the face of coordinated global development efforts (see Sachs, 2012). Bill Gates, in 2013, called the MDGs "the best idea for focusing the world on fighting global poverty that I've ever seen" (Gates in Browne, 2017, p. 89).

The first report of the UN System Task Team on the post-2015 UN development agenda, *Realizing the Future We Want for All: Report to the Secretary-General* (UNSTT, 2012) includes a section that seems to fit with the contemporary general consensus regarding the *métiers* of the MDGs. The first strength highlighted in the report comprises the framework's concrete goals and targets, which are thought to provide focus and a sense of priority to action, as well as transparency in progress. Further,

> the format of the MDG framework brought an inspirational vision together with a set of concrete and time-bound goals and targets that could be monitored by statistically robust indicators. This has not only helped keep the focus on results, but also motivated the strengthening of statistical systems and use of quality data to improve policy design and monitoring by national governments and international organizations.
>
> (UNSTT, 2012, p. 6)

Another positive feature was the success of MDG 8, which focused on building a global partnership for development. The total quantity of ODA had increased significantly throughout the timeframe, as had the quality of its allocation; trade was made easier and more favourable in the developing world, and the proportion of external debt service to export revenue was reduced.

However, there is little doubt that the MDGs were fraught with shortcomings. Most of the goals were never reached, and in some places, very far from it. Some (Vandemoortele, 2009) suggest that the goals of the MDGs were perhaps not realistically supposed to be reached but were rather to act as motivation and encouragement. The point was not to be entirely successful, but to successfully *identify* problems and subsequently *accelerate* progress towards reaching them, towards the idea of human development. Regardless, though significant progress had been made, the goals had largely not been fulfilled. In the aforementioned foreword to the *2015 MDG report*, Ban Ki-moon concedes that progress had been uneven and incomplete. Significant changes needed to be made in order for the *post-2015 agenda* to have a greater chance of succeeding (see Table 2.3 for one suggestion). While keeping with the spirit of the MDGs, these changes included aspects of framing, prioritisation, emphasis, process, content, and implementation.

## The foundational normative structure of the post-2015 agenda

As implied earlier, the transition from the MDG to SDG framework was not characterised by a paradigmatic normative shift comparable to the rather grand entrance of the ideas of human development that emerged and subsequently cascaded from the late 1980s throughout the 1990s (see Figure 4.1). Explicit signs of this normative stability can be found throughout the various publications and reports that emanated from the preparatory processes as well as from the outcome document for the summit for the adoption of the post-2015 development agenda in September of 2015, at which the SDGs were officially presented:

> The new Agenda is guided by the purposes and principles of the Charter of the United Nations, including full respect for international law. It is grounded

in the Universal Declaration of Human Rights, international human rights treaties, the Millennium Declaration and the 2005 World Summit Outcome. It is informed by other instruments such as the Declaration on the Right to Development. . . . *We reaffirm the outcomes of all major United Nations conferences and summits which have laid a solid foundation for sustainable development and have helped to shape the new Agenda.* These include the Rio Declaration on Environment and Development, the World Summit on Sustainable Development, the World Summit for Social Development, the Programme of Action of the International Conference on Population and Development, the Beijing Platform for Action and the United Nations Conference on Sustainable Development. We also reaffirm the follow-up to these conferences, including the outcomes of the Fourth United Nations Conference on the Least Developed Countries, the third International Conference on Small Island Developing States, the second United Nations Conference on Landlocked Developing Countries and the Third United Nations World Conference on Disaster Risk Reduction.

(UNGA, 2015, pp. 4–5, authors' emphasis)[1]

The clear dominance of human development–era outcome documents is illustrative of the extent to which the development norms of the human development paradigm had internalised within the UN system by the end of the MDG era. The norm pool had not changed significantly over the last decade and a half, nor was it completely the same. Most notably, poverty eradication, the *super-norm* of the MDGs (Fukuda-Parr & Hulme, 2009), was no longer the undisputed protagonist of the global development agenda. Other issues had – though always present beneath the surface – ascended to a position that warranted them significantly more attention than previously given. In terms of the contents of the new framework and its goals, the most salient of these for the general approach is the elevation of *sustainability* to the position of *super-norm* for the post-2015 development agenda. Further, the more specific sectors and subsectors of development also experienced reorganisation and the introduction of new classifications and approaches to goals and sub-goals. Some of these are related to sustainability, while others address shortcomings of the previous framework or issue areas that had grown in scope to the extent that their omission would be conspicuous – for example, the increasingly unambiguous effects of climate change. The area of health was no exception to this, and the normative shifts within its sphere are the main points of interest featured in this chapter.

Although sustainability entered the fray as a new main feature of the agenda, it did not appear from an extraneous source separate from, or in competition with, the human development paradigm. On the contrary, the two are complementary:

The literatures on human development and sustainable development, or sustainability for short, have long been separate. This is surprising. On a very fundamental level, human development is what sustainability proponents want to sustain and without sustainability, human development is not true human development. . . . If human development is about enabling people to lead long, healthy, educated and fulfilling lives, then sustainable human development is about making sure that future generations can do the same. But in some sense adding 'sustainable' as a prefix is superfluous, *since human development without being sustainable cannot be true human development.*

(Neumayer, 2012, pp. 561–562), authors' emphasis)

The other major normative injection in the new framework was that of *inclusivity*, a concept that affected the new agenda on two distinct levels. Aside from influencing the content of the new *post-2015 agenda* with an emphasis, the new priority on inclusivity also had an intended effect on the *process* of the construction of it, achieved by a heavy emphasis on including the input of all stakeholders to inform the policy end-product (i.e. the SDGs). Rather than top UN-representatives and their DAC colleagues agreeing on the global goals in a closed meeting, various mechanisms had been designed to collect contributions from members of all levels of society on a global scale – including experts, civil society representatives, government officials, academics, workers; from young to elderly, developed to developing, rich to destitute, the idea was that everyone's voice was to be accounted for. The motto of *Leaving No One Behind*, as is examined more closely in a subsequent section of this chapter, thus had meaning and influence not only in terms of the actual content of the development goals but also in the process facilitating the conception and formulation of them.

## Sustainable development – a comeback story

As established earlier, the *meta-norm* of human development is implicitly or explicitly pervasive in the documents that emanated from the post-2015 consultation process. Two major changes from the MDGs are, however, topical to normative introduction of the new framework and its effect on the formulation of its goals, including those specific to health. The first and most significant is the introduction of the concept of *sustainability* as an overarching motif. This section provides an exploration of norms and policies related to sustainability, and sustainable development more specifically, which is the most important contextual variable of the post-2015 development agenda.

While not replacing the MDG *super-norm* of poverty eradication (Fukuda-Parr & Hulme, 2009), the concept of sustainability had evolved to fill a similar role – a new super-norm woven into concentric coexistence with the original. Just as poverty eradication is the theme that brings the MDGs together and that accommodates the health norms included in them, sustainability does much the same with the SDGs – most conspicuously evident in the naming of the new goals. To reiterate: a *super-norm* is a cluster of norms that are interrelated and that, when viewed together, comprise utilities and meanings greater than that of the sum of its parts. While the MDGs are informed by discrete norms relating more specifically to each goal, they also relate in some way to the higher-level concern of poverty eradication, as there are feedback loops between poverty and all the other issues addressed by the various goals – feedback loops that had been heavily emphasised before and during the incumbency of the MDGs. *Sustainability* takes on a similar role in the *post-2015 agenda*, though its holistic approach has even greater and more widespread implications for the formation of development policy; it aims to facilitate improvements focused on *everyone*, not just the poor in developing countries – though the latter population group still hold the top priority. As suggested in Chapter 2, the concept permeates the literature *along with* the continued problem of poverty. This permeation takes place on a few different levels. Most plainly, the aforementioned inclusion of the word *sustainability* as the leading explicit characteristic of the new framework of development goals speaks to its internalisation within the agenda and to the frame in which the new goals operate. A feature in the name, however, is only the tip of the iceberg of sustainability's benevolent incursion into the UN's global development *ethos*.

Since the publication of *Our Common Future*, better known as the *Brundtland Report* (1987), sustainable development has been a component of the development conversation, influencing policies in developed and developing countries alike (Hosseini & Kaneko, 2012). Indeed, the norms that predominated the discourse at the Rio Earth Summit in 1992 were clearly visible in the MDGs, and MDG 7 was directly dedicated to ensuring environmental sustainability. Kofi Annan's reflections on the issue in *We the Peoples* illustrate that the situation was rather dire already before the turn of the millennium and the MDG era: "we must face up to an inescapable reality: the challenges of sustainability simply overwhelm the adequacy of our responses. With some honourable exceptions, our responses are too few, too little and too late" (Annan, 2000, p. 56). While MDG 7 was deemed largely successful in achieving the sub-goals it had set out, environmental problems had certainly not diminished in the interim. In spite of progress in important areas, such as reducing deforestation and improving water sources for a significant number of people, larger, unaddressed problems had actually increased. Global emissions of carbon dioxide, for example, had doubled in the period since 1990. The adverse effects of these progressions were becoming less doubtful and more severe with every relevant report, most famously those published by the UN's own Intergovernmental Panel on Climate Change (IPCC).

As suggested, it had become increasingly clear by the turn of the decade that the MDGs would not live up to their full potential and that the goals were unlikely to be achieved. MDG 7 had been relatively successful, but inadequate in conception and execution alike; it would need to be expanded upon – the rationale being that without sustainability, any progress on human development may be nullified by environmental consequences. This sentiment is clear, for example, in a commentary written shortly before the drafting of the SDGs: "[i]t is not enough simply to extend the MDGs, as some are suggesting, because humans are transforming the planet in ways that could undermine development gain" (Griggs et al., 2013, p. 305). 'Business as usual' not being an option for the future is also an oft-repeated phrase. Generally, this is how sustainability is framed in the post-2015 framework documents: sustainability needs to be prioritised in order for development to have any effect at all in the future.

> Efforts to ensure global environmental sustainability have shown mixed results throughout the last 15 years. Much work remains for the post-2015 period, particularly given the acute environmental challenges the world is facing, such as climate change, food and water insecurity, and natural disasters. One theme emerging from the debate on the successor agenda to the MDGs is the importance of true integration of environment into development ambitions. Environmental sustainability is a core pillar of the post-2015 agenda and a prerequisite for lasting socioeconomic development and poverty eradication. Healthy, well-managed and diverse ecosystems and resources can play a strong role in mitigating future environmental challenges and improving livelihoods everywhere. Therefore, it is crucial to ensure that the development agenda for the future reflects the links between socioeconomic and environmental sustainability and protects and reinforces the environmental pillar.
>
> (UN, 2015, p. 61)

Some clarification is warranted as to the exact meaning of *sustainability*. As Moore, Mascarenhas, Bain, and Straus (2017) suggest, there is little or no clear consensus about the meaning of the term. In a video released on the UN's official YouTube channel in the days leading up to the Sustainable Development Summit in 2015 – at which the SDGs were formally adopted – the operational definition of sustainable development utilised by the narrator was not a novel conception. Instead, it is nearly identical to that formulated in the oft-cited, almost three decades old, *Brundtland Report*, which states that "Humanity has the ability to make development sustainable – to ensure that it meets the needs of the present without compromising the ability of future generations to meet their own needs" (Brundtland, 1987, p. 8). In *Agenda 21*, the main outcome document of UNCED (UN, 1992), as well as in the *Rio Declaration* emanating from the same summit, this same definition underlies the enormous number of policy recommendations that *were* to facilitate its realisation. In *We the Peoples*, Annan similarly proposes that "our goal must be to meet the economic needs of the present without compromising the ability of the planet to provide for the needs of future generations" (2000, p. 55). The *Millennium Declaration* (2000) also refers back to UNCED and *Agenda 21* when referencing sustainable development.

In other words, the definition of *sustainable development*, at least as far as the UN is concerned, has not changed since 1987, nor have the main contents of the norms encapsulated within it. Indeed, the major change that came to the fore in the build-up to the 2015 agenda was its centrality, saliency, urgency, and vogueishness – all contributing to strengthen the status of the sustainable development *super-norm*. Its contents had been further solidified in the interim at the two relevant summits that punctuate the timeline: namely, the WSSD in 2002 and Rio + 20 in 2012. Symptomatic of the two summits, which were both follow-up summits to 1992's influential UNCED – along with the traditional reaffirmation of previous commitments – is an intention to scale up the intensity and the influence of a sustainable development imperative. One avenue through which this would be done, particularly in the Rio+20 documents, would be through connecting sustainable development with the already established super-norm of poverty eradication, and by extension to all its related areas of concern.

> Eradicating poverty is the greatest global challenge facing the world today and an indispensable requirement for sustainable development. In this regard we are committed to freeing humanity from poverty and hunger as a matter of urgency. . . . We therefore acknowledge the need to further mainstream sustainable development at all levels, *integrating economic, social and environmental aspects* and recognizing their interlinkages, so as to achieve sustainable development in all its dimensions. . . . We recognize that poverty eradication, changing unsustainable and promoting sustainable patterns of consumption and production and protecting and managing the natural resource base of economic and social development are the overarching objectives of and essential requirements for sustainable development.
>
> (UNGA, 2012a, pp. 1–2, authors' emphasis)[2]

One measure of success in mainstreaming sustainable development in the project of global development at large – in other words, its *norm internalisation* – is its current status as the *pièce de résistance* of the post-2015 development agenda. Again, it is often stated that sustainability is now the second essential component and 'overarching objective' *along with* alleviating poverty, though the latter component needs no such emphasis. This is perhaps because by this time, the super-norm of poverty eradication had also become super-internalised – its status so ingrained in the relevant *ethos* as to be almost taken for granted, a framework named the *Poverty Development Goals* may well have been considered rather redundant. Making sustainable development the explicit structure within which all development goals operate was an act of framing that helped strengthen the norm of sustainability as well as a sign of its internalisation. Indeed, as the problem of poverty persisted post-MDGs, it would have been considered inappropriate to deprioritise it in the successor agenda – particularly, one explicitly built on the same normative foundation. Furthermore, poverty eradication is considered an essential component of the social dimension of sustainable development, which is further elaborated upon below. Framing relies partly on invoking imagery that is designed to elicit an emotional response. While poverty eradication conjured images of the destitute and emotions of sympathy and responsibility, the sustainability frame evokes responsibility not only for the planet's most destitute, but also for *all* future generations. Instilled in the imagery was also a sense of urgency that strongly suggested that a shift towards sustainable patterns of behaviour had to begin as soon as possible, lest a window of opportunity be lost.

Sustainable development was an approach that was reborn, reframed, and repositioned rather than one emerging from the left field in the context of the UN development agenda. As Dodds et al. (2014) point out, sustainability and development had been connected at least since the aforementioned *Brundtland Report* (1987), a report that recommended the convening of a conference on environment and development – realised five years later in the form of UNCED of 1992. Five years later, a WHO report suggests urgency on the matter: "it is argued that the move towards the notion of sustainable development arises from a meta-crisis facing the world. This meta-crisis comprises a set of three core crises of development, environment and security" (WHO, 1997, p. 29). However, 'planet-focused development' had, at some point, been deprioritised by the (at the time) separate sphere of 'people-centred development' (i.e. the human development paradigm) and its pronounced focal point of poverty eradication (Dodds, Donoghue, & Roesch, 2017). Indeed, the norms of environmental sustainability that had featured at UNCED and subsequently been admonished by *Agenda 21* were rather marginal in the *Millennium Declaration* and constituted an arguably isolated part of the MDG framework, in spite of the relative successes of MDG 7. The MDGs had tended to take attention away from topics they did not explicitly cover; Dodds et al. argue that the marginalisation of sustainability was further exacerbated in the aftermath of 9/11 and the ensuing shift towards a global focus on peace, (inter)national security, and terrorism. The WSSD, held in 2002 and designed to take stock of and recommit to the messages of the now 10-year old *Agenda 21*, and perhaps even add to the MDGs, was followed up with little vigour; its plan of implementation characterised as being eventually "reduced . . . to an insignificant and perhaps forgotten piece of paper" (Mbeki, 2006, p. 3). Emblematic of the mire that sustainable development found itself in around this time, was that the CSD failed to agree on a single policy outcome for the first time in its history when convening in 2007.

However, a major turning point occurred that same year, courtesy of Brazilian President Lula da Silva. In short, Lula petitioned the UNGA for a summit that would address global social inequality, suggesting that equality is a prerequisite for a safer global climate and thus for sustainability. Invoking the institutional memories associated with UNCED, which was held in Brazil, he suggested that 'our common heritage' was at serious risk unless a recommitment to sustainability could be negotiated. This was an effective act of framing on the part of the Brazilian and one that resonated with the UNGA. In a sense, Lula acted as an early and seminal norm entrepreneur, starting off a process that would elevate sustainable development to its current, central position. After a process of deliberation and lobbying, Brazil itself was tasked with hosting the conference that would become Rio+20 five years later.

Antecedents for the elevation of this narrative can be found in the latter half of the MDG period. For Dodds et al. (2014, 2017), development and sustainable development were two separate spheres until a series of events – some contemporaneous with the preparatory process of Rio+20 – acted to bring the two closer together. First, the ripple effects of the GFC were such that the very future of development was questioned, as were the legitimacy and stability of its arbiters; the crisis also served to amplify the increasing confluence of the agendas of the various follow-up commitments attendant to the two respective spheres of people-centred and planet-centred development. It also led to an elevation of the G20, which was considered a more appropriate forum for handling the crisis than the previously authoritative G8,[3] notably increasing the clout of the BRICS countries with regard to global economic policies (Lai & Ravenhill, 2012). This gradual normative and institutional convergence was also enhanced by the increasing political relevance of the climate change negotiations – such as the 2009 Copenhagen Conference – and by the increasing realisation by policymakers and negotiators acting on their behalf that climate change cuts across the social, economic, and environmental priorities of any national development agenda (Dodds et al., 2017). The 2009 UN Conference on the World Financial and Economic Crisis and Its Impact on Development as well as the 2010 High-Level Plenary Meeting of the UNGA on the MDGs further highlighted the connections between the economic, social, and environmental aspects of development.

These developments were accompanied by related legislation and value statements more or less related to the UN system, often spearheaded by individual governments and individuals and/or groups – acting as *norm entrepreneurs* – within governments. While Brazil has had its appropriate share of the spotlight and platforms upon which to espouse norms regarding sustainability for several decades, two other South American states have been central in advocating a normative position most commonly referred to as the *right of nature*. This position views nature – also described by proponents as *Mother Earth* – as a subject with innate rights. In 2008, Ecuador held a general vote that successfully introduced a new constitution that granted the country's forests, rivers, islands, and air these rights. Similar to how all human beings are held to have inalienable rights in the UDHR, the Ecuadorian people and its government decided that nature is entitled to its right "to exist, flourish and evolve within Ecuador. Those rights shall be self-executing, and it shall be the duty and right of all Ecuadorian governments, communities, and individuals to enforce those rights" (Faulkner & Johanson, 2018, p. 9).

The same norms inspired the 2010 Bolivia World People's Conference on Climate Change and the Rights of Mother Earth in Bolivia, which resulted in the *Universal Declaration on the Rights of Mother Earth*. The previous year, Bolivia – with President Evo Morales at the head – had been the driving force behind the eventual UNGA proclamation of *International Mother Earth Day* (UNGA, 2009). While the proclamation does not directly refer to *rights*, it promotes what is referred to as 'harmony with nature', emphasising the interdependence between natural ecosystems and human life on the planet. This proclamation has been followed by annual UNGA resolutions on *Harmony with Nature*, which espouse a non-anthropogenic relationship with nature. These are further accompanied by an annual *Report of the Secretary-General on Harmony with Nature*.

### Inclusivity: leaving no one behind

Another significant shift influencing the normative structure of the post-2015 agenda was a general movement towards inclusivity. While *inclusivity* is closely related to the already described social dimension of *sustainable development*, the concept is discussed in more depth in this section because of its extraordinary number of normative concentricities with sustainable health development. This may be because the social dimension can be argued to be the most *detectably normative* of the sustainable development trio, particularly because it carries a package of hot-topic norms – most notably *inequality* and *human rights*. *Inclusivity* is also given extra consideration because of what this study characterises as its dual effect on the *post-2015 agenda* – namely, both *process* and *content*.

As for the processual aspect, the major divergence from the process that facilitated the creation of the MDGs is the major emphasis that the formulation and composition of the post-2015 development agenda should be an inclusive process.

> Several inputs are critical of the process that led to the MDGs: the selection of the MDGs emerged from a technocratic closed-door process that was poorly specified, influenced by special interests, and lacked a coherent conceptual design or rigorous statistical parameters. . . . Other related criticisms are that the MDGs did not have enough input from low- and middle-income countries, and that the intended beneficiaries of the MDGs – people and communities – had no opportunity for involvement in the development and implementation of MDG actions.
>
> (WHO, 2013c, p. 24)

The rationale behind this is manifold: first, it was important that the agenda reflected, as accurately as possible, the development desires and aspirations of the world's groups, organisations, individuals, and governments. Second, such a process would inspire a greater sense of ownership and would contribute to augmenting the legitimacy of the framework (UNDP, 2014).

Inclusivity's influence on the process is somewhat different from the influence of the overarching meta-norm of human development, the sustainability supernorm, or indeed individual health-norms. While largely unexplored in IR or development studies, the field of conflict mediation and peace negotiation has experienced a surge of studies concerning norms of inclusivity in the last few years (Lanz, 2011; von Burg, 2015; Zanker, 2014). As Hellmüller, Federer, and Pring (2017) explain, the UN's guidelines on mediation explicitly encourage inclusivity, defined as "the extent and manner in which the views and needs of conflict parties and other stakeholders are represented and integrated into the process and outcome of a mediation effort" (UN, 2012). Hellmüller, Federer, and Zeller (2015) separate norms into various categories with regard to their meaning for a mediation process. *Inclusivity* is placed in the category of *process-related norms*, which are distinguished from *content-related norms*. Another way of separating the two categories is that the former concerns itself with *how* matters are being negotiated, rather than the latter's focus on *what* is being negotiated, such as the health norms discussed in the previous chapter; this is further discussed later. In this case, however, the *inclusivity norm* acts in a double position as process- and content-influencing.

*Inclusivity* was not a particularly controversial idea with which to imbue the *post-2015 agenda*-setting process. This new imperative was first and foremost a practical challenge, and the quest to achieve it multifaceted. The process entailed several subprocesses, each designed to gauge the views and sentiments of the various stakeholders in the process. In principle, this included representatives from all layers of society, their opinions mined through the various processes described briefly in Chapter 2 (see Tables 2.2 and 2.3). In the end, the statements given in the respective reports of these separate input groups were convergent and largely homogenous with regard to the general approach of the new framework. In particular, the overarching consensus reflected an intention to redouble the efforts of the previous framework, keeping aspects deemed successful, while attempting to reinvent aspects that in hindsight were unsatisfactory; placing special emphasis on the spheres of sustainability and inequality. By and large, the major points of agreement mainly reflect the general sentiments found in the Rio+20 outcome document *The Future We Want* (UNGA, 2012a).

Inclusivity would also come to influence the *content* of the goals in a significant way. The issue of unequal distribution of goals-related development had been lamented in the vast majority of official and unofficial publications reflecting on the successes and failures of the MDGs in the years leading up to their temporal conclusion and would have to be addressed and approached very differently.

> As we embark on this great collective journey, we pledge that no one will be left behind. Recognizing that the dignity of the human person is fundamental, we wish to see the Goals and targets met for all nations and peoples and for all segments of society. And we will endeavor to reach the furthest behind first.
>
> (UNGA, 2015, p. 3)

These sentiments are most explicitly encapsulated in the slogan 'Leaving no one behind', a secondary *leitmotif* of the SDGs and the *post-2015 agenda*. While fully harmonious with foundational tenets of the human development paradigm, the norms of social inclusivity and participation had been more subdued in the previous development framework, perhaps for reasons of inexperience, perhaps for the purpose of keeping the goals clearly quantifiable. As Stuart and Samman (2017) suggest, this new intention was perhaps the only appropriate way to correct one of the most inimical aspects that short-circuited the success of the MDGs – namely, the unequal distribution of progress within and between regions, countries, and population groups.

> 'Leave no one behind' aims to address two related concerns: ending absolute poverty – in all its forms, and ensuring that those who have been 'left behind' (in relative terms or absolute terms) can 'catch up' with those who have experienced greater progress. . . . In part, 'leave no one behind' is an anti-discrimination agenda. But it also goes well beyond this. Indeed, it is a recognition that expecting progress to trickle-down the socioeconomic scale is naïve, and

that explicit and proactive attempts are needed to ensure populations at risk of being left behind are included from the start.

(Stuart & Samman, 2017, p. 2)

For an endeavour launched in order to help those most in need, this had been a glaring failure. The reality and consequences of this fault – or naïveté – of the MDG framework, and the subsequent attempts to rectify it, seems to have been one of the most significant lessons gleaned by the UN ahead of formulating the *post 2015-agenda.* In large part, 'leaving no one behind' is not normatively new in development. Indeed, the vast majority of the general sentiments found in recent publications that address the concept of 'leaving no one behind' can be found in the *Copenhagen Declaration of Social Development* (UN, 1995a), and again in the *Millennium Declaration* (UNGA, 2000b). However, these good intentions did not equal successful implementation and execution.

The most noticeable shift in the relevant publications regarding the SDGs is twofold. First, the language is more reflective of regret, urgency, and complexity, replacing some of the more optimistic tone employed in the documents and declaration of the 1990s. Second, there is recognition that a far more focused effort is required to mitigate inequalities and social exclusion. In a paragraph following one that bemoans the shortcomings just described, one ECOSOC publication sums up the current stance towards the issue:

> Against this backdrop, inclusiveness and shared prosperity have *emerged* as core aspirations of the 2030 Agenda for Sustainable Development. A central pledge contained in the 2030 Agenda is to ensure that no one will be left behind and to see all goals and targets met for all nations, peoples and for all parts of society, endeavouring to reach the furthest behind first.
>
> (UN-DESA, 2016, p. 1, authors' emphasis)

This broadening, highly interrelated with the social dimension of sustainability, necessitated an expansion of the goals that would cover far more holistic issue areas than, for instance, specific communicable diseases, as will be discussed later. While the normative basis for this emphasis was not emerging in the sense described in the first phase of the *norm life cycle* (Finnemore & Sikkink, 1998), the ascension of inclusiveness and the dedication to equitable distribution to become a 'core aspiration' was a novelty.

While mitigating the unequal distribution of the benefits produced by MDGs was a great motivation for the new framework to focus on inclusivity and quality, another factor that fuelled the rise of inclusivity as a central new tenet was the symptomatic characteristics it shared with a shifting world time-context, in which the related norms of equality, transparency, and democracy had become increasingly internalised. As suggested, IOs must maintain and reinforce their legitimacy through their actions and image. One of the most fundamental criticisms of the MDGs was process related, directed towards the heavily exclusive process leading up to their formation. The critique highlighted the lack of diverse participants as well as the lack of transparency during the negotiations. These shortcomings – aside from inherently transgressing increasingly widespread norms of transparency that increasingly apply to global governance (Bernstein, 2011) and non-exclusion/non-discrimination – may also have resulted in producing suboptimal goals. This was due to its lack of diverse perspectives. Some argue, for example, that the fact that there were no women's rights organisations present in this phase may explain "the striking absence of gender in many of the development targets" (Wisor, 2012, p. 119). The context at the beginning of the production of a *post-2015 agenda* was partly created by the previous agenda itself, as the fame and gravity gained by the MDGs over the course of the framework's timeline – during which progress reports provided a far stronger degree of transparency – helped accentuate the expectations of a transparent and more representative process in creating the new framework.

### The normative characteristics of sustainability and inclusivity

This is not the place for a full norm life cycle analysis of the norms of *sustainability* and *inclusivity*, if such an analysis is even possible with such a multi-faceted normative cluster as the sustainability *super-norm*. However, a detailed analysis of their normative attributes is helpful for understanding the context from which subsequent health norms were conceived. In this regard, there are several properties worth mentioning that are recognisable from Finnemore and Sikkink's (1998) description of characteristics that tend to be favourable for the success of an emerging norm. Sustainability is a global, sweeping issue, potentially affecting all members of society, every socioeconomic group, in every geographical location. This does not detract from the fact that some vulnerable demographics are extra exposed to the prospective consequences of the issue, a characteristic that serves further to strengthen the norm's legitimacy and saliency. Aside from being universalistic and concerned with protecting the most vulnerable (in the first instance; eventually everyone), sustainability's adjacency to established norms is nearly unparalleled. Indeed, the looming consequences of not addressing the issue involve eradicating everything that people tend to care about and that are perceived to deteriorate and minimise capabilities and/or to hinder or reverse progress towards their attainment in the present or future.

*Direct* causality between the existence of an undesirable issue and non-adherence to a potentially mitigating norm is important for that norm to garner legitimacy and subsequent widespread adoption. For example, the norm of washing your hands before preparing food directly mitigates the unwanted presence of germs. Conversely, non-response to climate change is an example of how tentative and non-visceral linkages can serve as impediments for the effective dissemination of a norm. However, as evidence has mounted over the last two decades, climate change has become an increasingly pressing issue, with samples of its consequences already affecting the present global population. The scientific consensus on the topic has become less ambiguous, and public access and understanding of the issue has grown exponentially – to some extent owing to the Internet partially eclipsing traditional media as a source of information (Spartz, Su, Griffin, Brossard, & Dunwoody, 2017) – and has resulted in a growing public concern about climate change worldwide (Capstick, Whitmarsh, Poortinga, Pidgeon, & Upham, 2015). This represents a shift in the relevant aspects of the *world time-context* (Finnemore & Sikkink, 1998). Perhaps even more importantly, and particularly in relation to the rise of the norms connected to sustainability, is the global interdependence and interconnectedness that have resulted from globalisation (Kakabadse & Khan, 2016).

Like the global effects of disease (real or imagined) and economic systems, climate is a global phenomenon and it is in every state and organisation's interest to preserve it. Though the links between *globalisation, interdependency*, and *cosmopolitanism* are ambiguous, one would be hard-pressed to find serious organisations that are *anti-environment*[4] or – in a similar vein – *pro-HIV/AIDS*. Indeed, much like the aspiration to eradicate poverty or specific diseases, striving towards a stable and sustainable environment is, by and large, an uncontroversial inclination. Therefore, the content of most mainstream norms surrounding sustainability have not truly been contested since their emergence in the 1970s and 1980s (Dodds et al., 2017). However, the evolution and cascade of the *super-norm* of sustainability has taken longer to manifest. The spread of the super-norm is at least circumstantially evidenced in a number of trends that have materialised after the turn of the millennium. For example, most actors in the automobile industry are currently moving towards the manufacture of increasingly 'eco-friendly' products (Calabrese, 2016), and advertisements for cars in the low-emission range often emphasise this point heavily. The 2015 Volkswagen emissions scandal, in which the German manufacturer was exposed as having doctored emissions results for laboratory tests in order to comply with regulations, while vastly overstepping the regulations in 'real-world' driving, is an example of norm-breaking behaviour, and the consequences were quite publicly severe – legally, financially, and reputationally.

Related is the tendency over the last decade and a half of major corporations to cultivate 'green' images:

> The consumer market for green products and services was estimated at $230 billion in 2009 and predicted to grow to $845 billion by 2015. At the start of 2010, professionally managed assets utilizing socially responsible investing strategies, of which environmental performance is a major component, were valued at $3.07 trillion in the U.S., an increase of more than 380 percent from $639 billion in 1995. More companies are now communicating about the greenness of their products and practices in order to reap the benefits of these expanding green markets. Green advertising has increased almost tenfold in the last 20 years and nearly tripled since 2006. As of 2009, more than 75 percent of S&P 500 companies had website sections dedicated to disclosing their environmental and social policies and performance.
>
> (Delmas & Burbano, 2011, p. 64)

Corporations that take great care to emphasise their 'green products', especially those representing particularly infamous industry sectors – such as extractors of fossil fuels – are often accused of selectively disclosing "positive environmental actions while concealing negative ones to create a misleadingly positive impression of overall environmental performance" (Marquis & Toffel, 2012, p. 2) in a process derogatorily referred to as 'greenwashing'. The hospitality industry has also ventured into this area, an example being the Scandinavian hotel chain Nordic Choice Hotels and their decision to cease the serving and selling of all food products containing palm kernel oil[5] not proven to be sustainably farmed, as assessed by the relevant authority. Some hotels are also choosing to move away from plastic room access cards and are promoting the use of a specialised mobile application instead. More recently, a significant number of restaurants and cafés in South Africa ceased giving plastic straws to patrons due to the concern of sea-polluting plastic waste. In May 2018, the EU proposed legislation for the total ban of 10 single-use plastic products, such as straws and plastic cutlery.

Much like poverty eradication had been before its elevation in prioritisation from the 1990s onward, sustainability had existed as a nascent super-norm since at least the 1970s.[6] But while sustainability can hardly be considered an emerging norm in the period preceding the preparatory process to the *post-2015 agenda*, its elevation to current prominence significantly accelerated in the wake of Rio+20. The outcome document of this particular summit is essential to the *post-2015 agenda*-setting process – for one, it is the progenitor of several processes related to the eventual conception of the SDGs, including the request to assemble the OWG and its subsequent subprocesses and reports. Second, it was also responsible for mandating a process known as 'mainstreaming the three dimensions of sustainable development throughout the UN system' (United Nations Economic and Social Council, 2015). International organisations can change over time as they adopt emergent norms (Katzenstein, 1996); these normative absorptions can have *constitutive* and *regulative* effects on the given organisation. As was the case of the UNDP and the incursion of the human development paradigm as described in Chapter 4, the integration of norms of sustainability and inclusivity had a double effect on the UN: the identity of the organisation had explicitly been redressed as one emphasising the imperatives of sustainable development. Though not responsible for a normative revolution, these imperatives serve as complementary additions to the organisation's foundational value system; they also prescribe behaviours deemed appropriate within the parameters of this refurbished identity, exemplified in a developmental context by the naming and substance of the SDGs.

Viewed from a perspective of normative progression and diffusion, the norm of sustainability grew in saliency and urgency over the course of the MDG years, driven in large part by increasingly unambiguous science, the continued warming of the planet's mean temperature and the prospective and present consequences.

> Although specific definitions vary, sustainable development embraces the so-called triple bottom line approach to human wellbeing. . . . The urgency of the triple bottom line arises from a new realisation brought to global awareness by

earth science and the yearly changes around us. The world has entered a new era, indeed a new geological epoch, in which human activity has come to play a central and threatening part in fundamental earth dynamics.

(Sachs, 2012, pp. 2206–2207)

Another essential factor is the public's aforementioned increased exposure to, understanding of, and concern about the risks of global warming and the unsustainability of current behaviour, brought about partly by increased coverage, increased access to information through non-traditional channels such as the Internet, and the intermittent reports such as those of IPCC as well as those by norm entrepreneurs[7] such as Al Gore (Jacobs, 2012). This endeavour was further bolstered by the norm entrepreneurship of Ecuador and Bolivia in promoting the *rights of nature* in 2008–2010.

"Norms in the sustainability discourses are both ethical and techno-scientific and relate to relevant actors and entities at different scales – from global and national institutions to local communities and individuals" (Schmieg et al., 2018, p. 786). The UN assumed most of the responsibility regarding global environmental protection after UNCED in 1992, where sustainability was first discussed on such a highly publicised level. The resulting UNFCCC and the 1997 *Kyoto Protocol* could be viewed as pivotal in the life cycle, as can sustainability's inclusion as a stand-alone goal in the MDG framework. While there were a large number of more specified environmental agreements (e.g. protecting endangered species and limiting damage to the ozone layer) that sprang up in the 1970s and 1980s, unified approaches only started appearing later. The EU established its own Climate Change Programme in 2000 and an Emissions Scheme in 2005, while different combinations of American states and Canadian provinces organised various climate change initiatives between 2001 and 2012.

As suggested by Finnemore and Sikkink (1998), 'world historical events' such as wars or financial crises have the potential to act as catalysts for the emergence of new sets of norms, partly by denouncing norms perceived as causing a crisis or as being fundamental values to the losing side of a conflict (i.e. national socialism). In these momentous contexts, the normative space is highly contested and arguably favours novel norms that replace those norms that have expired – analogous to the fertile soil of a burnt-out forest. Dodds et al. (2014) suggest the situation in the wake of the 2008 GFC "provided a golden chance for a growing number of developing countries to redouble their claims to a greater share of influence in international decision-making and coordination processes with a direct impact on their own national development perspectives" (Dodds et al., 2014, p. 25). The growth and expansion of the BRICS association and its growing influence in the time period is symptomatic of such an effort.

Lastly, forces described within the concept of *world time-context* also exerted an influence affecting this particular case. Finnemore and Sikkink (1998) extend the concept to refer to slower, more ambient processes and how these circumstances can facilitate norm diffusion – an example being globalisation. Processes like these affect the general likelihood of norm emergence because they alter the inherent mechanics of how norms diffuse. Globalisation is the archetypical example, considering the way it has transformed and streamlined essential aspects such as – most decisively – communication, and transportation. Reaching out to larger audiences, or travelling to meet audiences in person has become exponentially easier and more affordable than was the case in say, 1990, let alone 1950. Rather than analogous to burnt-out soil (but staying in the realm of crops), this aspect has more in common with fertiliser or a good irrigation system. There are several identifiable aspects of the time period between 2000 and 2015 that are markedly conducive to a strengthening of the norm of sustainability and that partially explain its mutation into a super-norm. This has to do with the symbiotic relationship between the aforementioned ethical and techno-scientific normative spheres. As has been suggested, norms have a better chance of reaching their potential *tipping point* if they are universalistic, and the universal consequences of non-sustainable behaviour – or 'business as usual' – have become increasingly clear. This is not only true for the heavily publicised and increasingly gloomy environmental dimension of sustainability in the eyes of countries, the general public, and the UN, but the problems with a lack of economic and social sustainability had become clearer to every stakeholder involved in global development – the latter two particularly illuminated by some of the shortcomings of the MDGs.

## The health SDG: one goal to heal them all

The combination of the holism of sustainability and the all-embracing imperatives of inclusivity make for a context in which health norms belonging to the categories of state security and human security – separately and in combination – have the opportunity to integrate. This section, and the remainder of the chapter, is dedicated to exploring the health norms that constitute health-related development in the SDG framework. It begins by introducing the SDG health goal, its targets, and the general sentiments that underpin them, before viewing health in relation to the larger normative context described earlier – namely, sustainable development and inclusivity. The final part of the section is dedicated to a detailed *norm life cycle* discussion of the emergence of the two most significant aspects new to the post-2015 framework. These are the inclusion and emphasis on (1) NCDs and (2) universal health coverage (UHC).

> The 2030 agenda recognizes that the many drivers of good health are interdependent; that they are part of a system that crosses the conceptual boundaries between professional disciplines and the administrative limits of government departments.
>
> (Dye & Acharya, 2017, p. 666)

Health is an essential part of human development and had been a standout feature of the MDGs, with three of eight goals assigned to the effort – each one dedicated to different sectors of health, commonly denominated by a focus on poverty-related issues, as described in the previous chapter. In the final and concluding MDG report (UN, 2015), statistical results illustrate whether or not the respective goals and sub-goals had been achieved, providing bite-sized paragraphs of qualitative explanations and additional information. As is the case with the majority of the MDGs, progress regarding the indicators defined for the sphere of health had been significant, yet inadequate and uneven (Buse & Hawkes, 2015; UN, 2015).

In early consultations on the *post-2015 agenda*, health was regarded in a relatively optimistic light:

> The health sector has led the development success of the MDG era and created an unprecedented opportunity to achieve even more after 2015. The health MDGs have raised the profile of global health to the highest political level, mobilized civil society, increased development assistance for health, and contributed to considerable improvements in health outcomes in low- and middle-income countries.
>
> (WHO, 2013c, p. 7)

Health's centrality had not diminished in the *post-2015 agenda*. Its dual role as a means and an end of development is widely acknowledged, and sentiments alluding to it are repeatedly emphasised in the reports of the respective preparation processes, as well as in the final outcome document of the Sustainable Summit (UN, 2015). The WHO, reflecting on the OWG's thematic session on health, concluded that health's position in development post-2015 seemed secure.

> Health is a contributor and outcome of development, and a key indicator of what a people-centred, rights-based equitable development seeks to achieve. Health is important as an end in itself and as an integral part of human wellbeing, which includes material, psychological, social, cultural, educational, work, environmental, political and security dimensions.
>
> (WHO, 2013c, p. 19)

The general approach to addressing health, however, had been significantly revised. Several aspects of the MDG health effort had come under scrutiny, and some of these aspects had been deemed clearly suboptimal in terms of results as well as in terms of approach. The first and most glaring amendment was one of quantity, connectedness, and integration. Instead of three separate goals, there is only one single health SDG. This goal – number 3 in the list – is expressed as '*Ensure healthy lives and promote wellbeing for all at all ages*' and is significantly more extensive than its three MDG predecessors combined. This decision was based on several reasons. Primarily, there was the sense that dividing the health goals had created an unnecessary and unproductive separation between occasionally interconnected problems and objectives.

> By not articulating the synergies between the individual goals, opportunities for coordination and efficiency were missed. Similarly, while the specificity of

the MDGs is widely seen as a strength, the selection of a few goals for health also contributed to fragmentation within the health systems in some low- and middle-income countries.

(WHO, 2013c, p. 25)

Another vein of criticism of the three goals was that this specificity had generated negative side effects in areas of concern that were *not* specifically mentioned in the framework, as they generally received less attention than the significance of the problems would indicate they needed. "For example, spending by bilateral agencies on tackling [NCDs] was lower in the late 2000s than it had been in the 1990s – the MDGs excluded the NCDs despite their significant and rising proportion of the burden of global disease" (Buse & Hawkes, 2015, p. 2).

Addressing this multifaceted flaw resulted in perhaps the largest paradigmatic shift in the transition from health MDGs to the health SDG. The new, more comprehensive goal includes nine targets and four additional sub-targets that, aside from addressing all the issue areas covered within the MDGs (including the reproductive health goals added in 2007), also includes auxiliary health-related realities such as NCDs, road traffic deaths, and UHC. Indeed, health is explicitly viewed far more holistically and more true to the WHO's prevailing definition, which rejects the notion that health is equivalent to merely the absence of physical disease (or death). It also emphasises the interconnectedness between various aspects of development as determinants of health.[8] In the new agenda, health is treated less as simply freedom from infirmity, but rather as a holistic concept affected by several, often ostensibly heterogeneous, variables, which have direct and indirect effects.

> Moreover, the SDGs are concerned with an extremely wide range of structural drivers, risk factors and diseases. Gone is the narrow focus of the MDGs with its overwhelming emphasis on maternal and child health and a small (but burdensome) number of infections. The SDGs, in contrast, reflect more of the epidemiological transitions that have occurred in the last 20 years and seek to address a much broader range of conditions limiting human well-being, including the non-communicable diseases, mental health, violence and environmental risks which contribute the bulk of the global burden of disease.
>
> (Hawkes & Buse, 2016, p. 338)

The health approach of the new framework received some applause from the WHO for the same reasons: "[a]ltogether, the SDGs more closely reflect the range of real world concerns that countries face, compared with the narrower agenda of the MDGs. It is a development agenda relevant to all countries, not just developing countries" (WHO, 2016, p. 3).

As the SDGs are most directly a product of the OWG deliberations, their health-specific thematic session reveals much of the underlying principles at work in the formation of SDG 3. A report (WHO, 2013c) on the place of health in the

OWG's post-2015 vision suggests that there were six main pillars around which their approach would be built:

1 Clearly state that health is a human right
2 Incorporate specific health-related targets as part of other development sector goals
3 Take a holistic, life-course approach to people's health with an emphasis on health promotion and disease prevention
4 Promote the provision of affordable, accessible, comprehensive, high-quality health care services
5 Integrate the concept of shared and differentiated responsibility for issues of global health
6 Allow countries to tailor target and indicators to their own health priorities and circumstance

The first pillar on the list is the most normatively significant, the realisation of which can be seen as the *end* to which the *means* described in the other five points on the list aim to contribute. This is because the association with human rights acts as a framing device that motivates the pursuit of the others.

The goal itself can be split into three categories. In general, four of the 13 health SDG targets and sub-targets are carryovers from the MDGs. These represent the unfinished, incomplete, and slightly revised goals that were addressed within the previous frameworks. These are:

3.1 Reduce maternal mortality
3.2 End preventable new-born and child deaths
3.3 End the epidemics of HIV, TB, malaria, and neglected tropical diseases, and combat hepatitis, waterborne, and other communicable diseases
3.7 Ensure universal access to sexual and reproductive health-care services[9]

The second category, and the focus of the remainder of this chapter, comprises five targets, each addressing a concern not included in the three health MDGs:

3.4 Reduce mortality from NCDs and promote mental health
3.5 Strengthen prevention and treatment of substance abuse
3.6 Halve global deaths and injuries from road traffic accidents
3.8 Achieve UHC
3.9 Reduce deaths from hazardous chemicals and air, water, and soil pollution and contamination

A final category consists of targets that aim to improve means of implementation:

3.a Strengthen the implementation of the WHO Framework Convention on Tobacco Control in all countries, as appropriate

**3.b** Support the research and development of vaccines and medicines for the communicable and non-communicable diseases that primarily affect developing countries; provide access to affordable essential medicines and vaccines, in accordance with the *Doha Declaration on the TRIPS Agreement and Public Health*, which affirms the right of developing countries to use to the full the provisions in the *Agreement on Trade-Related Aspects of Intellectual Property Rights* regarding flexibilities to protect public health and, in particular, provide access to medicines for all

**3.c** Substantially increase health financing and the recruitment, development, training, and retention of the health workforce in developing countries, especially in least developed countries and small island developing states

**3.d** Strengthen the capacity of all countries, in particular developing countries, for early warning, risk reduction, and management of national and global health risks[10]

In the following section, this new approach to health development is viewed in terms of its connections to the normative spheres of sustainable development and inclusivity.

### Health and sustainable development: the links

The introduction of the new super-norm of sustainability was, as had been the case for poverty eradication uniting the MDGs, partially contingent upon its ability to interconnect with other, established spheres of development. Poverty and health are connected in several ways, and the myriad consequences of poverty are considered to be some of the most salient social determinants of health. Similarly, the range of issues in which health's dual position as an outcome and an indicator of sustainable development coalescence is extensive. This 'super-position' allows for health norms that appeal to both state and human security as well as their areas of concentricity; it is partly responsible for enabling the emergence of health norms novel to the contemporary global development goal context. Many of these issues were emphasised in *The Future We Want*, the outcome document of Rio+20 (UNGA, 2012a) and were elaborated upon in the subsequent preparatory consultation processes. The connections can be divided into three categories, consonant with the aforementioned three dimensions of sustainable development: environmental, social, and economic.

Points of correlation between *environmental* factors and health have increased over the course of the last few decades and have perhaps become more visceral and commonsensical, in harmony with the increasing awareness of and concern about climate change and pollution that have evolved since the early part of the new millennium (Pouster & Manevich, 2017). The numbers have also increasingly warranted an amplified concern towards the environmental determinants of health. Indeed, the WHO's *Global Health Risks: Mortality and Burden of Disease Attributable to Selected Major Risks* (2009) found that nearly 10% of worldwide deaths were attributable to environmental risks.[11] A more recent study (Cohen et al., 2017) found that ambient air pollution[12] was ranked the fifth-highest mortality risk factor of 2015 and that exposure had a significant negative effect on life expectancy. Other studies (Haines & Dora, 2012) have shown how health can benefit from a 'green economy' – for example, by reducing greenhouse gas emissions.

*Social* sustainability is somewhat notorious for being less clearly defined and less tangible than its two counterpart dimensions in the sustainability triumvirate. This is illustrated by the relative popularity (in terms of citations) of articles such as *What is social sustainability: A clarification of concepts* (Vallance, Perkins, & Dixon, 2011), and the state of the concept is often referred to as 'chaotic'. This paucity of clarity is partly explained by the combination of tangible and intangible aspects of societal concepts and issues that the concept attempts to capture. While not explicitly mentioning social sustainability, the *Brundtland Report* states that "the distribution of power and influence within society lies at the heart of most development challenges" (Brundtland, 1987, p. 37). This characterisation can refer to issues such as:

> inter- and intra-generational equity, the distribution of power and resources, employment, education, the provision of basic infrastructure and services, freedom, justice, access to influential decision-making fora and general 'capacity-building'.
>
> (Vallance et al., 2011, p. 343)

A 1997 WHO report on city planning, health, and social sustainability suggests that the introduction of social sustainability into the discourse of sustainable development shifted that discourse "from reducing the environmental effects of economic development as an inherent objective to working towards human development being served by environmentally supportive and equitable economic development" (WHO, 1997, p. 31). Some lucidity can be drawn from Dempsey, Bramley, Power, and Brown's (2011) study on social sustainability in an urban context, in which they refer to a definition originating from the EU, of sustainable *communities* as:

> places where people want to live and work, now and in the future. They meet the diverse needs of existing and future residents, are sensitive to their environment, and contribute to a high quality of life. They are safe and inclusive, well planned, built and run, and offer equality of opportunity and good services for all.
>
> (Dempsey et al., 2011, p. 290)

Social sustainability encapsulates a wide range of physical and non-physical factors (see Table 6.1) that contribute to the extent to which a society can sustain itself over time. The idea is that these factors, when realised optimally, will create stable and thriving societies with minimal conflict and destitution, inhabited by fulfilled citizens free from want and fear, and rife with capabilities and functioning.

*Table 6.1* Some factors considered central to social sustainability

| Non-physical factors | Physical factors |
|---|---|
| Education | Infrastructure |
| Social inclusion, sense of community | Housing |
| Employment | Accessibility |
| Health and well-being | Urban planning |
| Civil society and democratic participation | Amenities |
| Safety | Recreational facilities |

(Source: The authors).

Furthermore, it is thought that citizens will be better able to address and mitigate environmental concerns once these factors are at least somewhat satisfied.[13]

From this, it becomes clear that social sustainability is highly congruent with the capabilities approach and, by extension, generally with human development. Indeed, these factors correspond as being identical to, or mechanisms conducive to, many of the *freedoms* in the form of capabilities featured in the work of Amartya Sen.

The *economic* dimension of sustainability is also connected to health. As has been suggested throughout the study, economic growth and health work in symbiosis, one benefitting from the success of the other. In the SDG framework, the economic dimension of sustainability is characterised by an emphasis on sustained and inclusive growth. In accordance with the objectives of social sustainability, this means that (1) economic growth should not occur at the expense of future economic growth (i.e. through the depletion of resources) and (2) growth should benefit all members of society, partly for the intrinsic social reasons outlined earlier and partly because inequality can act as an obstacle to economic growth. Further, sustainable economic growth is believed to have some prerequisites, all of which are treated in separate goals in the framework.

> Economic development requires sound foundations. *Universal access* to education and *health services*, access to financial services, new technologies and affordable bank loans, gender equality and more equal distribution of resources can all support economic development
> (UN Sustainable Development Knowledge Platform, n.d., para. 2., authors' emphasis).

The most direct impact this focus had on health policy was the target of achieving UHC, the emblem of a health norm returned to in greater detail below. The overarching idea is that economic growth should result in *shared* benefits and that inclusiveness should be the metric with which success in the area is measured. Another measure by which economic sustainability is connected with health is the positive instrumental effects associated with a healthy population:

> A healthier workforce is more productive and more resilient because workers tend to have more energy and better mental health, and there is less

absenteeism. . . . Healthy populations live longer and therefore have increased incentives to save for their future financial needs. An increase in national savings leads to a larger supply of capital, leading to further domestic investment, additional physical and human capital, and technological progress, all of which are classic drivers of economic growth. In addition, a country with a healthy workforce is likely to attract more foreign direct investment.

(WHO, 2013c, p. 31)

The three dimensions of sustainability often interrelate, and their connections with health are no exception. For example, social factors, particularly inequality, interact with the environment in ways that distribute negative health consequences that are skewed towards the most vulnerable populations:

92% of all pollution-related mortality is seen in low-income and middle-income countries, with the greatest numbers of deaths from pollution-related disease occurring in rapidly developing and industrialising lower-middle-income countries. In the most severely affected countries, pollution is responsible for more than one in four deaths.

(Landrigan et al., 2017, p. 13)

This is also a point at which poverty eradication intersects with health and sustainable development. It further informs and supports the overall attitude that the SDGs should, while benefitting everyone, prioritise the most marginalised and vulnerable demographics.

### Health, human rights, inclusivity, and 'Leaving no one behind'

As suggested, *Leaving no one behind* is an initiative that attempts to mitigate the unequal benefits produced by the MDG era. Just as is the case with the dimension of social sustainability, the focus on inclusivity in relation to health means that everyone has the right to enjoy a healthy life. Two main changes had been made to the health approach in the *post-2015 agenda*. First, the concept of health had been expanded to encapsulate a more holistic reality in which the absence of certain infectious diseases does not necessarily make for a healthy population; that the classically poverty-related diseases of HIV/AIDS, malaria, and tuberculosis are only the tip of the iceberg with regard to addressing global health issues – even in low- and middle-income countries (LMICs).

Second, norms connected with the *right to health* had been significantly amplified in the agenda. As Forman, Ooms, and Brolan (2015) suggest in their analysis of the consultative process preceding the SDGs, health had become increasingly connected with rights rather than being confined to discussing the feasibility of eradicating certain diseases.

The adoption in the Sustainable Development Goal (SDG) of an explicit human rights and right to health focus would sharply contrast with how human rights were dealt with in the MDGs. Although states affirmed their commitment to "upholding respect for human rights and fundamental freedoms" in the 2000 Millennium Declaration, the MDG process that followed showed little awareness or sustained engagement with human rights.

(Forman et al., 2015, p. 799)

As described in Chapter 3, the right to health is enshrined in several international agreements, most broadly in United Nations Economic and Social Council's *General Comment no. 14* (2000), and has roots all the way back to at least the 1940s. As a health norm in global health, the right to health was the underlying principle of the *Declaration of Alma-Ata* (WHO, 1978) and was invoked by the global activist movement that successfully advocated for affordable ARVs in the early 2000s – a campaign that contributed to a "sharpened awareness of the importance of health equity, gender equality and human rights – in their own right and for public health" (WHO, 2014, p. xii). Reflecting on this normative comeback in relation to the unsuccessful sentiments of the *Declaration of Alma-Ata*, Youde suggests that

[t]he emergence and apparent adoption of a new norm is, in and of itself, a remarkable event. Even more remarkably, this new norm emerged less than 30 years after an earlier attempt to promote universal health care for all failed to take hold within the international community.

(Youde, 2008, p. 416)

However, the rights-based health norm agenda had been rather subdued in the MDGs and in global development discourse generally, particularly until Rio+20 and UNGA's *Resolution 67/81* of the same year (UNGA, 2012c). In the latter, significant normative and factual statements are made that reaffirm the global right to health, including a strong emphasis on the effects of various economic and social determinants. Crucially, the resolution highlights the imposition of the poor who are, for various reasons, cut off from access to medicine and health care, and subsequently, it endorses a movement towards UHC. The focus on human rights was clear early on, particularly after the OWG's thematic session on health. An early analysis from the WHO suggested that

[p]romoting human rights in the post-2015 development framework is a principal argument running through most of the thematic consultations. The rationale is both normative and pragmatic since injustice and inequalities undermine the prosperity, health and stability of society. A human rights approach also grounds the post-2015 development framework in existing international laws and norms. In many ways, this reinforces the people-centred approach of the MDGs. Human rights, social protection and social determinants of health approach are each mutually reinforcing.

(WHO, 2013c, p. 13)

*Leaving no one behind* is an imperative that explicitly focuses on involving the most vulnerable and least empowered segments of the population, with the intention of providing equally distributed benefits of development. While representing a normative response to the most woeful shortcomings of the previous framework, this new imperative also directly contributes to facilitating the social dimension of sustainable development, with its emphasis on inclusiveness.

> Beyond the foundational role of inclusion and the moral imperative to correct imbalances in power, voice and influence, there are also practical reasons to ensure that no one is left behind. Inclusion strengthens not only the social, but also the economic and environmental dimensions of sustainable development.
>
> (UN-DESA, 2016, p. 6)

While *Leaving no one behind* prioritises those most excluded – namely, "all children, youth, persons with disabilities (of whom more than 80% live in poverty), people living with HIV/AIDS, older persons, indigenous peoples, refugees and internally displaced persons and migrants" (UNGA, 2015), it is also a universally sweeping notion that aims to benefit *all* people in *all* segments of society and to cover issue areas affecting large numbers of people, which were not included in the MDGs.

With sustainable development and inclusivity as a basis, the post-2015 development agenda was moving in the direction towards health norms associated with human security. However, as was the case for the HIV/AIDS in the MDGs, the frame of sustainable development allows for health norms related to state security to benefit simultaneously. In the final part of this chapter, the major normative novelties associated with the health SDG – separated into two categories – are explored more closely and viewed within the scope of the norm life cycle. The first category explores the integration of NCDs, while the second category examines the rise and internalisation of UHC.

## The newcomers, part 1: NCDs[14]

> The agenda for global health is changing in ways that influence how priorities for development will be defined in the future. The major change is the political recognition of the societal and economic impact of non-communicable diseases.
>
> (WHO, 2012b, p. 2)

One of the major defects identified with the health MDGs was that in the pursuit to mitigate the specific issue areas covered in the goals, other issue areas *not included* in the list were becoming disproportionately deprioritised in terms of the allocation of attention and resources, thereby leaving large portions of the global burden of disease comparatively unchecked. While 'other diseases' are included in MDG 6, these were limited to the category of communicable disease, while issues such as mental health and NCDs were excluded (Minas, Tsutsumi, Izutsu, Goetzke, & Thornicroft, 2015). As noted in Chapter 3, global health development has traditionally been relatively uninterested in NCDs, despite their being responsible for substantial proportions of the global disease burden, posing significant economic and social burdens within and among developing and developed countries alike. While steps towards addressing certain global NCDs have been taken (most notably 2003's FCTC), GHG had – until including it as an SDG 3 sub-target – mobilised an underwhelming response in proportion to the scope of the problem. As suggested in Chapter 3, the relative absence of NCDs in global health may be caused by their typical lack of suddenness, exogeny, and striking imagery often associated with communicable diseases such as Ebola (Benson & Glasgow, 2015).

That this omission would not be replicated in the post-2015 development agenda was clear from the earliest of the publications indicating the next framework's envisaged trajectory. The UN System Task Team's *Health in the post-2015 UN development Thematic Think Piece*, published as early as May 2012, identifies one side of the NCD problem when it notes that "The cost of inaction in relation to [NCDs] – estimated in trillions of dollars – is now recognized as a global risk requiring action in all countries that extends well beyond the health sector alone" (UNSTT, 2012, p. 6). A few months later, the first paragraph in the *Health and Population* section of the outcome document of Rio+20, *The Future We Want* (UNGA, 2012a), simultaneously positions health as integral to sustainable development *and* injects the substance of what would become the newly included health aspects that were to be presented three years later in the form SDG 3.

> We recognize that health is a precondition for and an outcome and indicator of all three dimensions of sustainable development. We understand the goals of sustainable development can only be achieved in the absence of a high prevalence of debilitating communicable and *non-communicable diseases*, and where populations can reach a state of *physical, mental and social well-being*. We are convinced that action on the social and environmental determinants of health, both for the poor and the vulnerable and for the entire population, is important to create inclusive, equitable, economically productive and healthy societies. We call for the full realization of the right to the enjoyment of the highest attainable standard of physical and mental health.
>
> (UNGA, 2012a, p. 37, authors' emphasis)

The wide range of focus areas mentioned in this statement differs from comparable statements in publications emanating from Rio+20's predecessors. *Agenda 21*, the outcome document of 2002's UNCED, mentions NCDs only once in its 14-page section on health, which deals overwhelmingly with reducing the effects of communicable disease; there is no mention of mental health. In the outcome document of its follow-up 2002 summit in Johannesburg, WSSD, one single paragraph reflects an agreement to develop programmes to address NCDs – including mental health – though no explicit relationship with sustainable development is explored. NCDs and mental health have also been conspicuously absent from explicit discussion in HDRs, even though these are variables that have massive implications for the HDI, most directly with regard to life expectancy – illustrated by the fact that around 52% of all deaths under the age of 70 are the result of preventable and/or curable NCDs each year.

The WHO was an early proponent of recognising the importance of mitigating NCDs globally and first recognised them as a global health challenge in its 1996 *Global Burden of Disease Study*. In 2000, the organisation began working on a strategy that would promote and support research that would contribute to the prevention and control of NCDs (WHO, 2000). At the WHA in 2008, this commitment was reaffirmed, now with greater urgency; it refers to the growing scope of the problem and the lacklustre responses to address it, particularly in LMICs. Though the severity of NCD mortality had been known since at least the early 1990s (Gribble & Preston, 1993), a significant "gap between information and action" (Strong, Mathers, Leeder, & Beaglehole, 2005, p. 1578) has characterised the response of global health governance in addressing it, illustrated, for example, by its complete omission from the MDGs. One seminal article (Strong et al., 2005) identified that a majority of annual deaths were related to ailments belonging to the classification of *chronic diseases* (70% of which were defined as noncommunicable), labelling the burden as a "neglected epidemic" (Strong et al., 2005). In the same publication, the authors also suggested a global goal for reducing the annual death toll of chronic diseases by 2% each year. Also in 2005, the WHO published a report titled *Preventing Chronic Diseases: A Vital Investment* (WHO, 2005c), which echoes many of these concerns.

The norm entrepreneurship that precipitated the position of NCDs as a priority area in the development agenda was a mixed effort that includes academic and governmental as well as non-governmental actors. In the years following the aforementioned article (Strong et al., 2005), several publications that featured various versions of 'calls to action', petitioned global health and/or development initiatives to address NCDs in a number of different capacities. These prescriptive articles, commentaries, and editorials presented data that demonstrated the scope and severity of the negative health effects of certain diseases, before stating the need to mitigate these severities. Among the specific ones mentioned are breast cancer (Coughlin & Ekwueme, 2009), salt intake, and tobacco use (Asaria, Chisholm, Mathers, Ezzati, & Beaglehole, 2007), as well as more general categories such as respiratory diseases (Bousquet, Dahl, & Khaltaev, 2007) and mental health (Prince et al., 2007). Others supported Strong et al.'s (2005) cause for the necessity of general initiatives to reduce the burden inflicted by general chronic and non-communicable disease (Abegunde, Mathers, Adam, Ortegon, & Strong, 2007; Beaglehole, Ebrahim, Reddy, Voute, & Leeder, 2007); still, others aimed to inform policy through suggesting determinants (Miranda, Kinra, Casay, Davey Smith, & Ebrahim, 2008).

The arguments presented in these commentaries are similar in their rationale and generally connect their specific or general issue with already established wisdoms, in effect amplifying their adjacency to internalised health norms. The diseases are described in the context of their scope, their death tolls, and other unpleasant consequences for the individuals affected. More specifically, these consequences include chronic or acute pain, the inability to work, and social exclusion. Their effects on a local and global societal level are also presented, particularly in economic terms. Another common thread in these publications is that they highlight that the reason for these epidemics is due partly to the unavailability of infrastructure and resources for prevention, treatment, and palliative care and that these problems are particularly prevalent in LMICs, suggesting the relevance of inequality and social development as central to the cause. In 2011, an article was published by the *Lancet NCD Action Group* (Beaglehole et al., 2011) that builds upon the evidence presented in some of these earlier publications to create a synthesised suggestion for priority areas.

The year 2009 saw the creation of the *NCD Alliance*, a subsequent ally of the *Lancet NCD Action Group*. The NCD Alliance is a global partnership that currently comprises around 2,000 organisations, whose common goals include the introduction of national action plans to combat NCDs and aspirations such as a 'tobacco free world'. The alliance was originally founded by Ann Keeling, the then CEO of the International Diabetes Federation, who invited its sister federations, the World Heart Federation and the Union for International Cancer Control (and the next year, the International Union against TB and Lung Disease), to form a new NGO, which would promote political action on NCDs in a concerted effort. At the WHA later that year, they appealed to the UN to hold a summit on NCDs, which was realised in the form of the UNGA's high-level meeting on NCD prevention and control in 2011.

As a result of efforts like these, the combined strength of the alliance proved to be among the most significant non-state influencers with regard to putting NCDs on the global health agenda. Next, the NCD Alliance "campaigned for a strong reference to NCDs at [Rio+20], and secured a stand-alone target on the NCDs and other NCD-related targets in the 2030 Agenda for Sustainable Development" (NCD Alliance, n.d., para. 7). In effect, the creation of the alliance was a strengthening of the organisational platform of communities and organisations that had various specific focus areas but shared a fundamental core interest. The vision of the NCD Alliance is simple: to make NCD prevention and control a priority, everywhere. The overarching frame – based firmly in reality and needing little embellishment – was to present NCDs as a significant contributor to poverty, as an obstacle for general development, and as a global health emergency. Important for the success of the NCD Alliance is that their membership is truly global, with member organisations representing 170 countries, thereby appealing to the inclusive imperative of the new framework.

The first major signs of *states* shifting focus towards addressing the NCD problem started in a regional multilateral scene. In Europe, 2006 saw the passing of the *Charter on Counteracting Obesity* (WHO, 2006). In 2007, heads of state and government of the Caribbean Community (CARICOM) agreed on the *Port-of-Spain Declaration: Uniting to Stop the Epidemic of Chronic Non-Communicable Diseases*

(CARICOM, 2007). The *Port-of-Spain Declaration* framed NCDs as a significant risk and problem for the region and was the first of its kind to give clear, intersectoral policy directions to address NCDs multilaterally (Chattu & Sakhamuri, 2018). As Samuels and Hospedales (2011) indicate, this declaration, and the subsequent work of CARICOM, provided a state's perspective on the matter and contributed to bringing the issue to the attention of the higher-ups in GHG. Most of all, CARICOM, by virtue of speaking on behalf of its 15 Caribbean member states, had a strong organisational platform from which they could diffuse their concerns and ideas to the UNGA.

The *Port-of-Spain Declaration* inspired other actors to take steps in the same direction. Within a few years, similar or equivalent plans of action had been agreed upon in various respective regional *fora*, indicating a period leading up to a *norm cascade*. In 2009, for example, the *Pacific NCD Forum* – convened collaboratively by the WHO and the Secretariat of the Pacific Community (SPC)[15] – made similar regional commitments in the attempt to mitigate the negative impacts of NCDs on the region. Two years later, at its second meeting, the forum referred to the current effects as a social and economic crisis (Tolley et al., 2016). In April 2011, a ministerial conference, jointly organised by the WHO and Russia, was held in Moscow. The meeting had the explicit intention of highlighting the scope and magnitude of the NCD problem and of amplifying the urgent need for global and national responses to address it – including its inclusion in national health plans in the global development discourse. Indeed, one of its stated objectives was "[t]o accelerate integration of the prevention and control of NCDs into the global development agenda" (WHO, 2011a, p. 6). These sentiments are enshrined in the resulting *Moscow Declaration* (WHO, 2011b).

Partly as a result of efforts by CARICOM (Patterson, 2018), the most significant event of this period was the September 2011 convening of an UNGA high-level meeting on NCD prevention and control. This was only the second time in the history of the forum that it was convened solely in order to address a health issue – the first instance being the previously discussed 2001 meeting on HIV/AIDS (UNGA, 2001). In the resolution document published in the wake of the meeting, the organisation's sentiments towards NCDs are made clear:

> the global burden and threat of non-communicable diseases constitutes one of the major challenges for development in the twenty-first century, which undermines social and economic development throughout the world and threatens the achievement of internationally agreed development goals;. . . . Recognize the urgent need for greater measures at the global, regional and national levels to prevent and control non-communicable diseases in order to contribute to the full realization of the right of everyone to the highest attainable standard of physical and mental health.
>
> (UNGA, 2011, pp. 1–2)

In addition to being a normative statement, this observation recognises how NCDs and mental health issues undermine current and future efforts towards realising the objectives of human development, a sentiment that would be further highlighted through the lens of sustainable development and that would come to permeate health-related discussions in the consultative process. Indeed, once these connections had been made, a *tipping point* had been reached. The *high-level meeting* was followed by other indications of a *norm cascade*. One point of criticism directed at the health approach of the MDGs highlighted in the first report of the UNSTT (UNSTT, 2012), for example, is the omission of NCDs – suggesting that the issue would merit inclusion in the *post-2015 agenda*.

The cascade culminated in the numerous mentions of NCDs in the Rio+20 outcome document: *The Future We Want* (UNGA, 2012a). This served as the first clear signal that the NCD health norm had *internalised* within the UN development agenda. Accentuating this internalisation process was the 2013 establishment of the *UN Interagency Task Force on the Prevention and Control of NCDs* (UNIATF). Its purpose is to coordinate efforts across the UN system and various other IOs in supporting government efforts to optimise endeavours towards NCD-related commitments and goals. The WHO, as a direct response to the newfound imperatives espoused by the 2011 high-level meeting, established the *NCD Global Monitoring Framework*, which provides concrete targets and indicators for governments to pursue; it was adopted by member states at the 2013 WHA.

The WHO also published its *Global Action Plan for the Prevention and Control of NCDs* that same year (WHO, 2013b). The *Action Plan* identifies policy areas and sets nine voluntary targets scheduled for fulfilment by 2020. The targets have met some criticism because of their focus on individual behaviour rather than on systemic inequities and vulnerabilities (Nulu, 2017; Patterson, 2018). In 2014, the WHO established the *Global Coordination Mechanism on the Prevention and Control of NCDs*, an institution meant to engage with NCD issues and coordinate responses among member states; its purpose is to accelerate progress towards the target set out in the *Action Plan*. The consensus among the various bodies of the post-2015 consultation process was also one that supported the inclusion of an NCD objective in the new agenda, and there was little or no controversy attached to the announcement of the four broadly NCD-related sub-targets when the SDGs were formally adopted in September of 2015 – a final and most definitive piece of evidence for its current internalisation (see Figure 6.1).

Some compounding key factors worked together to precipitate the institutionalisation of this health norm, leading to the expansion of the development agenda to include NCDs. First, the *intrinsic* properties partly found in the numbers, which had become increasingly noticeable to UN member states, unilaterally and regionally. NCDs are responsible for 70% of global deaths annually, a three-quarter majority of which occur in LMICs (Islam et al., 2014). Aside from the inherent human and social ramifications of these deaths, NCDs – as disease in general – prevent individuals, and commonly the people surrounding them, from achieving capabilities and exercising their functionings, or freedoms. By another metric, NCDs pose a massive economic burden globally and their substantial growth over the next two decades has been forecast (Bloom et al., 2012). Mental health issues that affect untold numbers of people in developing and developed

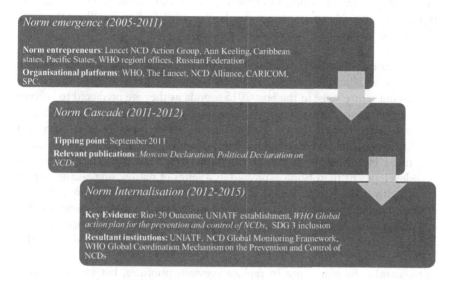

Norm emergence (2005-2011)

**Norm entrepreneurs**: Lancet NCD Action Group, Ann Keeling, Caribbean states, Pacific States, WHO regionl offices, Russian Federation
**Organisational platforms**: WHO, The Lancet, NCD Alliance, CARICOM, SPC.

Norm Cascade (2011-2012)

**Tipping point**: September 2011
**Relevant publications**: *Moscow Declaration, Political Declaration on NCDs*

Norm Internalisation (2012-2015)

**Key Evidence**: Rio+20 Outcome, UNIATF establishment, *WHO Global action plan for the prevention and control of NCDs*, SDG 3 inclusion
**Resultant institutions**: UNIATF, NCD Global Monitoring Framework, WHO Global Coordination Mechanism on the Prevention and Control of NCDs

*Figure 6.1* The norm life cycle of NCDs ahead of the SDG inclusion

countries alike had been another significant omission of the previous framework. For example, annual death rates attributed to suicide in 2016 were almost on par with deaths from HIV/AIDS and more than double the number of deaths resulting from malaria. Other statistics make similar impressions: "Just one of the major risk factors, tobacco use, claims nearly 6 million lives annually, and costs 1–2% of the global gross domestic product every year" (Clark, 2013, p. 510). Generally, the various adverse effects of NCDs on several interrelated aspects of society were becoming increasingly extensive, documented, and undeniable – as well as *universally* applicable.

A second aspect conducive to the expansion of the health SDG to accommodate a new health norm and to include NCDs was the general expansion of the post-2015 development agenda, spearheaded by the new normative imperatives discussed earlier: namely, sustainability and inclusivity. Recommencing the narrow approach that the MDGs had been criticised for would have been highly incongruous with the *post-2015 agenda*'s new focus on holism and of leaving no one behind. Such an approach would simply not do justice to the interrelated aspects of sustainable development that were in the process of being defined (Minas et al., 2015). The inclusion of NCDs, therefore, shared *adjacency* with the established imperatives of sustainability and inclusivity. As a result, conventional wisdom relating NCDs to development became internalised, and statements such as the following became commonplace in the last few years leading up to the SDG formulation: "[b]etter health outcomes from [NCDs] is a precondition for, an outcome of and an indicator of all three dimensions of sustainable development: economic development, environmental sustainability, and social inclusion" (WHO, 2013b, p. 15). Certain publications were particularly prophetic when describing the probable themes of health in the *post-2015 agenda*:

> Priorities in health will be influenced by demographic changes, disease burden shifts, and lifestyle changes. These transitions are likely to result in [NCDs] taking centre stage in the post-2015 agenda as they are predicted to become an even greater cause of mortality and disability in the future. While this does not mean that NCDs will 'replace' other disease priorities, it is likely that environmental and behavioural determinants of health will be better recognised. Health will be seen more as a means to achieving broader objectives of development than being expressed in a series of narrow single-issue targets. Health is likely to be included in terms of targets that take a more holistic life-course approach, with evidence-based, system-wide interventions that recognise environmental influences and see health as a human right.
>
> (Eaton, Kakuma, Wright, & Minas, 2014)

Significantly, the aim is not to replace previous priorities, but to complement them with a fuller understanding of health as something other than the absence of (communicable) disease. With poverty as the main framing agent of the MDGs, addressing health issues that were most viscerally related to the plight of the poor – HIV/AIDS and malaria – was appropriate. In the context of the SDGs and its holistically charged focus on sustainability and inclusivity, this was no longer viable.

> The [SDGs] are intended to be universal in the sense of embodying a universally shared common global vision of progress towards a safe, just and sustainable space for all human beings to thrive on the planet. They reflect the *moral principles* that no-one and no country should be left behind, and that everyone and every country should be regarded as having a common responsibility for playing their part in delivering the global vision.
>
> (Osborn, Cutter, & Ullah, 2015, p. 2)

As suggested, health has symbiotic effects with all three dimensions of sustainable development. It acts as a contributor, a beneficiary, and as a way of measuring the progress of its success.

> In addition to the fact that healthy people have stronger cognitive and physical capabilities and, in consequence, make more productive contributions to society, health policy contributes to poverty reduction through the financial protection inherent in universal health coverage. Changes in population growth rates, age structures and distribution of people are also closely linked to national and global development challenges. In addition, health is also a potential beneficiary of policies in a wide range of other sectors such as transport, energy and urban planning. And health metrics can measure

progress across the economic, social and environmental pillars of sustainable development.

(WHO, 2012a, p. 2)

NCDs are no exception; their connections to economic sustainability have already been established, as they are projected to be responsible for a cumulative loss of $40–$50 trillion by 2030. The social dimension of sustainability is also significantly affected by NCDs, as social determinants such as income, education, and housing all affect vulnerability and associated risk factors, leaving the people living in poverty disproportionately susceptible. The environmental dimension is also represented, as the links between the natural environment and health risks are becoming more and more salient, particularly in LMICs. These include, among others, the effects of air pollution and the degradation of land and biodiversity.

The *capabilities approach*, with which the meta-norm of human development shares so much of its fundamental philosophy, does not distinguish between health issues derived from communicable or non-communicable sources, and the inclusion of NCDs, therefore, needed little effort by way of normative persuasion. Rather, this was a case of realising faults and inconsistencies between the stated purpose of the dominant normative structure of human development and that of its implementation (embodied in the UN development agenda). "Unlike the laws of physics, which are free of inconsistencies, every man-made order is packed with internal contradictions. Cultures are constantly trying to reconcile these contradictions, and this process fuels change" (Harari, 2014, p. 142). In this context, this meant realising that if health were to have a significant position in the future of development, the scope of health issues addressed would have to be expanded.

With such a broad focus, NCDs have been brought into the limelight by countless individuals and organisations; pinpointing an exhaustive list of norm entrepreneurs in this context would inevitably lead to the unintentional omission of important contributors. However, the WHO and influential academic and medical communities, such as the *Lancet*, have been essential in positioning the issue on the global health agenda. Non-state actors such as the NCD Alliance and state-actors such as CARICOM were also significant protagonists bringing *prominence* to the issue. Relatedly, the WHO had the most central position of acting as an organisational platform for its member states and regional partners, such as the SPC. More direct state involvement also contributed to the institutionalisation of the need to address NCDs. As illustrated by the *Moscow Declaration* (WHO, 2011b), the scope of the problem had become significant in certain larger middle-income countries as well; multilateral fora such as the BRICS association and the countries unilaterally comprising it had become more included in the decision-making process than had previously been the case – particularly after the 2008 GFC (Dodds et al., 2014). The tendency of governments motivated to take action on NCDs because of their growing domestic relevance relates to the *non-intrinsic* variable of *legitimation* in norm absorption. Combining with the *intrinsic* content-specific characteristics described earlier, these considerations contributed to the strength of the NCD health norm underlying its success in internalising within the sustainable development agenda.

## The newcomers, part 2: universal health coverage

The second significant novel focus area for the health SDG is the inclusion of a target for achieving UHC. In short, *UHC* refers to a health care system that ensures health care for all citizens of a country, regardless of social status, income, race, gender, geographical location, or any other variable that may impede an individual's access. In other words, UHC is an approach "based on the principle that all individuals and communities should have access to quality essential health services without suffering financial hardship" (WHO, 2017b, p. 2). With this sub-target, the health SDG directs greater attention towards the problem of *accessibility* to health care and its increasingly apparent and clear far-reaching consequences to all three dimensions of sustainable development.

> Good quality health delivery systems with universal access protect individuals from illness, stimulate economic growth, and fight poverty by keeping people healthy. They also contribute to social harmony by providing assurance to the population that services are available in the event of illness. Yet more than a billion people cannot use the health services they need because they are either unavailable or they cannot afford to use them [UHC] requires that everyone can use the health services that they need.
>
> (Evans, Marten, & Etienne, 2012, p. 864)

The normative foundation of UHC is similar to that which admonishes action on NCDs, and this foundation is nested within the larger structure – the sustainability *super-norm*. Considering the numerous linkages and feedback loops between UHC, social inclusion, and (health) equality, the normative relationship that these concerns have with the *social dimension* of sustainable development is the most striking.

> It is undeniable that health care, especially when provided universally, promotes equality. With the introduction of universal care, for instance, disparities in service utilization and access across socioeconomic classes tend to decrease, although the health status gradient never completely disappears. Furthermore, UHC coverage implies a sense of solidarity and interconnectedness within a society as members agree to pool resources to guarantee at least an acceptable level of response to those in need.
>
> (Borgonovi & Compagni, 2013, p. 536)

As Vega (2013) suggests, UHC became a constant in the world of global health after the passing of *UNGA resolution 67/81* in December of 2012 (UNGA, 2012c). In the resolution, the *right to health* and the related general sentiments of the *Declaration of Alma-Ata* – by then over three decades old – are invoked, establishing the normative rationale upon which the matter of UHC is subsequently discussed (Abiiro & de Allegri, 2015).[16] In other words, the WHO, with Halfdan Mahler at the head, was perhaps the original *norm entrepreneur* that attempted to introduce primary health for all as a global health norm – though this attempt subsequently failed for a number of reasons, perhaps particularly in terms of *world-time context* (Finnemore & Sikkink, 1998).

To reiterate its normative position, the *Declaration of Alma-Ata* (WHO, 1978) framed health – defined broadly and not merely as the absence of disease – within the sphere of fundamental human rights, and specified that the realisation of these rights is inextricably linked with social and economic determinants that need to be addressed. This early rendition of the health norm that came to form the ideational crux of UHC advocacy influenced people such as Jonathan Mann and was based entirely on an *ethos* equivalent to that of human security – though it was conceived of well before alternative perspectives on security were part of the international/global health *zeitgeist*. Particularly, it directs attention to inequality and the fact that the poorest and most vulnerable populations are the furthest from realising this right, proclaiming it to be "politically, socially and economically unacceptable, and . . . therefore, of common concern to all countries" (1978, p. 1). The *Declaration* especially emphasises the need for a global implementation of primary health care. In *Resolution 67/81* (UNGA, 2012c), these sentiments are restated nearly verbatim, using a slightly different language and with slightly different emphases. It reaffirms the position of health as an essential human right, as an essential component of development, and as an outcome and indicator of all three dimensions of sustainable development.

The *Resolution* concludes with two central recommendations directly related to both the MDGs and the then-budding post-2015 development agenda:

> *Urges* Governments, civil society organizations and international organizations to promote the inclusion of universal health coverage as an important element on the international development agenda and in the implementation of the internationally agreed development goals, including the Millennium Development Goals, as a means of promoting sustained, inclusive and equitable growth, social cohesion and well-being of the population and achieving other milestones for social development, such as education, work income and household financial security. . . . *Recommends* that consideration be given to including universal health coverage in the discussions on the post-2015 development agenda in the context of global health challenges.
>
> (UNGA, 2012c, pp. 5–6, original emphasis)

This resolution, among the first indicators of *internalisation* for the UHC health norm, came about as a result of a process largely initiated by the WHO, along with other state and non-state organisations whose ambition it was to integrate UHC into the global development agenda that had begun in earnest the better part of a decade earlier. Certain central sentiments associated with UHC (such as universal access to treatment and medicine) re-emerged during the HIV/AIDS treatment campaigns throughout the early 2000s. These campaigns effectively framed the plight of HIV/AIDS-afflicted persons, and subsequently their access to essential medicines, within the normative spheres of human rights and health equality (Forman et al., 2015; WHO, 2014). The campaign for universal access to ARVs reinvigorated the normative connections between health and human rights in GHG discourse; the momentum created by the success of this global campaign was seized upon by the WHO in particular, allied with sympathetic academic and non-governmental actors. Concerns associated with state security were also fulfilled: Vieira (2007) argues that the *Doha Declaration* of 2001 was a clear sign of the securitisation of HIV/AIDS, and that this helped further to accelerate state absorption of norms related to the right to health and access to medicines.

In 2003, the Commission of Human Security[17] submitted its first report to the UN secretary-general, in which human security was partly framed as complementary to state security. The report provides a relatively early endorsement of universal access to health care, which is listed as *the* top priority in terms of health-related objectives (Aldis, 2008). In 2005, member states of the WHO committed to start developing their health systems towards the realisation of UHC. The *World Health Report* of that year (WHO, 2005d) also invokes norms associated with the right to health, along with equity and solidarity, and argues that any approach or response that takes seriously the social and economic ramifications of health (and by extension, development in general, particularly *sustainable development*) would be inadequate without an aim towards affordable UHC for all citizens. The MDG framework was one example of such an inadequate system, in which emphasis was placed on reducing occurrences of specified and narrow areas of health, and in which human rights existed as more of a side note, especially regarding implementation (Alston, 2005; Forman et al., 2015).

The Rockefeller Foundation launched its *Transforming Health Systems* (THS) initiative in 2008 (an initiative concluded in 2017) that explicitly promoted global implementation of UHC. The THS initiative had a global advocacy strategy of (1) disseminating information on UHC, (2) promoting dialogues on the issue, (3) identifying and supporting certain global and regional champions of UHC, and (4) mobilising individuals and organisations to muster support at country level. The fourth point is notable in a theoretical sense, as it indicates a partial *outsourcing of norm entrepreneurship*. The Rockefeller Foundation has since then been one of the most omnipresent funders and supporters of various UHC-related large-scale events and research projects as well as of advocacy groups. In an internal evaluation report, the THS initiative is thought to have exerted a direct influence on UHC's eventual inclusion in the health SDG:

> Through its highly adaptive, multicomponent and multilevel advocacy strategy, THS was able to influence the post-2015 agenda process, culminating in the inclusion of UHC in the SDGs. By maintaining a highly adaptive and flexible approach to grantmaking, and using multiple tools and vehicles for policy influence and agenda-setting at the global, regional, and country levels, the

Rockefeller Foundation was able to strengthen and shape the UHC move-ment, and ultimately influence the SDG process.

(Sattar & Smith, 2017, p. vi)

One example of advocacy groups directly funded by the Rockefeller Foundation is the UHC Coalition. Similar to the NCD Alliance, the UHC Coalition is a con-glomerate of various health and development organisations and institutions that have different specialities but share a larger, common goal – in this case, a global aspiration for the implementation of UHC. The UHC Coalition is, among other feats, responsible for the existence of an international UHC Day; its date – 12 December – is the anniversary of *UNGA Resolution 67/81*. The passing of this *Resolution* was, incidentally, also actively supported by the Rockefeller Foundation: "THS built relationships with well-placed country leaders willing to champion UHC within the UN arena, and provided strategic technical assistance to UN country missions, which key informants regarded as critical for facilitating the UN resolution process" (Sattar & Smith, 2017, p. vi).

In a speech given at a global health dialogue in Venice in 2009, the director-general of the WHO, Margaret Chan, bridged a significant gap hitherto present in global health, and more specifically global health development. This was the gap between the approach that focused largely on specific diseases *à la* the MDGs and one that shifted the emphasis to focus on systemic equity, so central to sustainable development:

> I think we can now let a long-standing and divisive debate die down. This is the debate that pits single-disease initiatives against the agenda for strength-ening health systems. As I have stated since taking office, the two approaches are not mutually exclusive. They are not in conflict. They do not represent a set of either-or options. It is the opposite. They can and should be mutually reinforcing. We need both. . . . This is the essence of the equity argument: people should not be denied access to life-saving interventions for unfair rea-sons, including an inability to pay.
>
> (Chan, 2009, para 3, 4;11)

This statement can also be seen as one that bridges concerns traditionally con-nected with the respective state and human security categories of health norms. Improved health systems act as preventative measures for the spread of EIDs, potentially reducing the need for reactive responses, which tend to create unnec-essary levels of fear and uncertainty, such as was the case during, for example, the H1N1 virus outbreak in 2009. At the same time, strengthening health sys-tems towards the goal of achieving UHC is the most effective tool to ensure the realisation of a universal right to health and of ensuring human security. The next year, the *World Health Report* amplified and reasserted the urgent need and ethical imperative of implementing UHC on a global basis:

> Promoting and protecting health is essential to human welfare and sustained economic and social development. This was recognized more than 30 years

ago by the Alma-Ata Declaration signatories, who noted that Health for All would contribute both to a better quality of life and also to global peace and security.

(WHO, 2010, p. 7)

The report urged member states to raise and prioritise funds that could support their respective health care systems as well as presenting practical pathways of financing. This report, considered seminal by some observers (see the Lancet, 2012), constituted a *tipping point*; it was followed up by a significant rally for the mainstreaming of UHC and for its connection to, and position within, the global development agenda – this rally comprised the *cascade* of the UHC health norm. According to its own evaluation report, the Rockefeller Foundation's THS initiative was included behind the scenes also in this case:

> Many are not aware of the Foundation's specific contributions to pivotal events in the history of the UHC movement, such as the WHO's 2010 World Health Report. . . . The THS team was able to influence institutions – such as WHO, World Bank, UNICEF, and the UN Secretary-General's office – to engage in the UHC movement, mainly due to the Foundation's legacy in the global health arena, as well as the reputation and connections of individual THS leaders. . . . The Foundation has not publicized its role or successes in the UHC arena, but instead empowered global and country actors to be UHC champions. The Foundation's website does not provide extensive information about UHC or the THS initiative or offer a central place for accessing the many research products and publications that have been generated under the THS initiative. As a result, the Foundation's role in the UHC movement is not well recognized or understood outside of the movement's inner circles.
>
> (Sattar & Smith, 2017, p. ix)

Later in 2010, the WHO and a number of partner organisations hosted the First Global Symposium on Health System Research, subtitled 'Science to accelerate UHC'. The event was funded by a diverse blend of private and state-affiliated health and development institutions, such as the Rockefeller Foundation, the GAVI Alliance, USAID, the Norwegian Agency for Development Cooperation, and numerous others. Its purpose was to improve the scientific basis of evidence required for policymakers and leaders to make important decisions in accelerating progress towards UHC. The event produced the *Montreux Statement*, which affirms the aim of future symposiums to create an international society for health systems research, and to further facilitate and encourage studies and investigations that support these stated purposes.

In late 2010, the *Lancet* published an article by a group of scientists titled *Education of Health Professionals for the 21st Century: a Global Independent Commission*. The commission advocates for a reform in health care and health education, and states twice over the course of the article that "[t]he ultimate purpose is to assure universal coverage of the high-quality comprehensive services that are essential to advance opportunity for health equity within and between countries" (Frenk et al., 2010, p. 6). The commission was funded, in part, by the Rockefeller Foundation. The WHO endorsement of UHC was again reaffirmed at the 2011 WHA through its *Resolution 64.9* on sustainable health financing structures and universal coverage (WHO, 2011c). *Inter alia*, the resolution "requested the Director General of the World Health Organization to convey to the Secretary-General of the United Nations the importance of [UHC] for discussion by a forthcoming session of the [UNGA]" (UNGA, 2012c, p. 3). The remainder of 2011 was a year in which the imminent plateau of the *norm cascade* built up to the full manifestation that was to follow in the next year.

WHO Director-General Margaret Chan had, by 2012, further intensified her resolve: "universal coverage is the single most powerful concept that public health has to offer. It is our ticket to greater efficiency and better quality. It is our saviour from the crushing weight of [NCDs] that now engulf the globe" (Chan, 2012, para 24–25). By this time, UHC's momentum within the spheres of global health and development had become irreversible. Indeed, 2012 was a watershed year for the broad-based institutionalisation of UHC in health governance within and outside the UN system. Three significant regional conferences cemented this trend. At the 2012 Prince Mahidol Award Conference in January,[18] the theme centred around moving towards UHC, with a focus on financing; its resultant *Bangkok Statement on Universal Health Coverage* proclaims that the attendees of the conference agree to cooperate, across sectors, to produce evidence-based policy intentions and recommendations that facilitate the effectuation of UHC in developing countries in particular. In April of the same year, the Mexico International Forum on universal health coverage brought together participants from every region to discuss and share experiences related to UHC and to work towards finding better solutions to facilitate progress.

The event produced the *Mexico City Political Declaration on Universal Health Coverage*, which reaffirms connections between health and human rights; it also emphasises that UHC is essential to successful sustainable development, before calling upon governments and organisations to "[w]ork to promote the inclusion of universal health coverage as an important element in the international development agenda and in the internationally agreed development goals, as a means to promote sustainable growth, social cohesion and population well-being" (WHO, 2012b, p. 3). African health and finance ministers convened in Tunis in July that year, resulting in the *Tunis Declaration on Value for Money, Sustainability and Accountability in the Health Sector*. The *Declaration* recognises the importance of UHC for the continent and recommends accelerated efforts to make it a reality – for example, by laying "the path to universal coverage for each country in particular establishing mechanisms to ensure equitable access to essential health services including social health insurance while ensuring effective safety nets to protect vulnerable individuals, households and communities" (African Bank Development Group, 2012, p. 2).

These multilateral efforts were further bolstered by the academic and scientific community, particularly in the latter half of 2012. Published in the time leading up to, during and after Rio+20, a dedicated *Lancet* series provided multiple per-spectives on the matter, one of which commented that: "[as] the world's nations gather for the UN meetings in September, 2012, real momentum on achievement of universal health coverage – aimed at giving everyone the health services they need without causing financial hardship – is no longer a distant dream" (Rodin & de Ferranti, 2012, p. 861). In the same article, the authors suggest that UHC has the potential to be the 'third global health transition', following the illustrious footsteps of (1) the introduction of basic sewage and sanitation in the late 18th century and (2) the epidemiological revolution of the 20th century, after which cures for major communicable diseases such as smallpox and polio were discov-ered. Other publications of the same article series similarly presented evidence arguing for the inherent and instrumental value of UHC (Frenk & De Ferranti, 2012), the ways in which UHC improves population health – especially in poorer countries (Moreno-Serra & Smith, 2012) – and how UHC is integral to successful human and sustainable development (Evans et al., 2012).

At the same time as publications emanated from the *Lancet* series, the Rio+20 summit outcome document, *The Future We Want* (UNGA, 2012a) offered similar sentiments, most succinctly presented in one paragraph under the subheading of *Health and Population*, thereby cementing the position of UHC within sustainable development:

> We also recognize the importance of universal health coverage to enhancing health, social cohesion and sustainable human and economic development. We pledge to strengthen health systems towards the provision of equitable universal coverage. We call for the involvement of all relevant actors for coordinated multisectoral action to address urgently the health needs of the world's population.
>
> (UNGA, 2012a, p. 37)

As mandated by the secretary-general, the HLP submitted their report in the first quarter of 2013, in which the panel supported and encouraged progress towards UHC and to ensure "equality in all the interconnected areas that contribute to health (social, economic and environmental)" (HLP, 2013, p. 38). The OWG the-matic session on health was held in June 2013. In the report that followed, it is clear that *health* was to be framed as a *human right*, treated far more holistically than previously, and that the interdependent dimensions at the nexus of sustain-able development and health would be central to the health goals of the new agenda – though not explicitly mentioning UHC (WHO, 2013c). In the mean-time, the 2013 *World Health Report* (WHO, 2013d) also focused on UHC, this time emphasising various avenues of research that would advance progress toward it – further mainstreaming the agendas such as the *Montreux Statement* and the *Bangkok Statement*. In 2013, World Bank President Jim Yong Kim indicated that achieving UHC and equity in health is central to the goals of his organisation, and that goals towards its realisation "should be firmly embedded in the emerging post-2015 global development agenda" (Kim, 2013, para. 7).

As a final piece to the puzzle, the OWG submitted its final report and its proposal for the SDGs in 2014 (OWG, 2014). In the case of health, the goal and sub-targets suggested in this proposal were identical to the final version passed in September 2015, with *Goal 3.8* aimed at the achievement of UHC. Now internalised, UHC has a special position in the development agenda for health: "[it] is the only target that underpins, and is key to the achievement of, all the others" (WHO, 2016, p. 41). This is because it embodies the normative and technical aspects conducive to attaining the full spectrum of health as it relates to sustainable development.

The inclusion of a UHC target in the health SDG was far from a surprise by the time the goals were first suggested by the OWG in 2014. Indeed, the lack of *antipreneurs* (Bloomfield, 2016) in the context of UHC is remarkable, though one outlier state remains the U.S. with regard to its ambiguity in dealing with its complicated domestic health care situation.

> Certain concepts resonate so naturally with the innate sense of dignity and justice within the hearts of men and women that they seem an insuppressible right. That health care should be accessible to all is surely one such concept. Yet in the past, this notion of has struggled against barriers of self-interest and poor understanding.
>
> (The Lancet, 2012, p. 859)

Although the sentiments incorporated in the quest for UHC seem familiar, the concept is a newcomer in the realm of coordinated global development. Normatively, this realm had changed significantly since the conception of the MDGs, and especially since the 1980s. Most pertinent to the inclusion of UHC is the re-emergent importance dedicated to sustainable development and its many implications. One of these implications is especially highlighted in this chapter as well as in most of the official SDG material available, namely *inclusivity*. Central to the social dimension of *sustainable development*, *inclusivity* ensures that benefits of development are distributed throughout society and that marginalised and vulnerable groups should be the first to enjoy these benefits. Once the several clear connections between UHC and sustainable developments had been made, its inclusion as a health target was the only appropriate response. The core normative basis that is most consistently invoked in this regard is the *right to health*, which itself is an indication of the increasing internalisation of human security and the human development paradigm. As with health in general, however, the instrumental value of UHC – and of socially sustainable development more generally – is not only a fortunate side effect, but a clear motivation more in line with the traditional notion of *hard politics* and the interests of states. However, this state ambiguity enables cooperation with less self-interested non-state actors, through IOs and otherwise, towards common objectives, exemplified by endeavours such as the Global Symposium on Health System Research.

Amid a plethora of individual and organisational actors who share responsibility for the successful introduction of UHC into the UN development agenda via the health SDG, there are two that stand out. The first is the Rockefeller Foundation, more specifically its THS initiative. Through the financial and reputational influence of the foundation as an *organisational platform*, this initiative was involved in nearly every event described in all three stages of the norm's *life cycle*. Convinced early on by the need for UHC to enter the mainstream of global health and health development, the THS was an important component of the movement that helped frame UHC within sustainable development and effectively emphasised these connections in order to accentuate UHC's centrality and appropriateness within the new development agenda. Though a connection with socially sustainable development entails much of what traditionally belongs to the category referred to as '*high politics*', the THS also had other arguments intended to persuade state actors to acquiesce.

> To foster their adoption, THS developed an economic argument for UHC, which it then presented to global leaders sympathetic to the need for health systems strengthening in LMICs. . . . During this period, THS also identified the UN system as a key vehicle to advance adoption of the UHC concept at the global and country levels. THS initially focused its UN advocacy efforts on achieving a UN resolution on UHC. Gaining enough support to pass a UHC resolution called for THS to shape and align UN delegates' messages on UHC.
>
> (Sattar & Smith, 2017, p. 13)

The THS had a willing and powerful ally in form of the WHO. Furthermore, the WHO is the site where the most significant individual candidate to attain the title *norm entrepreneur* held her position in the relevant timeframe. This norm entrepreneur is Margaret Chan, who on one occasion stated that UHC is "part of [her] DNA" (Chan in Holmes, 2012). Inspired in part by her own experiences – and in part by the efforts of people such as one of her predecessors as director-general of the WHO, Halfdan Mahler – Chan has long been a vehement supporter and advocate of UHC. Since she took office in 2006, the promotion of UHC and its importance for society and individuals has been unwavering. Her effective framing of the matter as common sense both in moral and instrumental terms contributed to the relatively quick cascade of UHC in the years surrounding 2010: *the tipping point* of the UHC norm (see Figure 6.2). In terms of organisational platform, Chan held what is perhaps the most advantageous position imaginable. The WHO has been a protagonist throughout this chapter as well as in previous ones; its position in global health, though diminished, is undoubtedly still at the very core. While no longer the normative hegemon, the organisation's stature was reaffirmed in the outcome document of Rio+20, *The Future We Want*: "[w]e support the leadership role of the [WHO] as the directing and coordinating authority on international health work" (UNGA, 2012a, p. 39). Further evidence for the WHO's continued clout is the fact that the organisation had some degree of involvement in most of the multilateral conferences and resultant agreements listed as part of the *norm cascade* of the UHC health norm. Chan's successor as director-general, Tedros

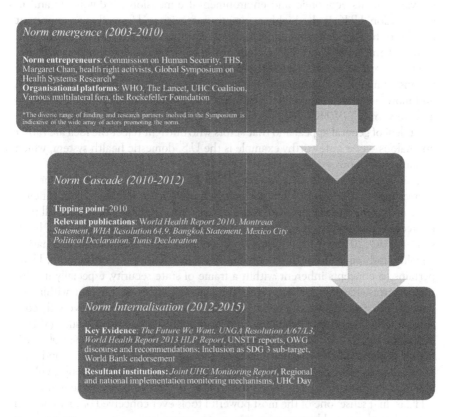

*Figure 6.2* The norm life cycle of UHC ahead of the SDG inclusion

Adhanom Ghebreyesus, is also an ardent supporter of UHC and has stated that its fulfilment is the top priority of the organisation (Ghebreyesus, 2017).

Further, the WHO is at the forefront in terms of assessing progress towards UHC achievement, chiefly through its annual *UHC Monitoring Report*, produced and published jointly with the World Bank. A substantial amount of work has been directed towards developing effective ways of measuring implementation and success, and several indices that attempt to capture the essentials of this have been suggested (Fullman & Lozano, 2018; Hogan, Stevens, Hosseinpoor, & Boerma, 2018; Wagstaff, Cotlear, Eozenou, & Buisman, 2016).

In terms of norm dynamics, the intrinsic characteristics of the UHC health norm benefited greatly from its clear adjacency with the super-norm of sustainability as well as with the *meta-norm* of human development. Indeed, this adjacency was perhaps its greatest advantage precipitating its successful emergence. As suggested, UHC is a natural component of sustainability; and while this is particularly true with regard to its social dimension, there is also extensive relevance to its economic and environmental dimensions, individually and in combination. UHC is also highly commensurate with and framed as an important enabler of human development. Other *non-intrinsic* characteristics that acted in favour of the success of UHC include those of *prominence* and *legitimation*. Still the most prominent GHG actor, the WHO has been at the forefront of endorsing the instrumental and inherent benefits of promoting UHC at least since 2005, and more assertively since 2010. In terms of legitimation, UHC is identified as a "vote winner" (WHO, 2013a). This is to say that the concept generally has a great deal of general appeal and that actors who outright reject the idea are rather anomalous – one noteworthy example is the U.S. domestic health system, which remains ambiguous.

This is connected to the content of the UHC health norm and its *intrinsic characteristics*. While UHC denotes complex intricacies, its underlying principle is clear. To reiterate the broadest sense of the term, "[UHC] exists when all people receive the quality health services they need without suffering financial hardship" (WHO, 2013a, p. 9); it is built upon a normative framework that emphasises equality and argues from a rights-based normative position. Furthermore, UHC pertains to concepts inherent within a frame of state security, especially in economic terms. Its universal appeal to the average citizen is inherent within the concept's first word and concept, while *health* is a core capability universally considered to be important: "for many UHC is literally a life or death issue" (WHO, 2013a, p. 10). While morally charged, arguments for UHC are increasingly fortified by evidence of its beneficial effects on general health, equality rates, and – via various tracks – the economy. While advantageous for all income groups, vulnerable and marginalised populations stand most to gain from its implementation. UHC is, in a sense, one of the most powerful tools ever conceived of to attain and ensure health-related human security.

Finally, the *world-time context* in which UHC institutionalised (that is, to say, the period after the 2008 GFC) was one characterised by an increasing sense of the impact of adverse environmental potentialities. Another contributing factor was a general normative movement toward an emphasis on inclusivity, participation, and scepticism[19] of the reticent hegemons of global political and economic governance.

## Conclusion

This chapter identified, described, and explained the emergence and institutionalisation of newly introduced health norms into the UN development agenda's current standard-bearer, the SDGs. The chapter was divided into three interrelated parts that gradually point the spotlight towards the specific health norms that comprise the focal point of analysis. The first part introduced the wider normative context in which the SDGs were conceived, beginning with the apparent trials and tribulations of the MDGs. The section continued with an account of the rise of *sustainability* and subsequently its ancillary imperative of *inclusivity* as the most central components of the post-2015 development agenda. Building on this, the next section introduced the details of the single health SDG; it also provided an exploratory account of the most salient connections between health, sustainability, and inclusivity. Against this backdrop, the final section analysed the normative incursions of NCDs (broadly defined) and UHC into the agenda, utilising the heuristic of the *norm life cycle* and its associated notions related to intrinsic and non-intrinsic norm characteristics.

The ambitious inclusion of NCDs and UHC in the SDG health goal were natural consequences of the UN's turn toward the imperatives of *sustainability* and their integration into its organisational identity. Norms set out to ensure sustainability are also framed within the higher-level constitutive norms that make up the organisation's *raison d'être*. Norms such as those related to sustainability refine an organisation's identity and subsequently set associated parameters for appropriate behaviour. Once the UN's adoption of sustainable development was explicitly internalised, particularly after the Rio+20 summit, the inclusion of UHC and NCDs in the upcoming development agenda was a logical next step.

This progression was further bolstered by state interest and support from NGOs, philanthropic foundations, and the scientific community. The WHO, in particular, played an important role in espousing both these related new ambitions and the human and state security-related norms connected with them. Motivated by concerns ranging from self-interest to rights-based magnanimity, well-positioned actors such as the Rockefeller Foundation, CARICOM, Margaret Chan, and the Commission on Human Security helped bring these causes to the forefront of GHG discourse and argued for their natural position within a post-2015 development agenda centred on sustainability.

\*

We completed this book in July 2020, as Covid-19 raged across the planet. In terms of global health governance, for those of us who support a multilateral, institutionalised response to health challenges, the Trump administration's attack on the World Health Organization is disquieting and destructive. Many GHG observers and practitioners are saddened by the reactionary global health and development politics coming out of Trump's United States, Bolsonaro's Brazil, Brexit UK, and Modi's India. However, we take heart in the multilateral health governance and diplomacy of states such as Merkel's Germany and the inclusive, cosmopolitan stance of many other countries. As international relations embarks on an intellectual reckoning of GHG in a time of Covid-19,[20] we remain confident that the vision of Mahbub ul Haq and Amartya Sen will persevere.

## Notes

1 Note that none of those conferences that were not considered to be follow-ups (this includes the 2005 World Summit, widely considered a follow-up to the Millennium Summit – particularly with regard to development), predate the year 2000.
2 The added emphasis corresponds with the *three pillars of sustainable development* as described in Chapter 2.

3  After Russia's expulsion from the group following its annexation of Crimea in 2014, the G8 has been reformatted to its current constellation, the G7.

4  Rowell (1996) describes how environmental activists occasionally face risks of violence and legal persecution at the behest of corporations or individuals associated with the industries demonstrated against. While this occurs on a grand scale, these actors are not representatives of an explicit anti-environmentalist organisation or corporation. On the contrary, these companies typically spend significant amounts of resources on cultivating responsible and 'green' images of themselves.

5  Palm oil became an environmental pariah in the mid-2000s, as it was becoming increasingly clear that plantations were often built on recently deforested tropical forestland. The palm oil industry is therefore thought to be partly responsible for shrinking carbon-sequestering forests, particularly in Indonesia. Furthermore, the industry has been linked to displacement of human settlements, as well as to the habitat destruction of animals, some of which are threatened with extinction. Other adverse environmental effects have also been documented as being partly derived from these plantations.

6  The 1972 Stockholm Conference on the Human Environment put environmental concerns on the global governance map. It also addressed social issues such as human rights, advocating, among other issues, for the end of the apartheid.

7  Gore's norm entrepreneurship does not fit neatly with the norm life cycle framework's linearity. As suggested, norms of sustainable development were present in the MDGs as well. The momentum from UNCED, which was still fresh in the memory of the UN, earned sustainable development a place in the *Millennium Declaration*. It also earned environmental sustainability its own development goal in the form of MDG 7. The most significant change had been the circumstances: the experience of the MDG failure and a related significant shift in terms of framing sustainability, the latter being instrumental in transforming it into a super-norm, which acted as a connector for the interrelated aspects of development that were enshrined in the goals.

8  One source of inspiration for such an approach is the success of health-in-all-policies, which advocates for intersectoral collaboration in order to properly address the indirect determinants of health, in the belief "that health is largely constructed in other sectors beyond the health sector" (Sihto, Ollila, & Koivusalo, 2006, p. 3). The approach was mainly professed by Finland, most notably during a period in which it held the EU presidency in the second half of 2006.

9  While the norms associated with reproductive health only translated into a retroactive inclusion into the MDGs after nearly a decade in which they were excluded from the framework, its inclusion in the health SDG is not treated as a novelty to the framework. The emphasis on *universal access*, however, is considered an integral part of the norms associated with UHC described later.

10  This sub-goal, though less of a quantifiable goal, is a 'means of implementation' that is relevant to global health security, particularly in relation to upholding the IHRs (see Chapter 3). While such a point does constitute a novelty in the context of the UN development agenda, it supposes optimisation and maintenance of the status quo rather than introducing new normative imperatives in global health.

11  The majority of deaths within these 10% are attributed to the subcategories of *unsafe water, sanitation,* and *hygiene* and *indoor smoke from solid fuels*.

12  According to the WHO, ambient air pollution refers to air pollutants emitted by industries, households, cars, and trucks. Fine particulate matter in these pollutants has been proven to have adverse effects on human health and is associated with various chronic and acute illnesses.

13  Certain schools of thought within economics believe in what is referred to as an *environmental Kuznets curve* (Shafik, 1994), which suggests that developing economies tend to initially cause deterioration of the environment and that a rise in GDP is correlated with an improvement in society's relationship with nature. This theory has largely been

disconfirmed by empirical evidence (Stern, 2004) but is still occasionally invoked in public discourse.

14 Although SDG 3 features five new targets in the category of new issue areas for the new development agenda, this study approaches the novel health norms in only two separate groups. One category clusters together four of the targets, all related to addressing neglected and significant sections of the global health burden more or less connected. These are NCDs and mental health, substance abuse, air pollution, and road-traffic accidents. The second category is UHC, which, while still related to the first category, sets itself apart because of its more systemic and rights-driven focus.

15 The SPC is the principal organisation that multilaterally coordinates development policy and research for the Pacific region, comprising 26 countries and territories.

16 Though the resolution lists a number of antecedent outcomes – in this case of "conferences and summits which have contributed to the advancement of the global health agenda" (UNGA, 2012c, p. 1) – the *Declaration* of *Alma-Ata* is not mentioned. Indeed, no summit or conference preceding the 1990s is included in the list.

17 The Commission on Human Security was established in 2001 to focus on a number of issues that are relevant to human security and to produce reports that present their findings. The aim of the report is to prove the validity and utility of the approach as an alternative security framework.

18 The Prince Mahidol Award for public health and medicine is a prestigious annual international health award. A conference linked to it is hosted by the Thai government and the Prince Mahidol Foundation, along with relevant IOs and NGOs. The conference is a forum for sharing and discussing ideas and evidence related to policies and commitments in health development. It is typically attended by significant numbers of health ministers and participants from academia, civil society, and the private sector.

19 This scepticism has been invoked and utilised for mobilisations in several contexts, and for various purposes. For example, Donald Trump's denouncement and intended abolishment of corrupt and malevolent elites – notably encapsulated in the slogan 'draining the swamp' – was an effective framing tool used in his campaign prior to the 2016 U.S. presidential election.

20 For instance, see several contributions in the July/August 2020 issue of *Foreign Affairs* (vol. 99, no. 4).

# Bibliography

Abegunde, D. O., Mathers, C. D., Adam, T., Ortegon, M., & Strong, K. (2007). The burden and costs of chronic diseases in low-income and middle-income countries. *The Lancet*, *370*(9603), 1929–1938.

Adler, E. (2002). Constructivism and international relations. In W. Karlsnaes, T. Risse, & B. A. Simmons (Eds.), *Handbook of international relations*. London: Sage.

Abiiro, G. A., & De Allegri, M. (2015). Universal health coverage from multiple perspectives: A synthesis of conceptual literature and global debates. *BMC International Health and Human Rights*, *15*(1), 17.

African Bank Development Group. (2012). *Tunis declaration on value for money, sustainability and accountability in the health sector*. Retrieved July 1, 2018, from www.afdb.org/fileadmin/uploads/afdb/Documents/Generic-Documents/Tunis%20declaration%20english%20july%206%20(2).pdf

Aldis, W. (2008). Health security as a public health concept: A critical analysis. *Health Policy and Planning*, *23*(6), 369–375.

Alkire, S. (2005). Why the capability approach? *Journal of Human Development*, *6*(1), 115–135.

Alston, P. (2005). Ships passing in the night: The current state of the human rights and development debate seen through the lens of the millennium development goals. *Human Rights Quarterly*, 755–829.

Amon, J. J. (2015). Health security and/or human rights? In S. Rushton & J. Youde (Eds.), *Routledge handbook of global health security*. Oxon: Routledge.

Amorim, C., Douste-Blazy, P., Wirayuda, H., Støre, J. G., Gadio, C. T., Dlamini-Zuma, N., & Pibulsonggram, N. (2007). Oslo ministerial declaration – global health: A pressing foreign policy issue of our time. *The Lancet*, *369*(9570), 1373–1378.

Amstutz, M. R. (2013). *Evangelicals and American foreign policy*. Oxford: Oxford University Press.

Anderson, W. (1995). Excremental colonialism: Public health and the poetics of pollution. *Critical Inquiry*, *21*(3), 640–669.

Annan, K. A. (2000). *We the peoples: The role of the United Nations in the 21st century*. New York, NY: United Nations.

Annan, K. A. (2005). *In larger freedom: Towards development, security and human rights for all*. Executive Summary. Retrieved October 20, 2015, from www.un.org/en/events/pastevents/pdfs/larger_freedom_exec_summary.pdf

Archer, M. S., & Elder-Vass, D. (2012). Cultural system or norm circles? An exchange. *European Journal of Social Theory*, *15*(1), 93–115. doi:10.1177/1368431011423592

Ariana, P., & Naveed, A. (2009). Health. In S. Deneulin & L. Shahani (Eds.), *An introduction to the human development and capability approach* (pp. 228–245). London: Earthscan, International Development Research Centre.

Arimah, B. (2004). Poverty reduction and human development in Africa. *Journal of Human Development, 5*(3), 399–415.

Arndt, H. W. (1978). *The rise and fall of economic growth: A study in contemporary thought.* Melbourne: Longman Cheshire.

Arnold, D. (1993). *Colonizing the body: State medicine and epidemic disease in nineteenth-century India.* Berkeley, CA: University of California Press.

Asaria, P., Chisholm, D., Mathers, C., Ezzati, M., & Beaglehole, R. (2007). Chronic disease prevention: Health effects and financial costs of strategies to reduce salt intake and control tobacco use. *The Lancet, 370*(9604), 2044–2053.

Ashe, J. W. (2013). *The post-2015 development agenda: Setting the stage! High-level events/ Thematic debates to be convened by the president of the general assembly: Note to member states.* Retrieved December 10, 2015, from www.un.org/en/ga/president/68/pdf/letters/12052013Post-2015_Development_Agenda.pdf

Asher, R. (1982). *Transcript of interview with Mahbub ul Haq.* The World Bank/IFC Archives. Oral History Program. World Bank. Retrieved October 20, 2017, from http://documents.worldbank.org/curated/en/538481468338976295/pdf/790280TRN0Haq00iew0December03001982.pdf

Baldwin, D. A. (1995). Security studies and the end of the cold war. *World Politics, 48*(1), 117–141.

Ban, K. M. (2008). *Committing to action: Achieving the millennium development goals. Background note by the secretary-general.* Retrieved October 30, 2015, from www.un.org/millenniumgoals/2008highlevel/pdf/commiting.pdf

Ban, K. M. (2010). *Keeping the promise: A forward-looking review to promote an agreed action agenda to achieve the millennium development by 2015.* Retrieved October 24, 2015, from https://reliefweb.int/sites/reliefweb.int/files/resources/62C31608D19F702C492576E9000634F0-Full_Report.pdf

Barnett, M. (1990). High politics is low politics: The domestic and systemic sources of Israeli security policy, 1967–1977. *World Politics, 42*(4), 529–562.

Barnett, M., & Finnemore, M. (1999). The politics, power, and pathologies of international organisations. *International Organisation, 53*(4), 699–732.

Beaglehole, R., Bonita, R., Horton, R., Adams, C., Alleyne, G., Asaria, P., . . . Cecchini, M. (2011). Priority actions for the non-communicable disease crisis. *The Lancet, 377*(9775), 1438–1447.

Beaglehole, R., Ebrahim, S., Reddy, S., Voute, J., & Leeder, S. (2007). Prevention of chronic diseases: A call to action. *The Lancet, 370*(9605), 2152–2157.

Becker, G. S. (1994). Human capital revisited. In *Human capital: A theoretical and empirical analysis with special reference to education* (3rd ed.). Chicago, IL: University of Chicago Press.

Behrman, G. (2004). *The invisible people.* New York, NY: Free Press.

Bell, J. (2013). *The world's Muslims: Religion, politics and society.* Pew Research Center Forum on Religion & Public Life. Washington, DC: Pew Research Center.

Bellamy, E. (1951). *Looking backward: 1887–2000.* New York, NY: Random House, Modern Library.

Benagiano, G., d'Arcangues, C., Requejo, J. H., Schafer, A., Say, L., & Merialdi, M. (2012). The special programme of research in human reproduction: Forty years of activities to achieve reproductive health for all. *Gynecologic and Obstetric Investigation, 74*(3), 190–217.

Benson, C., & Glasgow, S. M. (2015). Noncommunicable disease as a security issue. In S. Rushton & J. Youde (Eds.), *Routledge handbook of global health security*. Oxon: Routledge.

Berg, A., & Qureshi, Z. (2005). The MDGs: Building momentum. *Finance & Development, 42*(3), 21–23.

Bernstein, S. (2011). Legitimacy in intergovernmental and non-state global governance. *Review of International Political Economy, 18*(1), 17–51.

Besson, S. (2013). The legitimate authority of international human rights: On the reciprocal legitimation of domestic and international human rights. In A. Føllesdal, J. K. Schaffer, & G. Ulfstein (Eds.), *The legitimacy of international human rights regimes: Legal, political and philosophical perspectives*. Cambridge: Cambridge University Press.

Beyond 2015. (2011). *Towards a successor framework to the millennium development goals next steps for the United Nations*. Retrieved December 3, 2015, from www.together2030.org/archive/www.beyond2015.org/sites/default/files/Towards%20a%20successor%20framework%20to%20the%20MDGs.pdf

Bloom, D. E., Cafiero, E., Jané-Llopis, E., Abrahams-Gessel, S., Bloom, L. R., Fathima, S., ... O'Farrell, D. (2012). *The global economic burden of noncommunicable diseases*. PGDA Working Paper No. 8712. Programmeon the Global Demography of Aging. Retrieved from https://www.hsph.harvard.edu/pgda/working.htm

Bloomfield, A. (2016). Norm antipreneurs and theorising resistance to normative change. *Review of International Studies, 42*(2), 310–333.

Bode, I. (2015). *Individual agency and policy change at the United Nations: The people of the United Nations*. Oxon: Routledge.

Borgonovi, E., & Compagni, A. (2013). Sustaining universal health coverage: The interaction of social, political, and economic sustainability. *Value in Health, 16*(1), 34–38.

Bousquet, J., Dahl, R., & Khaltaev, N. (2007). Global alliance against chronic respiratory diseases. *Allergy, 62*(3), 216–223.

Boyle, K. (1995). Stock-taking on human rights: The world conference on human rights, Vienna 1993. *Political Studies, 43*(1), 79–95.

Braveman, P., & Gruskin, S. (2003). Defining equity in health. *Journal of Epidemiology & Community Health, 57*(4), 254–258.

Brown, G. W., & Stoeva, P. (2015). Reevaluating health security from a cosmopolitan perspective. In S. Rushton & J. Youde (Eds.), *Routledge handbook of global health security*. Oxon: Routledge.

Browne, S. (2017). *Sustainable development goals and UN goal-setting*. Oxon: Routledge.

Brundtland, G. (1987). *Report of the world commission on environment and development: Our common future*. Retrieved September 1, 2015, from www.un-documents.net/our-common-future.pdf

Brundtland, G. (1994). *Key note address to the international conference on population and development, Cairo, 5 September 1994*. Retrieved November 20, 2017, from www.un.org/popin/icpd/conference/gov/940905192242.html

Bumiller, E. (1998, April 14). Public lives; putting women's rights in population policy. *The New York Times*. Retrieved December 1, 2017, from https://archive.nytimes.com/www.nytimes.com/partners/aol/special/women/warchive/980414_921.html

Buse, K., & Hawkes, S. (2015). Health in the sustainable development goals: Ready for a paradigm shift? *Globalization and Health, 11*(1), 13.

Buzan, B. (1991). New patterns of global security in the twenty-first century. *International Affairs, 67*(3), 431–451.

Buzan, B. (1997). Rethinking security after the cold war. *Cooperation and Conflict, 32*(1), 5–28.

Buzan, B., & Gonzalez-Pelaez, A. (2005). *The middle East through English school theory: A regional international society.* WISC Conference Istanbul. Retrieved October 4, 2017, from www.bisa.ac.uk/files/Paper%20Archive/buzan05.pdf

Buzan, B., Wæver, O., & De Wilde, J. (1998). *Security: A new framework for analysis.* London: Lynne Rienner Publishers.

Caballero-Anthony, M., & Amul, G. C. (2015). Health and human security: Pathways to advancing a human-centered approach to health security in East Asia. In S. Rushton & J. Youde (Eds.), *Routledge handbook of global health security.* Oxon: Routledge.

Calabrese, G. (Ed.). (2016). *The greening of the automotive industry.* Basingstoke: Palgrave Macmillan.

Capstick, S., Whitmarsh, L., Poortinga, W., Pidgeon, N., & Upham, P. (2015). International trends in public perceptions of climate change over the past quarter century. *Wiley Interdisciplinary Reviews: Climate Change, 6*(1), 35–61.

Caribbean Community. (2007). *Port-of-Spain declaration: Uniting to stop the epidemic of chronic non-communicable diseases.* Retrieved May 19, 2018, from www.paho.org/hq/dmdocuments/2009/cmn09day1pres6.pdf?ua=1

Chan, M. (2009). *Why the world needs global health initiatives.* Address at the high-level dialogue on maximizing positive synergies between health systems and global health initiatives. Retrieved June 22, 2018, from www.who.int/dg/speeches/2009/global_health_initiatives_20090622/en/

Chan, M. (2012). *Universal coverage is the ultimate expression of fairness.* Acceptance speech at the Sixty-fifth World Health Assembly, Geneva, Switzerland. Retrieved June 13, 2018, from www.who.int/dg/speeches/2012/wha_20120523/en/

Chang, S. S., Stuckler, D., Yip, P., & Gunnell, D. (2013). Impact of 2008 global economic crisis on suicide: Time trend study in 54 countries. *BMJ: British Medical Journal, 347,* f5239.

Chattu, V. K., & Sakhamuri, S. (2018). Port-of-Spain declaration for global NCD prevention. *The Lancet, 391*(10131), 1682.

Chen, L., & Narasimhan, V. (2003). Human security and global health. *Journal of Human Development, 4*(2), 181–190.

Chigwedere, P., Seage, G. R., Gruskin, S., Lee, T. H., & Essex, M. (2008). Estimating the lost benefits of antiretroviral drug use in South Africa. *Journal of Acquired Immune Deficiency Syndromes, 49*(4), 410–415.Clark, H. (2013). NCDs: A challenge to sustainable human development. *The Lancet, 381*(9866), 510–511.

Clemens, M. A., Kenny, C. J., & Moss, T. J. (2007). The trouble with the MDGs: Confronting expectations of aid and development success. *World Development, 35*(5), 735–751.

Cohen, A. J., Brauer, M., Burnett, R., Anderson, H. R., Frostad, J., Estep, K., . . . Feigin, V. (2017). Estimates and 25-year trends of the global burden of disease attributable to ambient air pollution: An analysis of data from the global burden of diseases study 2015. *The Lancet, 389*(10082), 1907–1918.

Cohen, S. P. (2004). *The idea of Pakistan.* Washington, DC: Brookings Institution Press.

Commission on Human Security. (2003). *Human security now.* Retrieved May 2, 2016, from https://reliefweb.int/sites/reliefweb.int/files/resources/91BAEEDBA50C6907C1256D19006A9353-chs-security-may03.pdf

Commission on Social Determinants of Health. (2008). *Closing the gap in a generation: Health equity through action on the social determinants of health.* Final Report of the Commission on Social Determinants of Health. Geneva, Switzerland: World Health Organization.

Cornia, G. A., Jolly, R., & Stewart, F. (1987). *Adjustment with a human face, vol. I: Protecting the vulnerable and promoting growth.* Oxford: Clarendon Press for UNICEF.

Cornwall, A., & Brock, K. (2005). *Beyond buzzwords: "Poverty reduction", "participation" and "empowerment" in development policy.* United Nations Research Institute for Social Development, Overarching Concerns Programme – Paper No. 10. Geneva, Switzerland: UNRISD.

Cortell, A. P., & Davis, J. W. (2005). When norms clash: International norms, domestic practices, and Japan's internalisation of the GATT/WTO. *Review of International Studies, 31*(1), 3–25.

Coughlin, S. S., & Ekwueme, D. U. (2009). Breast cancer as a global health concern. *Cancer Epidemiology, 33*(5), 315–318.

Cruz, I., Stahel, A., & Max-Neef, M. (2009). Towards a systemic development approach: Building on the human-scale development paradigm. *Ecological Economics, 68*(7), 2021–2030.

Dabla-Norris, E., Minoiu, C., & Zanna, L. F. (2015). Business cycle fluctuations, large macroeconomic shocks, and development aid. *World Development, 69*, 44–61.

Davies, D. S., & Verde, E. S. (2013). Antimicrobial resistance. *Search of a Collaborative Solution, World Innovation Summit for Health, Doha*, 1–36.

Davies, S. (2010a). *Global politics of health.* Cambridge: Polity Press.

Davies, S. (2010b). What contribution can international relations make to the evolving global health agenda? *International Affairs, 86*(5), 1167–1190.

Davies, S., Elbe, S., Howell, A., & McInnes, C. (2014). Global health in international relations: Editors' introduction. *Review of International Studies, 40*(5), 825–834.

Davies, S., Kamradt-Scott, A., & Rushton, S. (2015). *Disease diplomacy: International norms and global health security.* Baltimore, MD: Johns Hopkins University Press.

de Carvalho, B., & Neumann, I. B. (Eds.). (2014). *Small state status seeking: Norway's quest for international standing.* Oxon: Routledge.

DeLaet, D. (2015). Whose interests is the securitisation of health serving?? In S. Rushton & J. Youde (Eds.), *Routledge handbook of global health security.* Oxon: Routledge.

Delmas, M. A., & Burbano, V. C. (2011). The drivers of greenwashing. *California Management Review, 54*(1), 64–87.

Dempsey, N., Bramley, G., Power, S., & Brown, C. (2011). The social dimension of sustainable development: Defining urban social sustainability. *Sustainable Development, 19*(5), 289–300.

Der Derian, J., & Shapiro, M. (Eds.). (1989). *International/intertextual relations: Boundaries of knowledge and practice in world politics.* Lexington, KY: Lexington Books.

Diethelm, P., & McKee, M. (2009). Denialism: What is it and how should scientists respond? *The European Journal of Public Health, 19*(1), 2–4.

DiMaggio, P. J., & Powell, W. W. (Eds.). (1991). *The new institutionalism in organizational analysis.* Chicago, IL: University of Chicago Press.

Dodds, F., Donoghue, D., & Roesch, J. L. (2017). *Negotiating the sustainable development goals.* Oxon: Routledge.

Dodds, F., Laguna-Celis, J., & Thompson, L. (2014). *From Rio+ 20 to a new development agenda: Building a bridge to a sustainable future.* New York, NY: Routledge.

Dodgson, R., Lee, K., & Drager, N. (2002). *Global health governance: A conceptual overview.* Discussion Paper No.1: Key issues in Global Health Governance. Department of Health and Development. Geneva, Switzerland: World Health Organization.

Dunn, D. H. (Ed.). (1996). *Diplomacy at the highest level: The evolution of international summitry.* Basingstoke: Palgrave Macmillan.

Dye, C., & Acharya, S. (2017). How can the sustainable development goals improve global health? A call for papers. *Bulletin of the World Health Organization, 95*(10), 666.

Easterly, W. (2001). *The elusive quest for growth: Economists' adventures and misadventures in the tropics.* Cambridge, MA: MIT Press.

Eaton, J., Kakuma, R., Wright, A., & Minas, H. (2014). A position statement on mental health in the post-2015 development agenda. *International Journal of Mental Health Systems, 8*(1), 28.

Ekwempu, C. C., Maine, D., Olorukoba, M. B., Essien, E. S., & Kisseka, M. N. (1990). Structural adjustment and health in Africa. *The Lancet, 336*(8703), 56–57.

Elbe, S. (2011). Pandemics on the radar screen: Health security, infectious disease and the medicalisation of insecurity. *Political Studies, 59*(4), 848–66.

Elder-Vass, D. (2015). Developing social theory using critical realism. *Journal of Critical Realism, 14*(1), 80–92. doi:10.1179/1476743014Z.00000000047

Escobar, A. (1995). *Encountering development: The making and unmaking of the third world.* Princeton, MA: Princeton University Press.

Esteva, G., & Prakash, M. S. (1998). *Grassroots post-modernism: Remaking the soil of cultures.* London: Palgrave Macmillan.

Evans, D. B., Marten, R., & Etienne, C. (2012). Universal health coverage is a development issue. *The Lancet, 380*(9845), 864–865.

Evans, G. (2013). Commission diplomacy. In A. Cooper, J. Heine, & R. Takur (Eds.), *The Oxford handbook of modern diplomacy.* Oxford: Oxford University Press.

Faulkner, N., & Johanson, P. (2018). *Nonrenewable resources and you.* New York, NY: The Rosen Publishing Group, Inc.

Feachem, R. G. A. (2000). Poverty and inequity: A proper focus for the new century. *Bulletin of the World Health Organization, 78*(1), 1.

Ferreira, L. (2002). Access to affordable HIV/AIDS drugs: The human rights obligations of multinational pharmaceutical corporations. *Fordham Law Review, 71*, 1133.

Fidler, D. P. (1997). The globalization of public health: Emerging infectious diseases and international relations. *Indiana Journal of Global Legal Studies*, 11–51.

Fidler, D. P. (2002). *Global health governance: Overview of the role of international law in protecting and promoting global public health.* Discussion paper No. 3: Key issues in Global Health Governance. Department of Health and Development. Geneva, Switzerland: World Health Organization.

Fidler, D. P. (2003). Public health and national security in the global age: Infectious diseases, bioterrorism, and realpolitik. *George Washington International Law Review, 35*, 787–856.

Fidler, D. P. (2004). Germs, governance, and global public health in the wake of SARS. *The Journal of Clinical Investigation, 113*(6), 799–804.

Fidler, D. P. (2005). From international sanitary conventions to global health security: The new international health regulations. *Chinese Journal of International Law, 4*(2), 325–392.

Fidler, D. P. (2009). Health in foreign policy: An analytical overview. *Canadian Foreign Policy Journal, 15*(3), 11–29.

Fidler, D. P. (2010). *The challenges of global health governance.* Working Paper. New York, NY: Council of Foreign Relations.

Fidler, D. P. (2011). *Assessing the foreign policy and global health initiative: The meaning of the Oslo process.* Briefing Paper. Center on Global Health Security. London: Chatham House.

Finnemore, M. (1996). Norms, culture, and world politics: Insights from sociology's institutionalism. *International Organisation, 50*(2), 325–347.

Finnemore, M., & Sikkink, K. (1998). International norm dynamics and political change. *International Organisation, 52*(4), 887–917.

Food and Agriculture Organization of the United Nations. (1996). *World food summit plan of action*. Retrieved December 12, 2015, from www.fao.org/docrep/003/w3613e/w3613e00.htm

Ford, J. D. (2012). Indigenous health and climate change. *American Journal of Public Health, 102*(7), 1260–1266.

Forman, L., Ooms, G., & Brolan, C. E. (2015). Rights language in the sustainable development agenda: Has right to health discourse and norms shaped health goals? *International Journal of Health Policy and Management, 4*(12), 799.

Fourie, P. (2013). Turning dread into capital: South Africa's AIDS diplomacy. *Globalization and Health, 9*(1), 8.

Fourie, P. (2015). Aids as a security threat: The emergence and the decline of an idea. In S. Rushton & J. Youde (Eds.), *Routledge handbook of global health security*. Oxon: Routledge.

Fourie, P., & Schönteich, M. (2001). Africa's new security threat: HIV/AIDS and human security in Southern Africa. *African Security Review, 10*(4), 29–42.

Frank, A. G. (1966). The development of underdevelopment. *Monthly Review, 18*(4), 17–31.

Frank, A. G. (1967). *Capitalism and underdevelopment in Latin America* (Vol. 93). New York, NY: Monthly Review Press.

Frenk, J., Chen, L., Bhutta, Z. A., Cohen, J., Crisp, N., Evans, T., . . . Kistnasamy, B. (2010). Health professionals for a new century: Transforming education to strengthen health systems in an interdependent world. *The Lancet, 376*(9756), 1923–1958.

Frenk, J., & De Ferranti, D. (2012). Universal health coverage: good health, good economics. *The Lancet, 380*(9845), 862–864.

Frenk, J., & Moon, S. (2013). Governance challenges in global health. *New England Journal of Medicine, 368*(10), 936–942.

Fukuda-Parr, S. (2003). The human development paradigm: Operationalizing Sen's ideas on capabilities. *Feminist Economics, 9*(2–3), 301–317.

Fukuda-Parr, S. (2016). Equality as a valued social norm, inequality as an injustice. In ISSC, IDS, & UNESCO (Eds.), *Challenging inequalities: Pathways to a just world, world social science report 2016* (pp. 263–264). Paris, France: UNESCO Publishing.Fukuda-Parr, S. and Hulme, D. (2009). *International Norm Dynamics and 'the End of Poverty': Understanding the Millennium Development Goals (MDGs)*. BWPI Working Paper No. 96, University of Manchester: BWPI.

Fukuyama, F. (1989, Summer). The end of history? *The National Interest, 16*, 3–18.

Fullman, N., & Lozano, R. (2018). Towards a meaningful measure of universal health coverage for the next billion. *The Lancet Global Health, 6*(2), 122–123.

Garnett, J. C. (1996). European security after the cold war: Security issues in the post-cold war world. In M. J. Davis (Ed.), *Security issues in the post-cold war world* (pp. 12–39). Cheltenham: Edward Elgar.

Gasper, D. (2000). Development as freedom: Taking economics beyond commodities—The cautious boldness of Amartya Sen. *Journal of International Development, 12*(7), 989–1001.

Gasper, D. (2002). Is Sen's capability approach an adequate basis for considering human development? *Review of Political Economy, 14*(4), 435–461.

Gasper, D. (2005). Securing humanity: Situating human security as concept and discourse. *Journal of Human Development, 6*(2), 221–245.

Geertz, C. (1973). *The interpretation of cultures: Selected essays*. New York, NY: Basic Books.

Germain, A. (2018). The global movement for sexual and reproductive health and rights: Intellectual underpinnings. In C. O'Manique & P. Fourie (Eds.), *Global health and security: Critical feminist perspectives*. London: Routledge.

Ghebreyesus, T. A. (2017). All roads lead to universal health coverage. *The Lancet Global Health*, 5(9), e839–e840.

Gleditsch, N. P., Pinker, S., Thayer, B. A., Levy, J. S., & Thompson, W. R. (2013). The forum: The decline of war. *International Studies Review*, 15(3), 396–419.

Global Burden of Disease Collaborative Network. (2017). *Global burden of disease study 2016*. Seattle, WA: Institute for Health Metrics and Evaluation.

Gollin, D., & Zimmermann, C. (2007). *Malaria: Disease impacts and long-run income differences*. IZA Discussion Paper No. 2997. Bonn, Germany: IZA.

Gore, C. (2000). The rise and fall of the Washington consensus as a paradigm for developing countries. *World Development*, 28(5), 789–804.

Gostin, L. O. (2001). Public health, ethics, and human rights: A tribute to the late Jonathan Mann. *The Journal of Law, Medicine & Ethics*, 29(2), 121–130.

Gostin, L. O., Sridhar, D., & Hougendobler, D. (2015). The normative authority of the world health organization. *Public Health*, 129(7), 854–863.

Greig, A., Hulme, D., & Turner, M. (2007). *Challenging global inequality: Development theory and practice in the 21st century*. New York, NY: Palgrave Macmillan.

Gribble, J. N., & Preston, S. H. (Eds.). (1993). *The epidemiological transition: Policy and planning implications for developing countries*. Washington, DC: National Academy Press.

Griffith-Jones, S., & Ocampo, J. A. (2009). *The financial crisis and its impact on developing countries*. Working Paper No. 53. Brasilia, Brazil: International Policy Centre for Inclusive Growth.

Griggs, D., Stafford-Smith, M., Gaffney, O., Rockström, J., Öhman, M. C., Shyamsundar, P., . . . Noble, I. (2013). Policy: Sustainable development goals for people and planet. *Nature*, 495(7441), 305.

Groom, A. J. R. (2013). Conference diplomacy. In A. Cooper, J. Heine, & R. Takur (Eds.), *The Oxford handbook of modern diplomacy*. Oxford: Oxford University Press.

Grubb, M. (1993). *The earth summit agreements: A guide and assessment*. London: Earthscan.

Guzzini, S. (2000). A reconstruction of constructivism in international relations. *European Journal of International Relations*, 6(2), 147–182.

Haas, P. M., Levy, M. A., & Parson, E. A. (1992). How should we judge UNCED's success? *Environment: Science and Policy for Sustainable Development*, 34(8), 6–33.

Haines, A., & Dora, C. (2012). How the low carbon economy can improve health. *BMJ: British Medical Journal (Online)*, 344.

Hall, J. J., & Taylor, R. (2003). Health for all beyond 2000: The demise of the Alma-Ata declaration and primary health care in developing countries. *The Medical Journal of Australia*, 178(1), 17.

Hammonds, R., & Ooms, G. (2014). The emergence of a global right to health norm – the unresolved case of universal access to quality emergency obstetric care. *BMC International Health and Human Rights*, 14(1), 4.

Haq, K. (Ed.). (2017). *Economic growth with social justice: Collected writings of Mahbub ul Haq*. New Delhi: Oxford University Press.

Haq, K., & Kirdar, U. (1986). *Human development: The neglected dimension*. North-South Roundtable. Retrieved November 20, 2017, from https://nsrt.lums.edu.pk/sites/all/themes/nsrt/books/Human_Development.pdf

Haq, M. (1963). *Strategy of economic planning: A case study of Pakistan*. Karachi, Pakistan: Oxford University Press.

Haq, M. (1995). *Reflections on human development*. New York, NY: Oxford University Press.

Harari, Y. N. (2014). *Sapiens: A brief history of humankind*. New York, NY: Harper.

Hawkes, S., & Buse, K. (2016). Searching for the right to health in the sustainable development agenda: Comment on "rights language in the sustainable development agenda: Has right to health discourse and norms shaped health goals?" *International Journal of Health Policy and Management, 5*(5), 337.

Hein, W., & Kohlmorgen, L. (2009). Transnational norm-building in global health: The important role of non-state actors in post-Westphalian politics. In S. MacLean, S. Brown, & P. Fourie (Eds.), *Health for some: The political economy of global health governance*. London: Palgrave Macmillan.

Hellmüller, S., Federer, J. P., & Pring, J. (2017). *Are mediators norm entrepreneurs? Exploring the role of mediators in norm diffusion*. Bern, Switzerland: Swisspeace.

Hellmüller, S., Federer, J. P., & Zeller, M. (2015). *The role of norms in international peace mediation*. Bern, Switzerland: Swisspeace, NOREF.

Hettne, B. (2010). Development and security: Origins and future. *Security Dialogue, 41*(1), 31–52.

High-Level Panel of Eminent Persons on the Post-2015 Development Agenda. (2013). *A new global partnership: Eradicate poverty and transform economies through sustainable development*. Retrieved December 13, 2015, from https://sustainabledevelopment.un.org/content/documents/8932013-05%20-%20HLP%20Report%20-%20A%20New%20Global%20Partnership.pdf

Hirai, T. (2017). *The creation of the human development approach*. Basingstoke: Palgrave Macmillan.

Hoen, E. T., Berger, J., Calmy, A., & Moon, S. (2011). Driving a decade of change: HIV/AIDS, patents and access to medicines for all. *Journal of the International AIDS Society, 14*(1), 15.

Hofferberth, M., & Weber, C. (2015). Lost in translation: A critique of constructivist norm research. *Journal of International Relations and Development, 18*(1), 75–103.

Hoffman, S. J. (2010). The evolution, etiology and eventualities of the global health security regime. *Health Policy and Planning, 25*(6), 510–522.

Hoffman, S. J., Cole, C. B., & Pearcey, M. (2015). *Mapping global health architecture to inform the future*. London: Chatham House.

Hogan, D. R., Stevens, G. A., Hosseinpoor, A. R., & Boerma, T. (2018). Monitoring universal health coverage within the sustainable development goals: Development and baseline data for an index of essential health services. *The Lancet Global Health, 6*(2), 152–168.

Holmes, D. (2012). Margaret Chan: Committed to universal health coverage. *The Lancet, 380*(9845), 879.

Hopkins, M. (1991). Human development revisited: A new UNDP report. *World Development, 19*(10), 1469–1473.

Horton, R. (2007). Health as an instrument of foreign policy. *The Lancet, 369*(9564), 806–807.

Hosseini, H. M., & Kaneko, S. (2012). Causality between pillars of sustainable development: Global stylized facts or regional phenomena? *Ecological Indicators, 14*(1), 197–201.

Hulme, D. (2007). *The making of the millennium development goals: Human development meets results based management in an imperfect world*. Brooks World Poverty Institute Working Paper 16. Manchester: The University of Manchester.

Hulme, D. (2009). *Global poverty reduction and the millennium development goals: A short history of the world's biggest promise*. Brooks World Poverty Institute Working Paper 100. Manchester: The University of Manchester.

Hulme, D. (2010a). *Global poverty: How global governance is failing the poor*. New York, NY: Routledge.

Hulme, D. (2010b). Lessons from the making of the MDGs: Human development meets results-based management in an unfair world. *IDS Bulletin, 41*(1), 15–25.

Hyde-Price, A. (1991). *European security beyond the cold war: Four scenarios for the year 2010.* London: Sage.

Islam, S. M. S., Purnat, T. D., Phuong, N. T. A., Mwingira, U., Schacht, K., & Fröschl, G. (2014). Non-communicable diseases (NCDs) in developing countries: A symposium report. *Globalization and Health, 10*(1), 81.

Jackson, R., & Sørensen, G. (2013). *Introduction to international relations: Theories and approaches.* Oxford: Oxford University Press.

Jacobs, I. M. (2012). *The politics of water in Africa: Norms, environmental regions and transboundary cooperation in the Orange-Senqu and Nile rivers.* New York, NY: Continuum.

Jamison, D. T., Summers, L. H., Alleyne, G., Arrow, K. J., Berkley, S., Binagwaho, A., . . . Ghosh, G. (2013). Global health 2035: A world converging within a generation. *The Lancet, 382*(9908), 1898–1955.

Jolly, R., Emmerij, L., Ghai, D., & Lapeyre, F. (2004). *UN contributions to development thinking and practice.* Bloomington, IN: Indiana University Press.

Johri, M., Chung, R., Dawson, A., & Schrecker, T. (2012). Global health and national borders: The ethics of foreign aid in a time of financial crisis. *Globalization and Health, 8*(1), 19.

Joint United Nations Programme on HIV/AIDS. (2008). *UNAIDS: The first 10 years, 1996–2006.* Retrieved February 5, 2018, from http://data.unaids.org/pub/report/2008/jc1579_first_10_years_en.pdf

Jolly, R. (2007). Society for international development, the North – South roundtable and the power of ideas. *Development, 50*(1), 47–58.

Jones, S. (2015). Aid supplies over time: Addressing heterogeneity, trends, and dynamics. *World Development, 69,* 31–43.

Kakabadse, N. K., & Khan, N. (2016). Cosmopolitanism or globalisation. *Society and Business Review, 11*(3), 234–241.

Katzenstein, P. J. (Ed.). (1996). *The culture of national security: Norms and identity in world politics.* New York, NY: Columbia University Press.

Katzenstein, P. J., Keohane, R. O., & Krasner, S. D. (1998). International organisation and the study of world politics. *International Organisation, 52*(4), 645–685.

Keohane, R. O., & Nye, J. S. (2011). *Power and interdependence* (4th ed.). London: Pearson Longman.

Keukeleire, S., & Raube, K. (2013). The security – development nexus and securitization in the EU's policies towards developing countries. *Cambridge Review of International Affairs, 26*(3), 556–572.

Kickbusch, I., & Kökény, M. (2013). Global health diplomacy: Five years on. *Bulletin of the World Health Organization, 91*(3), 159.

Kim, Y. (2013). *Speech by world bank group.* Government of Japan-World Bank Conference on Universal Health Coverage. Retrieved June 17, 2018, from http://documents.worldbank.org/curated/en/165141468194971410/text/101913-WP-Box393267B-PUBLIC-2013-12-06-JK-Speech-at-the-Government-of-Japan-WB-Conference-on-Universal-Health-Coverage.txt

Kingdon, J. W. (2014). *Agendas, alternatives, and public policies* (2nd ed.). Essex: Pearson.

Koplan, J. P., Bond, T. C., Merson, M. H., Reddy, K. S., Rodriguez, M. H., Sewankambo, N. K., & Wasserheit, J. N. (2009). Towards a common definition of global health. *The Lancet, 373*(9679), 1993–1995.

Krasner, S. D. (1982). Structural causes and regime consequences: Regimes as intervening variables. *International Organization, 36*(2), 185–205.

Kroenig, M., McAdam, M., & Weber, S. (2010). Taking soft power seriously. *Comparative Strategy*, 29(5), 412–431.

Lai, J., & Ravenhill, J. (2012). Asia's multi-level response to the global financial crisis. *Asia Europe Journal*, 9(2–4), 141–157.

Lakoff, A. (2010). Two regimes of global health. *Humanity: An International Journal of Human Rights, Humanitarianism, and Development*, 1(1), 59–79.

Lancet. (2012). The struggle for universal health coverage: Editorial. *The Lancet*, 380(9845), 859.

Landrigan, P. J., Fuller, R., Acosta, N. J., Adeyi, O., Arnold, R., Baldé, A. B., . . . Chiles, T. (2017). The Lancet Commission on pollution and health. *The Lancet*, 391.

Lanz, D. (2011). Who gets a seat at the table? A framework for understanding the dynamics of inclusion and exclusion in peace negotiations. *International Negotiation*, 16(2), 275–295.

Lawn, J. E., Rohde, J., Rifkin, S., Were, M., Paul, V. K., & Chopra, M. (2008). Alma-Ata 30 years on: Revolutionary, relevant, and time to revitalise. *The Lancet*, 372(9642), 917–927.

Lederberg, J., Shope, R. E., & Oaks, S. C. (Eds.). (1992). *Emerging infections: Microbial threats to health in the United States*. Washington, DC: National Academy Press.

Lee, K., & Kamradt-Scott, A. (2014). The multiple meanings of global health governance: A call for conceptual clarity. *Globalization and Health*, 10(1), 28.

Lee, K., & Pang, T. (2014). WHO: Retirement or reinvention? *Public Health*, 128(2), 119.

Loewenson, R. (1993). Structural adjustment and health policy in Africa. *International Journal of Health Services*, 23(4), 717–730.

Lo Yuk-Ping, C., & Thomas, N. (2010). How is health a security issue? Politics, responses and issues. *Health Policy and Planning*, 25(6), 447–453.

Lyman, P. N., & Wittels, S. B. (2010). No good deed goes unpunished: the unintended consequences of Washington's HIV/AIDS programs. *Foreign Affairs* 89(4), 74-84.

MacLean, S., Black, D., & Shaw, T. (2006). *A decade of human security: Global governance and new multilateralism*. London: Routledge.

Magnus, G. (2012). *The age of aging: How demographics are changing the global economy and our world*. Singapore: John Wiley & Sons.

Mahler, H. (1981). The meaning of 'Health for All by the Year 2000'. *World Health Forum*, 2, 5–22.

Mandela, N. (2000). *Closing address by Nelson Mandela at 13th international aids conference, Durban*. Retrieved October 20, 2017, from www.mandela.gov.za/mandela_speeches/2000/000714_aidsconf.htm

March, J. G., & Olsen, J. P. (1998). The institutional dynamics of international political orders. *International Organisation*, 52(4), 943–969.

Marmot, M., & Wilkinson, R. (Eds.). (2005). *Social determinants of health*. Oxford: Oxford University Press.

Marquis, C., & Toffel, M. W. (2012). *When do firms greenwash? Corporate visibility, civil society scrutiny, and environmental disclosure*. Boston, MA: Harvard Business School.

Mbeki, T. (2006). *Statement by H.E. Mr. Thabo Mbeki on the occasion of the general debate of the 61st session of the United Nations general assembly*. Retrieved March 20, 2018, from www.un.org/webcast/ga/61/pdfs/south_africa-e.pdf

McCaw-Binns, A., & Hussein, J. (2012). The millennium development goals. In J. Hussein, A. McCaw-Binns, & R. Webber (Eds.), *Maternal and perinatal health in developing countries*. Oxford: CABI.

McDonald, M. (2008). Securitization and the construction of security. *European Journal of International Relations*, 14(4), 563–587.

McGillivray, M. (1991). The human development index: Yet another redundant composite development indicator? *World Development*, 19(10), 1461–1468.

McInnes, C. (2015). The many meanings of health security. In S. Rushton & J. Youde (Eds.), *Routledge handbook of global health security*. Oxon: Routledge.

McInnes, C., Kamradt-Scott, A., Lee, K., Reubi, D., Roemer-Mahler, A., Rushton, S., . . . Woodling, M. (2015). Framing global health: The governance challenge. In C. McInnes & K. Lee (Eds.), *Framing global health governance*. Oxon: Routledge.

McInnes, C., & Lee, K. (2006). Health, security and foreign policy. *Review of International Studies*, 32(1), 5–23.

McInnes, C., & Lee, K. (2012). *Global health and international relations*. Cambridge: Polity Press.

McInnes, C., & Rushton, S. (2010). HIV, AIDS and security: Where are we now? *International Affairs*, 86(1), 225–245.

McIntosh, C. A., & Finkle, J. L. (1995). The Cairo conference on population and development: A new paradigm? *Population and Development Review*, 223–260.

McMichael, A. J. (2013). Globalization, climate change, and human health. *New England Journal of Medicine*, 368(14), 1335–1343.

McMichael, A. J., & Woodruff, R. E. (2005). Climate change and human health. In *Encyclopedia of world climatology* (pp. 209–213). Heidelberg, Germany: Springer.

Melissen, J. (2003). *Summit diplomacy coming of age*. Clingendael, Netherlands: Netherlands Institute of International Relations.

Michaud, J. (2015). Health security and foreign policy. In S. Rushton & J. Youde (Eds.), *Routledge handbook of global health security*. Oxon: Routledge.

Michaud, J., & Kates, J. (2013). Global health diplomacy: Advancing foreign policy and global health interests. *Global Health: Science and Practice*, 1(1), 24–28.

Minas, H., Tsutsumi, A., Izutsu, T., Goetzke, K., & Thornicroft, G. (2015). Comprehensive SDG goal and targets for non-communicable diseases and mental health. *International Journal of Mental Health Systems*, 9(1), 12.

Miranda, J. J., Kinra, S., Casas, J. P., Davey Smith, G., & Ebrahim, S. (2008). Non-communicable diseases in low-and middle-income countries: Context, determinants and health policy. *Tropical Medicine & International Health*, 13(10), 1225–1234.

Moore, J. E., Mascarenhas, A., Bain, J., & Straus, S. E. (2017). Developing a comprehensive definition of sustainability. *Implementation Science*, 12(1), 110.

Moravcsik, A. (1995). Explaining international human rights regimes: Liberal theory and Western Europe. *European Journal of International Relations*, 1(2), 157–189.

Moreno-Serra, R., & Smith, P. C. (2012). Does progress towards universal health coverage improve population health? *The Lancet*, 380(9845), 917–923.

Mourens, D., & Fauci, A. (2015). Emerging infectious diseases in 2012: 20 years after the institute of medicine report. In *Emerging viral diseases: The one health connection*. Workshop Summary. Washington, DC: The National Academies Press, Institute of Medicine.

Murphy, C. N. (2006). *The United Nations development programme: A better way?* Cambridge: Cambridge University Press.

Murray, C. J. (2007). Towards good practice for health statistics: Lessons from the millennium development goal health indicators. *The Lancet*, 369(9564), 862–873.

NCD Alliance. (n.d.). *About the NCD alliance*. Retrieved April 29, 2018, from https://ncdalliance.org/who-we-are/about-ncd-alliance

Neumann, I. B. (2002). Returning practice to the linguistic turn: The case of diplomacy. *Millennium*, *31*(3), 627–651.

Neumayer, E. (2012). Human development and sustainability. *Journal of Human Development and Capabilities*, *13*(4), 561–579.

Newman, E. (2001). Human security and constructivism. *International Studies Perspectives*, *2*(3), 239–251.

Norwegian Ministry of Foreign Affairs. (2012). *Global health in foreign policy and development policy*. Oslo. Retrieved July 4, 2016, from www.regjeringen.no/en/dep/ud/documents/propositions-and-reports/reports-to-the-storting/2011-2012/meld-st-11-2011-2012.html?id=672110

Nulu, S. (2017). Neglected chronic disease: The WHO framework on non-communicable diseases and implications for the global poor. *Global Public Health*, *12*(4), 396–415.

Nussbaum, M. C. (1997). Capabilities and human rights. *Fordham Law Review*, *66*(2), 273–300.

Nussbaum, M. C. (1999). In defense of universal values. *Idaho Law Review*, *36*, 379.

Nussbaum, M. (2000). Women's capabilities and social justice. *Journal of Human Development*, *1*(2), 219–247.

Nussbaum, M. (2001). *Women and human development: The capabilities approach*. Cambridge: Cambridge University Press.

Nussbaum, M. C. (2004). Beyond the social contract: Capabilities and global justice. An Olaf Palme lecture, delivered in Oxford on 19 June 2003. *Oxford Development Studies*, *32*(1), 3–18.

Nussbaum, M. C. (2011). Capabilities, entitlements, rights: Supplementation and critique. *Journal of Human Development and Capabilities*, *12*(1), 23–37.

O'Manique, C. (2005). The "securitisation" of HIV/AIDS in sub-Saharan Africa: A critical feminist lens. *Policy and Society*, *24*(1), 24–47.

Open Working Group. (2014). *Progress report of the open working group of the general assembly on sustainable development goals*. Retrieved December 10, 2015, from https://sustainabledevelopment.un.org/content/documents/3238summaryallowg.pdf

Organisation of African Unity. (2001). *Abuja declaration on HIV/AIDS, tuberculosis, and other related infectious diseases*. Retrieved May 29, 2018, from www.un.org/ga/aids/pdf/abuja_declaration.pdf

Osborn, D., Cutter, A., & Ullah, F. (2015, May). *Universal sustainable development goals: Understanding the transformational challenge for developed countries*. Report of Study by Stakeholder Forum. Retrieved from https://sustainabledevelopment.un.org/content/documents/1684SF_-_SDG_Universality_Report_-_May_2015.pdf

Osmani, S., & Sen, A. (2003). The hidden penalties of gender inequality: Fetal origins of ill-health. *Economics & Human Biology*, *1*(1), 105–121.

Outcomes on Least Developed Countries. (n.d.). Retrieved August 31, 2015, from www.un.org/en/development/devagenda/ldc.shtml

Palmer, S. (2010). *Launching global health: The Caribbean Odyssey of the Rockefeller foundation*. Ann Arbor, MI: The University of Michigan Press.

Paris, R. (2001). Human security: Paradigm shift or hot air? *International Security*, *26*(2), 87–102.

Patterson, A. S. (2018). *Africa and global health governance: Domestic politics and international structures*. Baltimore, MD: JHU Press.

Patz, J. A., Campbell-Lendrum, D., Holloway, T., & Foley, J. A. (2005). Impact of regional climate change on human health. *Nature*, *438*(7066), 310.

Peabody, J. W. (1996). Economic reform and health sector policy: Lessons from structural adjustment programmes. *Social Science & Medicine, 43*(5), 823–835.

Peet, R., & Hartwick, E. (2009). *Theories of development: Contentions, arguments, alternatives.* New York, NY: Guilford Press.

Peters, D. H., Garg, A., Bloom, G., Walker, D. G., Brieger, W. R., & Rahman, M. H. (2008). Poverty and access to health care in developing countries. *Annals of the New York Academy of Sciences, 1136*(1), 161–171.

Piketty, T. (2014). *Capital in the twenty-first century.* Cambridge, MA: Harvard University Press.

Piot, P. (2005, February 8). *Why AIDS is exceptional.* Speech given at the London School of Economics. London: UNAIDS. Retrieved February 2, 2018, from http://data.unaids.org/media/speeches02/sp_piot_lse_08feb05_en.pdf

Pérez-Casas, C. (2001). HIV/AIDS medicines pricing report. Setting objectives: Is there a political will? *BETA: Bulletin of Experimental Treatments for AIDS: A Publication of the San Francisco AIDS Foundation, 13*(4), 17.

Pogge, T. (2001). Priorities of global justice. *Metaphilosophy, 32*(1–2), 6–24.

Porras, I. M. (1992). The Rio declaration: A new basis for international co-operation. *Review of European, Comparative & International Environmental Law, 1*(3), 245–253.

Pouster, J., & Manevich, D. (2017). *Globally, people point to ISIS and climate change as leading security threats: Concern about cyberattacks, world economy also widespread.* Pew Research Center. Retrieved May 18, 2017, from www.pewglobal.org/wp-content/uploads/sites/2/2017/07/Pew-Research-Center_2017.07.13_Global-Threats_Full-Report.pdf

President's Emergency Plan for AIDS Relief. (2018, September 28). *PEPFAR: the first 15 years.* Retrieved 22 October, 2019, from https://www.unaids.org/en/resources/presscentre/featurestories/2018/september/pepfar-the-first-15-years

Pressman, S., & Summerfield, G. (2000). The economic contributions of Amartya Sen. *Review of Political Economy, 12*(1), 89–113.

Price-Smith, A. T. (2002). *The health of nations. Infectious disease, environmental change and their effects on national security and development.* Cambridge, MA: The MIT Press.

Prince, M., Patel, V., Saxena, S., Maj, M., Maselko, J., Phillips, M. R., & Rahman, A. (2007). No health without mental health. *The Lancet, 370*(9590), 859–877.

Qureshi, Z. M. (2005). The millennium development goals and the Monterrey consensus: From vision to action. In F. Bourguignon, B. Pleskovic, & A. Sapir (Eds.), *Are we on track to achieve the millennium development goals?* (pp. 223–253). New York: Oxford University Press.

Rist, G. (2008). *The history of development: From Western origins to global faith.* London: Zed Books.

Robeyns, I. (2005). The capability approach: A theoretical survey. *Journal of Human Development, 6*(1), 93–117.

Robeyns, I. (2006). The capability approach in practice. *Journal of Political Philosophy, 14*(3), 351–376.

Rodin, J., & de Ferranti, D. (2012). Universal health coverage: The third global health transition? *The Lancet, 380*(9845), 861–862.

Ronsmans, C., Graham, W. J., & Lancet Maternal Survival Series Steering Group. (2006). Maternal mortality: Who, when, where, and why. *The Lancet, 368*(9542), 1189–1200.

Rosenau, J. (1992). Governance, order, and change in world politics. In J. Rosenau & E. Czempiel (Eds.), *Governance without government: Order and change in world politics.* Cambridge: Cambridge University Press.

Rostow, W. W. (1956). The take-off into self-sustained growth. *The Economic Journal*, 66(261), 25–48.

Rowell, A. (1996). *Green backlash: Global subversion of the environment movement*. New York, NY: Routledge.

Ruger, J. P. (2013). A global health constitution for global health governance. *Proceedings of the ASIL Annual Meeting*, 107, 267–270.

Ruggie, J. G. (1998). What makes the world hang together? Neo-utilitarianism and the social constructivist challenge. *International Organisation*, 52(4), 855–885.

Rushton, S. (2010). Framing AIDS: Securitization, development-ization, rights-ization. *Global Health Governance*, 4(1).

Rushton, S. (2011). Global health security: Security for whom? Security from what? *Political Studies*, 59(4), 779–796.

Rushton, S., & Youde, J. (Eds.). (2015). *Routledge handbook of global health security*. Oxon: Routledge.

Sachs, J. D. (2005). *Investing in development: A practical plan to achieve the millennium development goals*. New York, NY: UNDP.

Sachs, J. D. (2012). From millennium development goals to sustainable development goals. *The Lancet*, 379(9832), 2206–2211.

Sachs, W. (1992). *The development dictionary: A guide to knowledge as power*. London: Zed Books.

Sai, F. T. (1997). The ICPD programme of action: Pious hope or a workable guide? *Health Transition Review*, 7, 1–5.

Samuels, T. A., & Hospedales, C. J. (2011). From Port-of-Spain summit to United Nations high level meeting: CARICOM and the global non-communicable disease agenda. *West Indian Medical Journal*, 60(4), 387–391.

Sattar, S., & Smith, K. (2017). *Global advocacy for universal health coverage*. Monitoring and evaluation office. Rockefeller Foundation. Retrieved July 2, 2018, from https://assets.rock efellerfoundation.org/app/uploads/20180116194108/Global-Advocacy-for-Universal-Health-Coverage.pdf

Schmieg, G., Meyer, E., Schrickel, I., Herberg, J., Caniglia, G., Vilsmaier, U., . . . Lang, D. (2018). Modeling normativity in sustainability: A comparison of the sustainable development goals, the Paris agreement, and the papal encyclical. *Sustainability Science*, 13(3), 785–796.

Sen, A. (1980). Equality of what? In S. McMurrin (Ed.), *Tanner lectures on human values*. Cambridge, MA: Cambridge University Press.

Sen, A. (1992). *Inequality reexamined*. New York, NY: Clarendon Press.

Sen, A. (1999a). *Development as freedom*. New York, NY: Knopf.

Sen, A. (1999b). Health in development. *Bulletin of the World Health Organization*, 77(8), 619.

Sen, A. (2000). A decade of human development. *Journal of Human Development*, 1(1), 17–23.

Sen, A. (2002). Why health equity? *Health Economy*, 11, 659–666.

Sen, A. (2005). Human rights and capabilities. *Journal of Human Development*, 6(2), 151–166.

Sen, A. (2009). *The idea of justice*. Cambridge, MA: Harvard University Press.

Sending, O. J. (2004). Policy stories and knowledge-based regimes: The case of international population policy. In M. Bøås & D. McNeill (Eds.), *Global institutions & development: Framing the world?* London: Routledge.

Seyfang, G. (2003). Environmental mega-conferences – from Stockholm to Johannesburg and beyond. *Global Environmental Change, 13*(3), 223–228.

Shafik, N. (1994). Economic development and environmental quality: An econometric analysis. *Oxford Economic Papers, 46*, 757–773.

Shiffman, J. (2009). A social explanation for the rise and fall of global health issues. *Bulletin of the World Health Organization, 87*, 608–613.

Sihto, M., Ollila, E., & Koivusalo, M. (2006). Principles and challenges of health in all policies. In T. Ståhl, M. Wismar, E. Ollila, E. Lahtinen, & K. Leppo (Eds.), *Health in all policies. Prospects and potentials.* Helsinki: Finnish Ministry of Social Affairs and Health.

Skolnik, R. (2012). *Global health 101.* Burlington, VT: Jones & Bartlett.

Smith, J. H., Buse, K., & Gordon, C. (2016). Civil society: The catalyst for ensuring health in the age of sustainable development. *Globalization and Health, 12*(1), 40.

Smith, J. H., & Whiteside, A. (2010). The history of AIDS exceptionalism. *Journal of the International AIDS Society, 13*(1), 47.

Smith, R. A., & Siplon, P. D. (2006). *Drugs into bodies: Global AIDS treatment activism.* Westport, CT: Preager.

Society for International Development. (n.d.). *SID in brief.* Retrieved November 20, 2017, from www.sidint.net/content/sid-brief

Spartz, J. T., Su, L. Y. F., Griffin, R., Brossard, D., & Dunwoody, S. (2017). YouTube, social norms and perceived salience of climate change in the American mind. *Environmental Communication, 11*(1), 1–16.

Standing, H. (2004). Towards reproductive health for all? In R. Black & H. White (Eds.), *Targeting development: Critical perspectives on the millennium development goals.* London: Routledge.

St. Clair, A. L. (2004). The role of ideas in the United Nations development programme. In M. Bøås & D. McNeill (Eds.), *Global institutions & development: Framing the world?* London: Routledge.

Stern, D. I. (2004). The rise and fall of the environmental Kuznets curve. *World Development, 32*(8), 1419–1439.

Stevenson, M. A., & Moran, M. (2015). Health security and the distortion of the global health agenda. In S. Rushton & J. Youde (Eds.), *Routledge handbook of global health security.* Oxon: Routledge.

Strauss, J., & Thomas, D. (1998). Health, nutrition, and economic development. *Journal of Economic Literature, 36*(2), 766–817.

Streeten, P. (1981). *Development perspectives.* Basingstoke: Palgrave Macmillan.

Streeten, P. (2000). Freedom and welfare: A review essay on Amartya Sen, development as freedom. *Population and Development Review, 26*(1), 153–162.

Strong, K., Mathers, C., Leeder, S., & Beaglehole, R. (2005). Preventing chronic diseases: How many lives can we save? *The Lancet, 366*(9496), 1578–1582.

Stuart, E., & Samman, E. (2017). *Defining leave no one behind.* Briefing Note. London: Overseas Development Institute.

Symons, J., & Altman, D. (2015). International norm polarization: Sexuality as a subject of human rights protection. *International Theory, 7*(1), 61–95.

Talmon, S. (2005). The security council as world legislature. *American Journal of International Law, 99*(1), 175–193.

Thomas, C. (1989). On the health of international relations and the international relations of health. *Review of International Studies, 15*(3), 273–280.

Tolley, H., Snowdon, W., Wate, J., Durand, A. M., Vivili, P., McCool, J., . . . Richards, N. (2016). Monitoring and accountability for the Pacific response to the non-communicable diseases crisis. *BMC Public Health*, 16(1), 958.

United Nations. (1990a). *World declaration on the survival, protection and development of children*. Retrieved November 30, 2017, from www.unicef.org/wsc/declare.htm

United Nations. (1990b). *Major goals for child survival, development and protection*. Retrieved November 30, 2017, from www.unicef.org/wsc/goals.htm

United Nations. (1992). *United Nations conference on environment & development: Agenda 21*. Retrieved September 23, 2015, from https://sustainabledevelopment.un.org/content/documents/Agenda21.pdf

United Nations. (1993). *Vienna declaration and programme of action*. Retrieved September 5, 2015, from www.ohchr.org/Documents/ProfessionalInterest/vienna.pdf

United Nations. (1995a). *Copenhagen declaration on social development*. Retrieved September 15, 2015, from www.un.org/en/development/desa/population/migration/generalassembly/docs/globalcompact/A_CONF.166_9_Declaration.pdf

United Nations. (1995b). *From Cairo to Beijing: Women's conference amplifies ICPD*. Retrieved October 30, 2017, from www.un.org/popin/unfpa/taskforce/icpdnews/icpdnews9510/cairo.html

United Nations. (1995c). *Report of the fourth world conference on women*. Retrieved November 3, 2017, from www.un.org/esa/gopher-data/conf/fwcw/off/a-20.en

United Nations. (1996). *Istanbul declaration on human settlements*. Retrieved September 20, 2015, from www.un-documents.net/ist-dec.htm

United Nations. (1997). *World summit for children*. Retrieved August 2, 2015, from www.un.org/geninfo/bp/child.html

United Nations. (2007). *The United Nations development agenda: Development for all*. Retrieved May 2, 2015, from www.un.org/esa/devagenda/UNDA1.pdf

United Nations. (2008). *MDG action points: Addendum to the background note by the secretary-general on committing to action: Achieving the millennium development goals*. Retrieved October 5, 2015, from www.un.org/millenniumgoals/2008highlevel/pdf/addendum.pdf

United Nations. (2010). *The millennium development report goals 2010*. Retrieved October 20, 2015, from www.un.org/millenniumgoals/pdf/MDG%20Report%202010%20En%20r15%20-low%20res%2020100615%20-.pdf

United Nations. (2012). *Guidance for effective mediation*. Retrieved April 8, 2018, from https://peacemaker.un.org/sites/peacemaker.un.org/files/GuidanceEffectiveMediation_UNDPA2012%28english%29_0.pdf

United Nations. (2014). *Open working group proposal for sustainable development goals*. Retrieved December 12, 2015, from https://sustainabledevelopment.un.org/content/documents/1579SDGs%20Proposal.pdf

United Nations. (2015). *The millennium development goals report 2015*. Retrieved February 20, 2016, from www.un.org/millenniumgoals/2015_MDG_Report/pdf/MDG%202015%20rev%20(July%201).pdf

United Nations. (n.d.a). *AIDS as a security issue*. Retrieved October 25, 2017, from www.un.org/ga/aids/ungassfactsheets/html/fssecurity_en.htm

United Nations. (n.d.b). *Monterrey conference*. Retrieved October 2, 2015, from www.un.org/esa/ffd/overview/monterrey-conference.html

United Nations Economic and Social Council. (2000). *General comment no. 14: The right to the highest attainable standard of health (art. 12)*. Retrieved May 15, 2016, from www.refworld.org/pdfid/4538838d0.pdf

United Nations Economic and Social Council. (2014a). *Framework of actions for the follow-up to the programmed of action of the ICPD beyond 2014: Report of the general-secretary.* Retrieved October 10, 2018, from www.unfpa.org/sites/default/files/pub-pdf/ICPD_beyond2014_EN.pdf

United Nations Economic and Social Council. (2014b). *Ministerial declaration of the high-level political forum on sustainable development convened under the auspices of the Council on the theme "achieving the millennium development goals and charting the way for an ambitious post-2015 development agenda, including the sustainable development goals.* Retrieved January 10, 2016, from www.un.org/ga/search/view_doc.asp?symbol=E/2014/L.22&Lang=E

United Nations Economic and Social Council. (2015). *Mainstreaming of the three dimensions of sustainable development throughout the United Nations system.* Retrieved May 11, 2018, from www.un.org/ga/search/view_doc.asp?symbol=A/70/75&Lang=E

United Nations Department of Economic and Social Affairs. (2016). *Leaving no one behind: The imperative of inclusive development.* Report on the World Social Situation 2016. Retrieved May 10, 2018, from www.un.org/esa/socdev/rwss/2016/full-report.pdf

United Nations Development Programme. (1990). *Human development report 1990.* Retrieved April 22, 2015, from http://HDR.undp.org/en/reports/global/HDR1990

United Nations Development Programme. (1991). *Human development report 1991.* Retrieved August 3, 2015, from http://HDR.undp.org/en/reports/global/HDR1991

United Nations Development Programme. (1993). *Human development report 1993.* Retrieved August 5, 2015, from http://HDR.undp.org/en/reports/global/HDR1993

United Nations Development Programme. (1994). *Human development report 1994.* Retrieved August 10, 2015, from http://HDR.undp.org/en/content/human-development-report-1994

United Nations Development Programme. (1995). *Human development report 1995.* Retrieved August 11, 2015, from http://HDR.undp.org/en/content/human-development-report-1995

United Nations Development Programme. (1996). *Human development report 1996.* Retrieved August 16, 2015, from http://HDR.undp.org/en/content/human-development-report-1996

United Nations Development Programme. (1997). *Human development report 1997.* Retrieved August 20, 2015, from http://HDR.undp.org/en/content/human-development-report-1997

United Nations Development Programme. (1998). *Human development report 1998.* Retrieved August 25, 2015, from http://HDR.undp.org/en/content/human-development-report-1998

United Nations Development Programme. (1999). *Human development report 1999.* Retrieved August 30, 2015, from http://HDR.undp.org/en/content/human-development-report-1999

United Nations Development Programme. (2000). *Human development report 2000.* Retrieved October 20, 2017, from http://HDR.undp.org/sites/default/files/reports/261/HDR_2000_en.pdf

United Nations Development Programme. (2004). *Ideas, innovation, impact: How human development reports influence change* [PDF File]. New York, NY: Mwangi, Burd-Sharps, & Kurukulasuriya. Retrieved from http://HDR.undp.org/sites/default/files/impact_publication.pdf

United Nations Development Programme. (2014). *Delivering the post-2015 development agenda: Opportunities at the national and local levels.* Retrieved May 14, 2018, from https://

sustainabledevelopment.un.org/content/documents/1909UNDP-MDG-Delivering-Post-2015-Report-2014.pdf

United Nations Development Programme. (2016, November 23). *William Draper interview – 50th anniversary* [Video File]. Retrieved from www.youtube.com/watch?v=ILHkEfRAHxo

United Nations Development Programme. (n.d.). *What is human development?* Retrieved March 20, 2018, from http://HDR.undp.org/en/content/what-human-development

United Nations General Assembly. (1961). *General assembly resolution A/RES/1710 (XVI): United Nations development decade.* Retrieved April 16, 2015, from www.un.org/en/ga/search/view_doc.asp?symbol=A/RES/1710%20(XVI)

United Nations General Assembly. (1970). *Resolution 2625 (XXV): Declaration on principles of international law concerning friendly relations and co-operation among states in accordance with the charter of the United Nations.* Retrieved May 30, 2016, from https://documents-dds-ny.un.org/doc/RESOLUTION/GEN/NR0/348/90/IMG/NR034890.pdf?OpenElement

United Nations General Assembly. (1981). *General Assembly resolution A/RES/35/56: Third United Nations development decade.* Retrieved April 17, 2015, from www.un.org/en/ga/search/view_doc.asp?symbol=A/RES/35/56

United Nations General Assembly. (1986). *General assembly resolution 41/128: Declaration on the right to development.* Retrieved September 4, 2015, from www.un.org/documents/ga/res/41/a41r128.htm

United Nations General Assembly. (1989). *General assembly resolution 44/228: United Nations conference on environment and development.* Retrieved September 1, 2015, from www.worldiii.org/int/other/UNGA/1989/313.pdf

United Nations General Assembly. (1990). *General Assembly resolution 45/199: International development strategy for the fourth United Nations development decade.* Retrieved April 17, 2015, from www.un.org/en/ga/search/view_doc.asp?symbol=A/RES/45/199

United Nations General Assembly. (1998). *Resolution 53/202: The millennium assembly of the United Nations.* Retrieved October 2, 2015, from http://repository.un.org/bitstream/handle/11176/222277/A_RES_53_202-EN.pdf?sequence=3&isAllowed=y

United Nations General Assembly. (1999). *Resolution 2–21/2: Key actions for the further implementation of the programme of action of the international conference on population and development.* Retrieved March 30, 2018, from www.unfpa.org/sites/default/files/event-pdf/key_actions_en.pdf

United Nations General Assembly. (2000a). *Resolution 55/162: Follow-up to the outcome of the millennium summit.* Retrieved October 15, 2015, from http://undocs.org/en/A/RES/55/162

United Nations General Assembly. (2000b). *United Nations millennium declaration.* Retrieved October 16, 2015, from www.un.org/millennium/declaration/ares552e.pdf

United Nations General Assembly. (2001). *Resolution S-26/2: Declaration of commitment on HIV/AIDS.* Retrieved November 20, 2017, https://www.hivlawandpolicy.org/resources/declaration-commitment-hivaids-ga-res-s-262-un-doc-aress-262

United Nations General Assembly. (2005). *Resolution 60/1: 2005 world summit outcome.* Retrieved February 12, 2018, from www.un.org/en/development/desa/population/migration/generalassembly/docs/globalcompact/A_RES_60_1.pdf

United Nations General Assembly. (2006). *Resolution 60/262: Political declaration on HIV/AIDS.* Retrieved July 20, 2018, from http://data.unaids.org/pub/report/2006/20060615_hlm_politicaldeclaration_ares60262_en.pdf

United Nations General Assembly. (2009). *Resolution 63/278: International mother earth day.* Retrieved January 10, 2019, from https://undocs.org/A/RES/63/278

United Nations General Assembly. (2010). *Resolution 65/1: Keeping the promise: United to achieve the millennium development goals.* Retrieved November 30, 2015, from www.un.org/en/mdg/summit2010/pdf/outcome_documentN1051260.pdf

United Nations General Assembly. (2011). *Resolution 66/2: Political declaration of the high-level meeting of the general assembly on the prevention and control of non-communicable diseases.* Retrieved May 31, 2018, from www.who.int/nmh/events/un_ncd_summit2011/political_declaration_en.pdf

United Nations General Assembly. (2012a). *Resolution 66/288: The future we want.* Retrieved December 3, 2015, from www.un.org/en/development/desa/population/migration/generalassembly/docs/globalcompact/A_RES_66_288.pdf

United Nations General Assembly. (2012b). *Resolution 67/634: Initial input of the secretary-general to the open working group on sustainable development goals.* Retrieved December 4, 2015, from http://undocs.org/en/A/67/634

United Nations General Assembly. (2012c). *Resolution 67/81: Global health and foreign policy.* Retrieved May 22, 2018, from www.un.org/en/ga/search/view_doc.asp?symbol=A/RES/67/81

United Nations General Assembly. (2013a). *Resolution 67/290: Format and organizational aspects of the high-level political forum on sustainable development.* Retrieved December 15, 2015, from http://undocs.org/A/RES/67/290

United Nations General Assembly. (2013b). *Resolution 68/202: A life of dignity for all: Accelerating progress towards the millennium development goals and advancing the United Nations development agenda beyond 2015: Report of the secretary-general.* Retrieved December 10, 2015, from https://undocs.org/A/68/202

United Nations General Assembly. (2013c). *Summary of the first meeting of the high-level political forum on sustainable development: Note by the president of the general assembly.* Retrieved December 17, 2015, from www.un.org/ga/search/view_doc.asp?symbol=A/68/588&Lang=E

United Nations General Assembly. (2014a). *The road to dignity by 2030: Ending poverty, transforming all lives and protecting the planet.* Synthesis Report of the Secretary-General on the Post-2015 Agenda. Retrieved March 25, 2015, from https://undocs.org/A/69/700

United Nations General Assembly. (2014b). *Report of the open working group on sustainable development goals: Addendum.* Retrieved December 9, 2015, from http://undocs.org/A/68/970/Add.1

United Nations General Assembly. (2014c). *Resolution 68/309: Report of the open working group on sustainable development goals established pursuant to general assembly resolution 66/288.* Retrieved December 13, 2015, from www.un.org/en/ga/search/view_doc.asp?symbol=A/RES/68/309

United Nations General Assembly. (2014d). *Concept note for the high-level stocktaking event on the post-2015 development agenda: Contributions to the secretary-general's synthesis report.* Retrieved December 12, 2015, from www.un.org/en/ga/president/68/pdf/stocktaking/7172014%20stocktaking%20approved%20concept%20note_1.pdf

United Nations General Assembly. (2015). *Resolution 70/1: Transforming or world: The 2030 agenda for sustainable development.* Retrieved February 20, 2016, from www.un.org/en/development/desa/population/migration/generalassembly/docs/globalcompact/A_RES_70_1_E.pdf

United Nations General Assembly. (n.d.). *Committees*. Retrieved November 15, 2015, from www.un.org/ga/61/background/committees.shtml

United Nations Security Council. (2000). *Resolution 1308: On the responsibility of the security council in the maintenance of international peace and security: HIV/AIDS and international peace-keeping operations*. Retrieved October 20, 2017, from www.unaids.org/sites/default/files/sub_landing/files/20000717_un_scresolution_1308_en.pdf

United Nations Sustainable Development Knowledge Platform. (n.d.). *Sustained and inclusive economic growth*. Retrieved April 13, 2018, from https://sustainabledevelopment.un.org/index.php?page=view&type=9502&menu=1565&nr=7

United Nations System Task Team on the Post-2015 UN Development Agenda. (2012). *Realizing the future we want for all: Report to the secretary-general*. Retrieved November 20, 2015, from www.un.org/millenniumgoals/pdf/Post_2015_UNTTreport.pdf

United Nations System Task Team on the Post-2015 UN Development Agenda. (2013). *A renewed global partnership for development*. Retrieved December 1, 2015, from www.un.org/en/development/desa/policy/untaskteam_undf/glob_dev_rep_2013.pdf

Vallance, S., Perkins, H. C., & Dixon, J. E. (2011). What is social sustainability? A clarification of concepts. *Geoforum, 42*(3), 342–348.

Vandemoortele, J. (2009). The MDG conundrum: Meeting the targets without missing the point. *Development Policy Review, 27*(4), 355–371.

Vandemoortele, J. (2011). The MDG story: Intention denied. *Development and Change, 42*(1), 1–21.

Vandemoortele, J. (2012). *Advancing the global development agenda post-2015: Some thoughts, ideas and practical suggestions*. Background Paper prepared for the Experts Group Meeting to support the advancement of the Post-2015 UN Development Agenda. New York. Retrieved from https://www.un.org/en/development/desa/policy/untaskteam_undf/j_vandemoortele.pdf

Van Der Gaag, J., & Barham, T. (1998). Health and health expenditures in adjusting and non-adjusting countries. *Social Science & Medicine, 46*(8), 995–1009.

Vega, J. (2013). Universal health coverage: The post-2015 development agenda. *The Lancet, 381*(9862), 179–180.

Venkatapuram, S. (2011). *Health justice: An argument from the capabilities approach*. Cambridge: Polity Press.

Vieira, M. A. (2007). The securitization of the HIV/AIDS epidemic as a norm: A contribution to constructivist scholarship on the emergence and diffusion of international norms. *Brazilian Political Science Review (Online), 2*(SE), 137–181.

Vieira, M. A. (2011). Southern Africa's response (s) to international HIV/AIDS norms: The politics of assimilation. *Review of International Studies, 37*(1), 3–28.

Vizard, P., Fukuda-Parr, S., & Elson, D. (2011). Introduction: The capability approach and human rights. *Journal of Human Development and Capabilities, 12*(1), 1–22.

von Burg, C. (2015). *On inclusivity: The role of norms in international peace mediation*. Bern, Switzerland: Swisspeace.

Wagstaff, A., Cotlear, D., Eozenou, P. H. V., & Buisman, L. R. (2016). Measuring progress towards universal health coverage: With an application to 24 developing countries. *Oxford Review of Economic Policy, 32*(1), 147–189.

Weir, L. (2015). Inventing global health security, 1994–2005. In S. Rushton & J. Youde (Eds.), *Routledge handbook of global health security*. Oxon: Routledge.

Wendt, A. (1992). Anarchy is what states make of it: The social construction of power politics. *International Organisation, 46*(2), 391–425.

Wendt, A. (1999). *Social theory of international politics*. Cambridge: Cambridge University Press.

Whiteside, A. (2008). *HIV & AIDS: A very short introduction*. Oxford: Oxford University Press.

Wilmshurst, P. (1997). Scientific imperialism. *BMJ: British Medical Journal, 314*(7084), 840.

Wisor, S. (2012). After the MDGs: Citizen deliberation and the post-2015 development framework. *Ethics & International Affairs, 26*(1), 113–133.

World Bank. (1980). *World development report 1980*. Washington, DC: The World Bank.

World Bank. (1990). *World development report 1990*. New York, NY: Oxford University Press.

World Bank. (1993). *World development report 1993*. New York, NY: Oxford University Press.

World Health Organization. (1948). *Constitution of the world health organization*. Retrieved April 20, 2016, from www.searo.who.int/about/about_searo_const.pdf

World Health Organization. (1978). *Declaration of Alma-Ata*. Retrieved April 20, 2015, from www.who.int/publications/almaata_declaration_en.pdf

World Health Organization. (1986). *The Ottawa charter for health promotion*. Retrieved December 3, 2017, from www.euro.who.int/__data/assets/pdf_file/0004/129532/Ottawa_Charter.pdf

World Health Organization. (1992). *International conference on nutrition: Final report of the conference*. Retrieved September 2, 2015, from http://apps.who.int/iris/bitstream/handle/10665/61254/a34812.pdf?sequence=1

World Health Organization. (1996). *World health report 1996*. Retrieved May 23, 2016, from www.who.int/whr/1996/en/whr96_en.pdf

World Health Organization. (1997). *City planning for health and sustainable development*. European Sustainable Development and Health Series: 2. Retrieved August 10, 2018, from www.euro.who.int/__data/assets/pdf_file/0008/101060/wa38097ci.pdf

World Health Organization. (1998). *World health report 1998*. Retrieved May 30, 2016, from www.who.int/whr/1998/en/whr98_en.pdf

World Health Organization. (2000). *Resolution A51/4: Global strategy for the prevention and control of noncommunicable diseases*. Retrieved May 12, 2018, from http://apps.who.int/gb/archive/pdf_files/WHA53/ea14.pdf

World Health Organization. (2005a). *Health and the millennium development goals*. Retrieved April 27, 2015, from www.who.int/hdp/publications/mdg_en.pdf

World Health Organization. (2005b). *International health regulations 2005*. Retrieved April 20, 2016, from http://apps.who.int/iris/bitstream/handle/10665/43883/9789241580410_eng.pdf?sequence=1

World Health Organization. (2005c). *Preventing chronic diseases: A vital investment*. Retrieved May 2, 2018, from http://apps.who.int/iris/bitstream/handle/10665/43314/9241563001_eng.pdf?sequence=1

World Health Organization. (2005d). *World health report 2005*. Retrieved June 2, 2018, from www.who.int/whr/2005/whr2005_en.pdf

World Health Organization. (2006). *Charter on counteracting obesity*. Retrieved May 14, 2018, from www.euro.who.int/__data/assets/pdf_file/0009/87462/E89567.pdf

World Health Organization. (2007). *World health report 2007*. Retrieved April 30, 2016, from www.who.int/whr/2007/whr07_en.pdf

World Health Organization. (2009). *Global health risks: Mortality and burden of disease attributable to selected major risks*. Geneva, Switzerland: World Health Organization.

World Health Organization. (2010). *World health report 2010*. Retrieved June 28, 2018, from www.who.int/whr/2010/10_summary_en.pdf

World Health Organization. (2011a). *First ministerial conference on healthy lifestyles and non-communicable disease control*. Retrieved May 23, 2018, from https://www.who.int/nmh/events/moscow_ncds_2011/conference_documents/conference_report.pdf?ua=1

World Health Organization. (2011b). *Moscow declaration*. Retrieved May 23, 2018, from www.un.org/en/ga/president/65/issues/moscow_declaration_en.pdf

World Health Organization. (2011c). *World health assembly resolution 64.9: Sustainable health financing structures and universal coverage*. Retrieved June 17, 2018, from www.aho.afro.who.int/networks/sites/default/files/13._wha_resolution_64_9_sustainable_health_financing_structures_and_universal_health_coverage_uhc_0.pdf

World Health Organization. (2012a). *Mexico city political declaration on universal health coverage*. Retrieved June 19, 2018, from www.who.int/healthsystems/topics/financing/MexicoCityPoliticalDeclarationUniversalHealthCoverage.pdf

World Health Organization. (2012b). *Positioning health in the post-2015 development agenda*. Who Discussion Paper. Retrieved May 30, 2018, from www.who.int/topics/millennium_development_goals/post2015/WHOdiscussionpaper_October2012.pdf

World Health Organization. (2013a). *Arguing for universal health coverage*. Retrieved July 10, 2018, from www.who.int/health_financing/UHC_ENvs_BD.PDF

World Health Organization. (2013b). *Global action plan for the prevention and control of NCDs*. Retrieved April 30, 2018, from http://apps.who.int/iris/bitstream/handle/10665/94384/9789241506236_eng.pdf?sequence=1

World Health Organization. (2013c). *Health in the post-2015 agenda: Report on global thematic consultation on health*. Retrieved April 4, 2018, from www.who.int/pmnch/media/press_materials/pr/2013/health_post-2015_agenda.pdf

World Health Organization. (2013d). *World health report 2013*. Retrieved June 28, 2018, from http://apps.who.int/iris/bitstream/handle/10665/85761/9789240690837_eng.pdf?sequence=2

World Health Organization. (2014). *Global update on the health sector response to HIV, 2014*. Retrieved May 9, 2018, from www.who.int/hiv/pub/progressreports/update2014/en/

World Health Organization. (2016). *Health in the sustainable development goals: Where are we now in the South-East Asia region? What next?* Retrieved April 30, 2018, from www.aidsdatahub.org/sites/default/files/publication/WHO-SEARO_Health_in_the_Sustainable_Development_Goals_where_we_are_now_in_the_South-East_Asia_Region_What_next_2016.pdf

World Health Organization. (2017a). *Evaluation of WHO's normative function: Corporate evaluation commissioned by the WHO evaluation office*. Retrieved May 10, 2018, from www.who.int/about/evaluation/who_normative_function_report_july2017.pdf

World Health Organization. (2017b). *Universal health coverage on the journey towards healthy Islands in the Pacific*. Retrieved May 14, 2018, from www.wpro.who.int/southpacific/pic_meeting/2017/documents/12thphmm_session02_uhc_16august.pdf

World Trade Organization. (2001). *Ministerial declaration of 14 November 2001*. WTO Doc. WT/MIN(01)/DEC/1, 41 ILM 746.

Worrall, E., Basu, S., & Hanson, K. (2005). Is malaria a disease of poverty? A review of the literature. *Tropical Medicine & International Health, 10*(10), 1047–1059.

Youde, J. (2008). Is universal access to antiretroviral drugs an emerging international norm? *Journal of International Relations and Development, 11*(4), 415–440.

Youde, J. R. (2012). *Global health governance*. Cambridge: Polity Press.

Zanker, F. (2014). Legitimate representation: Civil society actors in peace negotiations revisited. *International Negotiation, 19*(1), 62–88.

# Index

Note: Page numbers in *italics* indicate a figure and page numbers in **bold** indicate a table on the corresponding page. Page numbers followed by 'n' indicate a note.

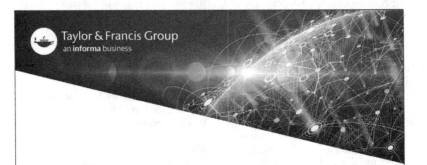

Printed in the USA
by Bookmasters

Printed in the United States
By Bookmasters